# The Hackett Introduction to Medical Ethics

A Guide for Students, Clinicians, and Ethics Committees

# The Hackett Introduction to Medical Ethics

A Guide for Students, Clinicians,
and Ethics Committees

Matthew C. Altman and Cynthia D. Coe

Hackett Publishing Company
Indianapolis

Copyright © 2025 by Hackett Publishing Company, Inc.

All rights reserved
Printed in the United States of America

28 27 26 25        1 2 3 4 5 6 7

For further information, please address
    Hackett Publishing Company, Inc.
    P.O. Box 44937
    Indianapolis, Indiana 46244-0937

    www.hackettpublishing.com

Cover design by Liz Wilson
Interior design by Laura Clark
Composition by Aptara, Inc.

Library of Congress Control Number: 2024948086

ISBN-13: 978-1-64792-218-4 (pbk.)
ISBN-13: 978-1-64792-219-1 (PDF ebook)
ISBN-13: 978-1-64792-220-7 (epub)

The paper used in this publication meets the minimum requirements of American National Standard for Information Sciences—Permanence of Paper for Printed Library Materials, ANSI Z39.48–1984.

∞

# CONTENTS

| | |
|---|---|
| *Acknowledgments* | xi |
| **Introduction** | 1 |
| **Chapter 1: Moral Reasoning in a Medical Context** | 7 |
| Introduction | 7 |
| Common Morality | 8 |
| Principle 1: Respect for Autonomy | 9 |
| Principle 2: Nonmaleficence | 13 |
| Principle 3: Beneficence | 15 |
| Principle 4: Justice | 19 |
| Ethics, Professional Codes, and the Law | 22 |
| Sample Applications | 24 |
| Moral Character | 26 |
| Moral Status | 28 |
| Objections to Principlism | 31 |
|    1. Methodological concerns | 31 |
|    2. Ethics of care objection | 32 |
|    3. Moral imperialism objection | 33 |
| Alternatives to Principlism | 35 |
| Conclusion: The Impact of Principlism | 37 |
| References | 37 |
| Further Reading | 40 |
| **Chapter 2: Collective Responsibility in Medicine** | 43 |
| Introduction | 43 |
| The Concept of Collective Responsibility | 44 |
| Case Study: RaDonda Vaught and VMC | 48 |
| Diffusion of Responsibility in the Vaught Case | 52 |
| Conclusion: The Collective Responsibility to Reduce Harm | 55 |
| References | 56 |
| Further Reading | 57 |

## Chapter 3: Paternalism and Patient Autonomy — 61
Introduction — 61
Medical Paternalism — 62
The Value of Autonomy — 66
Informed Consent — 70
Liberty versus Autonomy — 73
Deliberation and Practical Reasoning — 77
Relational Autonomy — 79
Conclusion: The Power and Limits of Autonomy — 80
References — 82
Further Reading — 86

## Chapter 4: Clinicians' Obligations to Patients and Themselves — 89
Introduction — 89
Truth-Telling, Autonomy, and Beneficence — 90
Disclosure of Medical Errors — 93
Confidentiality — 95
Conscientious Refusal — 99
Moral Distress, Moral Injury, and Burnout — 101
Conclusion: Moral Tensions in the Patient Encounter — 105
References — 105
Further Reading — 112

## Chapter 5: The Ethics and Legality of Abortion — 115
Introduction — 115
Common Arguments on the Morality of Abortion — 117
Constitutional Interpretation and the Legality of Abortion in the U.S. — 121
  1. Dworkin's interpretivism — 122
  2. *Roe v. Wade* (1973) — 125
  3. Scalia's textualism and originalism — 127
  4. *Dobbs v. Jackson Women's Health Organization* (2022) — 128
  5. Outstanding legal issues post-*Roe* — 130
Clinicians' Professional and Legal Obligations — 131
  1. Hippocratic Oath — 131
  2. American Medical Association — 132
  3. What counts as a threat to the pregnant woman's life? — 133
The Legality of Abortion outside the U.S. — 138

    Conclusion: The Challenge of Polarization    140
    References    141
    Further Reading    145

## Chapter 6: Pregnancy and Reproductive Technologies    149
    Introduction    149
    The Criminalization of Pregnancy    150
    In Vitro Fertilization    155
    Surrogate Motherhood    160
    Disability-Selective Abortion    167
    Genetic Enhancement    175
    Stem Cell Research    179
    Conclusion: Politics of the Body    183
    References    184
    Further Reading    193

## Chapter 7: Advance Directives and Decision-Making for Incapacitated Patients    197
    Introduction    197
    Legal Competence versus Medical Capacity    197
    Substituted Judgment and Best Interests Standards    199
    Case Study: Terri Schiavo    202
    The History of Advance Directives    205
    Substantive Directives and Proxy Directives    207
    Problems with Substantive Directives    211
    Problems with Proxy Directives    216
    Conclusion: What Advance Directives Can and Cannot Do    218
    References    219
    Further Reading    221

## Chapter 8: Medical Aid in Dying    224
    Introduction    224
    Terminology    224
    The History of Medical Aid in Dying Legislation in the U.S.    228
    Global Comparisons    230
    Arguments against Medical Aid in Dying    232
        1. The physician's role as healer    233
        2. Theoretical and empirical slippery slopes    235

Arguments for Medical Aid in Dying — 239
   1. Respect for autonomy — 240
   2. Beneficence — 242
Passive Euthanasia and Its Implications for Medical Aid in Dying — 245
Conclusion: Normative Commitments within the Debate — 247
References — 248
Further Reading — 252

## Chapter 9: Healthcare and Social Justice — 255
Introduction — 255
Allocation versus Rationing — 256
Types of Healthcare Systems — 257
   1. Single-payer — 257
   2. Free market — 258
   3. Arguments against a purely free market — 260
   4. Multi-payer — 261
The Right to Healthcare — 263
How Much Healthcare Do We Deserve? — 268
Conclusion: Who Controls Healthcare? — 270
References — 271
Further Reading — 274

## Chapter 10: Allocating Scarce Medical Resources — 278
Introduction — 278
Case Study: The "God Committee" — 279
Principles of Allocation — 280
Principlism — 285
QALYs and DALYs — 286
Organ Transplants: UNOS Points System — 289
Triage during the COVID-19 Pandemic — 292
Distribution of COVID-19 Vaccines — 298
Conclusion: The Dialogue between Theory and Practice — 302
References — 302
Further Reading — 306

## Chapter 11: Racial Disparities in Healthcare — 310
Introduction — 310
Health Outcomes — 311

| | |
|---|---|
| Medical Experimentation | 314 |
| Public Health Campaigns | 320 |
| Clinician-Patient Relationships | 321 |
| Weathering | 326 |
| Conclusion: Addressing Medical Racism | 327 |
| References | 329 |
| Further Reading | 335 |

## Chapter 12: Pediatric Ethics — 338

| | |
|---|---|
| Introduction | 338 |
| Beneficence and Emerging Autonomy | 339 |
| The Roles of Parents and Clinicians | 340 |
| Resolving Ethical Conflicts | 344 |
| Mature Minors | 347 |
| Childhood Vaccination and Screening | 349 |
| Medical Responses to Intersex | 351 |
| Other Elective Genital Surgeries | 354 |
| Healthcare for Transgender Minors | 355 |
| Pediatric Research | 359 |
| Race and Pediatric Ethics | 363 |
| End-of-Life Care | 365 |
| Conclusion: Respect for Emerging Autonomy | 366 |
| References | 367 |
| Further Reading | 372 |

## Chapter 13: Nursing Ethics — 376

| | |
|---|---|
| Introduction | 376 |
| The Gendered History of Nursing | 377 |
| Codes of Ethics | 382 |
| Advantages and Disadvantages of the Concept of Care | 383 |
| From Intelligent Machines to Moral Agents | 386 |
| Moral Problems Central to Nursing Ethics | 388 |
| Moral Distress and Compassion Fatigue | 393 |
| Conclusion: Nursing as a Moral Profession | 396 |
| References | 397 |
| Further Reading | 402 |

**Chapter 14: Experimentation on Human Subjects**     **405**
  Introduction     405
  Early Moral Discussions of Medical Experimentation     406
  Nazi Medical Experiments and the Nuremberg Code     408
  Post-war Experiments in the U.S.     412
       1. Tuskegee syphilis study (1932–1972)     412
       2. Willowbrook hepatitis study (1956–1971)     414
       3. Jewish Chronic Disease Hospital cancer study (1963)     415
       4. Other unethical research     416
  The Belmont Report and the Common Rule     418
  Contemporary Issues     423
  Conclusion: The Legacy of Paternalism     426
  References     427
  Further Reading     429

**Conclusion: Reflective Equilibrium, between Medicine and Philosophy**     **433**

*Index*     *437*

**For additional resources and updated cases or studies, please visit**
https://hackettpublishing.com/medical-ethics-online-resources

# ACKNOWLEDGMENTS

This book is better than it otherwise would be because of input from a community of supportive friends, colleagues, and professional acquaintances. Early versions of some chapters and parts of chapters were presented at meetings of the Association of Practical and Professional Ethics and the Northwest Philosophy Conference, where audience members offered constructive comments. Gavin Enck, Pam Kohlmeier, Dave Schwan, and Elizabeth Wise provided valuable feedback on the whole manuscript. Sandy Martinez and Deanna "Dede" Utley gave useful suggestions on specific chapters relevant to their areas of expertise. We appreciate how generous all these people were with their time in helping us to improve the book. Any remaining errors are, of course, our own.

Lucy and Sam inspire us and give us hope for the future. Matt's parents, Doug and Sheryl, and Cindy's parents, Bob and Jane, have been constant sources of encouragement.

We also thank Jeff Dean, senior editor at Hackett, for shepherding the book from initial concept to publication.

A note from Dr. Coe: While writing this book, I was diagnosed with cancer, followed by surgery and five months of chemotherapy. In unexpected ways, the subjective experiences of patients became immediate: the anxiety of receiving a diagnosis and trying to sort through alternative treatments, the difficulty of communicating with multiple healthcare professionals, the challenges of dealing with insurance companies, and above all the feeling of impaired autonomy. I became "a patient" whose life as a philosopher, parent, spouse, and child of aging parents had to be reprioritized. I had to attempt to make rational decisions in the midst of confusion and fear. These experiences brought home the importance of treating the patient as a whole person. Patients who are fatigued, wounded, or otherwise physically distressed are also going to be psychologically and cognitively impacted. And even if patients show up alone to appointments, they are immersed in communities and institutions that shape their medical decision-making and outcomes (in both positive and negative ways). I have continually wondered how people navigate these medical challenges without the privileges that I had, including English fluency, health insurance, paid medical leave, childcare, and reliable transportation. I am grateful for the intense support of family and friends who have helped me emerge from this dark forest.

# INTRODUCTION

Medical ethics is one of the most exciting and interesting areas of academic inquiry. It analyzes foundational philosophical concepts such as what makes someone morally considerable, the meaning and limits of autonomous self-determination, the value of health and happiness, obligations of the individual to the community and the community to its members, what makes a just institution, and the definitions of life and death. It also touches on deeply personal questions that confront almost everyone: How much should I reveal to my doctor, and will they keep my information private? How much input should my child have in their own healthcare decisions, and at what age or level of understanding? What are my medical and life priorities, and when should I refuse life-sustaining treatment? When should I stop life-sustaining treatment for an incompetent relative? Medical ethicists also address important social and political issues, including abortion, medical aid in dying, healthcare policy, and the allocation of resources during public health emergencies. The field is inherently interdisciplinary, involving not only philosophy but also natural science, law, economics, politics, history, psychology, and sociology. And the field constantly confronts new problems as cutting-edge medical technologies become available and as healthcare professionals' engagement with patients becomes more complicated.

This area of philosophy is called bioethics, medical ethics, or biomedical ethics. Bioethics, or the ethics of life, is sometimes defined broadly to include not only human life but also animals and the environment. By contrast, medical ethics is sometimes defined narrowly to cover issues that arise only in a clinical setting, mainly around the relationship between practitioners and patients. This narrow interpretation excludes theoretical questions, such as when life begins, and topics outside of ordinary medical interactions, such as the ethics of human experimentation. In this book, we adopt a middle position between these two poles: medical ethics is the study of moral issues that arise in providing healthcare to people, including clinical practice, social policies, and medical experimentation.

Medical ethics is one focus of applied ethics, which is a branch of ethics, which itself is a subfield within philosophy. Western philosophy has been around for about 2,600 years, and ethical issues in medicine have been raised at least since the Hippocratic Oath in 400 BCE. However, medical ethics has only recently become a distinct field of academic study. Most scholars trace the beginning of medical ethics to the Nuremberg Code in 1947, which set out basic principles governing human subjects research in the aftermath of World War II, and the ethical issues raised by the so-called "God Committee" in 1961, which decided how to allocate a limited number of dialysis machines to patients with kidney failure, an otherwise terminal condition. Although they have roots in the Hippocratic tradition, the values of informed consent, concern for patient well-being, and just allocation of risks and benefits were more formally recognized in the wake of these two developments.

In some ways, "applied ethics" is a misnomer. It gives the impression that we should first adopt a normative ethical theory, such as Immanuel Kant's deontological (duty-based) theory or John Stuart Mill's utilitarianism, and then simply apply that theory to actual cases (even if applying ethical theory is rarely a simple matter). But medical ethics is more complex than that. It is true that, when a theory makes sense, it should inform our decisions. For instance, the general commitment to promote patient well-being shapes countless ordinary choices on the part of clinicians, such as washing their hands, making prompt referrals, and checking drug interactions. However, we also react to specific cases with moral intuitions about what is right and wrong. Moral intuitions are immediate, but unlike fleeting emotions, they can be strong and stable over time since, ideally, they reflect a web of deep moral values informed by thoughtful evaluation. For example, we think that medical professionals should try to maximize patient well-being by extending life. But when terminal patients refuse aggressive treatment, our intuitions may make us revise our conception of well-being, considering not only quantity but quality of life. Concrete cases test and complicate our abstract principles. Through this back-and-forth process, where theory and practice mutually inform one another, we arrive at a state of reflective equilibrium.

Capturing this process, the most common analytical framework in medical ethics is Tom Beauchamp and James Childress's principlism.

Rather than devising an alternative theory from which moral conclusions could be derived, Beauchamp and Childress propose four principles—rooted in what they call the common morality—that should be used as a starting point for reflection and deliberation: respect for autonomy, nonmaleficence, beneficence, and justice. On this view, moral reasoning is a process by which tentative conclusions are reached and often later revised and refined in light of new scientific and social developments. Notably, two of the most promising alternatives to principlism—the casuistical approach and the care-based approach—have us focus on the specifics of cases and the particularity of individual patients. Medical ethics, then, is applied in the sense that any abstract moral concepts must engage constantly with medical practice.

In keeping with the nature of the field, this book emphasizes not only the theoretical underpinnings of various positions in medical ethics but also their practical implications—for public policy and the law, personal decision-making, and how clinicians treat patients. It is intended for a variety of readers, including philosophy students, medical students, healthcare professionals, hospital ethics committees, and institutional review boards. Indeed, we have endeavored to make the book accessible for anyone, inside or outside of academia, with an interest in the field. Although we refer to ethical theories and philosophical concepts, the book presupposes no specialized knowledge. We use boldface type when first explaining key philosophical, medical, and legal terms. We also include historical and contemporary case studies to illustrate ethical problems that have challenged practitioners and bioethicists. Our goal is to provide a concise introduction to medical ethics, but with a breadth of coverage that addresses most of the field's major topics.

The first two chapters examine theoretical concepts that are crucial for understanding specific issues in medical ethics—namely, what standards should we use to make moral judgments, and who is morally responsible? Chapter 1 focuses on principlism and its critics, including related issues such as how ethics differs from professional codes and the law, the virtues clinicians ought to develop, and what gives someone or something moral status. Chapter 2 defends the notion of collective responsibility in the healthcare setting and shows how it intersects with personal responsibility, using medical error as an illustrative example.

Chapters 3 and 4 look at the relationship between clinicians and patients. This relationship is defined by two poles: paternalistic concern for patient well-being on the one side and respect for patient autonomy on the other. How we prioritize these two values generates different models of medical decision-making. This tension raises theoretical questions about what it means for the patient to be freely self-determining and practical questions about the information clinicians ought to disclose to patients (including medical errors), patients' right to control their private medical information, and whether clinicians may refuse to fulfill professional responsibilities to which they have personal moral objections.

We then turn our attention to moral questions around human reproduction. Such questions are especially difficult because it is not obvious when an embryo or fetus becomes morally considerable or, to put it another way, when a pregnant woman's body ceases to be fully hers and becomes a growing person's habitat. We cover the perennial ethical issue of abortion in Chapter 5, including some pro- and anti-abortion arguments that depend on answering the personhood question and some that do not. We also examine the legality of abortion, particularly in the United States, where different theories of constitutional interpretation lead to opposite conclusions about the right to privacy and the right to abortion. Chapter 6 examines other issues in reproductive ethics, including the criminalization of pregnancy in the U.S. and moral quandaries raised by modern reproductive technologies, specifically in vitro fertilization, surrogate motherhood, disability-selective abortion, genetic enhancement, and stem cell research.

Chapters 7 and 8 focus on ethics at the end of life: how to control one's own healthcare decisions with advance directives, how to choose for incapacitated patients who have no clear directives, and whether clinicians ought to assist (or be allowed to assist) terminally ill patients in bringing about their own deaths. Such issues again raise questions about the extent of patient autonomy, how we can respect patients' choices while also promoting their well-being, and the broader social implications of how we treat people who are dying.

The chapters that follow remind us that medical ethics concerns not only personal medical decisions but also public policies, such as the allocation of healthcare and the provision of health insurance (Chapter 9) and the distribution of scarce medical resources such as transplantable organs, medical treatment, and vaccines (Chapter 10). Chapter 11 reveals how social attitudes impact the patient experience. In the U.S. especially, the presence of racial bias affects everything from the clinician-patient relationship to public health campaigns, resulting in statistically worse health outcomes for people of color.

The final three chapters consider three distinct subfields in medical ethics, each of which raises unique ethical issues: pediatric ethics (Chapter 12), nursing ethics (Chapter 13), and research ethics (Chapter 14). With pediatric patients, the issue of consent comes to the fore. How do we make healthcare decisions for minors? Should we disregard what they want in favor of doing what their parents and clinicians think is best for them, or should we take their opinions seriously, even though they are incapable of fully autonomous decision-making? Nursing poses other moral challenges. Nurses must navigate a system that privileges the judgments of physicians while advocating for patients under their care. This can lead to difficult choices about how best to fulfill their moral obligations, sometimes leading to a phenomenon called moral distress. Finally, in authorizing medical research, institutional review boards are bound by the same principles as medical professionals: respecting the autonomy of test subjects, looking out for their well-being, and allocating benefits and burdens justly. But those principles place different demands on medical researchers, as do the complex legal regulations that govern experimentation on human subjects.

Some of our most pressing political controversies concern topics in medical ethics: for example, whether basic healthcare should be guaranteed for all citizens or residents, whether there is a right to abortion, whether we ought to modify our children's genes, and whether there is a right to die. This book considers such issues philosophically. Among other things, philosophy makes us more comfortable with perplexity. Medical ethics deals with questions that are not easily answered, and innovations in medical science and technology continue to raise new problems. Within that perplexity, however, philosophy provides a method to recognize and articulate the morally salient points of an issue. It helps us cultivate critical thinking skills so we can draw more consistent conclusions, listen for what is legitimate even in judgments with which we disagree, and recognize the underlying principles and assumptions at work in our moral reasoning. Even if absolute truth is unattainable, we can reason our way to positions that are better than the alternatives and good enough to guide us in our personal decisions and public policies.

**For additional resources and updated cases or studies, please visit https://hackettpublishing.com/medical-ethics-online-resources**

# CHAPTER 1
# Moral Reasoning in a Medical Context

**Key topics in this chapter:**
- The four principles that make up the dominant approach in medical ethics: respect for autonomy, nonmaleficence, beneficence, and justice
- How the four principles articulate common moral intuitions, including intuitions about who is morally considerable
- How ethics is related to professional codes and the law
- Virtues that healthcare professionals should develop
- Objections and alternatives to principlism

## Introduction

The most widely accepted form of reasoning in medical ethics is Tom Beauchamp and James Childress's principle-based approach, or **principlism**. Academic philosophy courses, medical school ethics curricula, and hospital ethics committees typically use it as a way to pick out what is morally salient in theoretical debates, hypothetical scenarios, and concrete clinical cases. Because of the prevalence of this approach, this chapter will take this form of moral reasoning as its starting point and then consider objections and alternatives to it.

The U.S. National Commission for the Protection of Human Subjects of Biomedical and Behavioral Research was formed in 1974, composed of physicians, scientists, lawyers, and ethicists. Beauchamp served as one of the professional commission staff members. The Commission summarized its findings in the Belmont Report, published in 1979. It lists three ethical principles—respect for persons, beneficence, and justice—as the basis for protecting human research subjects. That same year, Beauchamp and Childress released *Principles of Biomedical Ethics*, now in its eighth edition, which justifies and expands on these concepts. Often known as "the Georgetown mantra" (because of where they worked at the time), the framework developed by Beauchamp and Childress articulates not only the principles that ought to guide moral decisions but also the character traits that healthcare professionals ought to develop and the qualities that determine moral status.

## Common Morality

Although Beauchamp and Childress draw on many ethical theories—utilitarianism, **deontological ethics** (duty-based ethics), rights ethics, and virtue theory, among others—they are not proposing another version of these theories, let alone an alternative to them. Instead, they develop a framework of moral principles to guide deliberation. The framework is based on what they call "the **common morality**," a set of "universally valid rules" that "is applicable to all persons in all places, and we appropriately judge all human conduct by its standards" (Beauchamp and Childress 2019, 3). They believe that the common morality is justified empirically because it converges with people's professed moral norms; theoretically because it follows from normative ethical theories, including appeals to what is rational or pragmatic; and conceptually because of the very definition of what makes such norms moral (as opposed to, say, strategic) (449–56). The common morality provides the content of the principles Beauchamp and Childress propose, but the principles do not exhaust the common morality. Instead, the four principles are the part of the common morality that is most relevant to medical practice, public health policy, and research on human subjects.

Beauchamp and Childress argue that, at least in the context of medicine, we are all committed to four basic moral principles: respect for autonomy, nonmaleficence, beneficence, and justice. These are not listed in order of importance, as if autonomy should always take priority. Instead, the different principles are given different weights in different situations. Their relative importance is established by means of deliberation (with oneself or others) and moral judgment. Like W. D. Ross, who proposed a theory of non-absolute duties, Beauchamp and Childress claim that the principles have only **prima facie standing**, meaning that we ought to act as each principle dictates unless some more pressing moral obligation overrides it. We should, for example, respect a patient's autonomous choice unless it endangers public health (Beauchamp and Childress 2019, 105). Because there is no algorithm for decision-making—no step-by-step instructions for arriving at the right answer—people can disagree even when they apply the same principles. So, while the four principles are widely held, people can come to different conclusions depending on which obligation they think is most pressing in a specific case (and also because people have different conceptions of moral status, which we discuss later). As Ross says, moral judgments are more like aesthetic claims than mathematical deductions. The reasons we have are better or worse, not true or false (Ross 2002, 19–20, 31). And even when we agree on what is right, we can disagree about the strength of the obligation. Beauchamp and Childress say that an action may be strictly obligatory, weakly obligatory, or supererogatory (beyond what we are obligated to do, such as heroic actions). The common morality has "indeterminate boundaries of what is required" (Beauchamp and Childress 2019, 47–49).

Despite the potential for disagreement, principlism provides a common vocabulary with which to engage one another in moral discussion. That is, when deciding what to do, we are supposed to invoke the four principles and explain how they are relevant. Beauchamp and Childress believe that we should use the principles to guide our decisions (top-down) and that our considered moral intuitions in particular cases should affect the relative weight that we give the different principles (bottom-up) until we achieve a state of **reflective equilibrium**—a coherence between our general principles and our particular judgments.

## Principle 1: Respect for Autonomy

The first principle, **respect for autonomy**, obligates us to acknowledge and support people's ability to make important decisions for themselves. Although they are often only implicit, each person has their own scale of values and priorities. Respect for autonomy means that we ought to allow people to act in accordance with those values, even if we have different values and even if we think a decision they make is wrong. Imagine someone is paralyzed after a spinal injury and demands that they be removed from the ventilator. Studies show that most people eventually adapt to their paralyses and go on to live happy and fulfilling lives. Despite clinicians' efforts, the patient is unconvinced. Honoring that decision respects their right to bodily self-determination. There is a generally accepted right to refuse medical treatment that is grounded in the respect for autonomy, even if it conflicts with what doctors recommend.

Beauchamp and Childress set out three conditions for autonomy: liberty, understanding, and agency (2019, 100–102). **Liberty**, which they also call voluntariness or noncontrol, is "independence from controlling influences" (100). One may lack liberty because of either internal constraints, such as mental illness, or external constraints, such as physical coercion by others (102). **Understanding** requires having "pertinent information and . . . relevant beliefs about the nature and consequences of [one's] actions," although it need not be perfect or complete comprehension (131). One may lack understanding because of language barriers or cognitive disabilities. **Agency**, which they also call intentionality, is the capacity to deliberate upon a plan of action (decisional autonomy) and to carry out that plan (executional autonomy) (139). One of the difficulties with progressive dementia is that people typically lose the ability to deliberate rationally before they lose the physical capacity to act, so they may wander away from a care facility without knowing where to go. In many practical situations, diminished autonomy arises when one is lacking in all three dimensions. Someone in an acute mental health crisis is suffering from internal constraints on liberty, cannot understand their situation, and cannot participate in decision-making about treatment.

In the history of ethics, Immanuel Kant is the most important proponent and strongest defender of the value of autonomous self-determination. According to Kant, **humanity**, defined as the ability to set one's own ends (or goals), distinguishes us from the rest of nature (1996b, 6:387, 392). It is by virtue of our humanity that we have "unconditional, incomparable worth" or "dignity" (1996a, 4:434–36), so we are necessarily and universally bound (by the categorical imperative) to respect people's humanity: "*So act that you use humanity, whether in your own person or in the person of any other, always at the same time as an end, never merely as a means*" (1996a, 4:429). In other words, all moral agents have an absolute duty to treat themselves and other people as rational end-setters rather than instruments they can manipulate to produce some desired state of affairs, such as maximizing happiness. When someone violates the categorical imperative, they sacrifice what is good without qualification for what is only conditionally good, based on what they happen to want. For Kant, then, we are fully autonomous only when we act rationally and for the sake of the moral law. True freedom is not only independence from constraints (both external and internal) and the capacity to choose but also using that capacity rightly to do what reason demands. Beauchamp and Childress, however, have a lower standard for what constitutes rational agency. For them, autonomy is uncoerced, deliberative decision-making rather than fully rational self-determination.

In medicine, we tend to emphasize the autonomy of patients and research subjects, and we only secondarily apply this principle to clinicians. Patients have a right to know their diagnosis, to control their confidential medical information, and to consent to treatment—provided that they are cognitively capable and legally competent. For at least the last fifty years, the pendulum has swung from having the physician paternalistically decide on the appropriate treatment to (in simplified form) having the physician present the patient with the available options from which the patient can choose. If a doctor fails to give all the viable treatment options (undermining liberty), presents explanations that are too complicated or jargon-filled (undermining understanding), or allows someone in severe emotional distress to make important medical decisions (undermining agency), then the resulting choice is not fully free.

In the clinical and research contexts, respect for autonomy requires obtaining **informed consent** from patients and test subjects. Beauchamp and Childress (2019) identify seven elements of informed consent. The first two are background conditions that make fully free and informed consent possible:

I. Threshold elements (preconditions)

   1. Competence (ability to understand and decide)
   2. Voluntariness (in deciding) (122)

These are the characteristics of the patient that often depend on factors outside of their control, such as their age, maturity level, or degree of cognitive ability, as well as the circumstances in which they are making decisions. Someone who is threatened or otherwise coerced is usually not acting voluntarily. But there are degrees of coercion, and it is a matter of judgment whether encouragement or pressure from others is great enough to constitute "undue influence."

II. Information elements
  3. Disclosure (of material information)
  4. Recommendation (of a plan)
  5. Understanding (of 3 and 4) (122)

In a clinical context, a physician is not required to mention every therapeutic alternative, only those that meet the appropriate standard of disclosure—what is customary in the profession, what a reasonable person would consider, or what the individual patient needs to understand their situation (124–25). A clinician does not have to remain neutral on which treatment is best as long as they do not pressure the patient to conform to the recommendation (or else it would not be voluntary). In human subjects research, informed consent requires explaining the purpose and methods of the experiment, disclosing foreseeable risks and benefits, describing how confidentiality will be protected, providing contact information for the researchers, and stating that subjects can withdraw at any time without penalty.

III. Consent elements
  6. Decision (in favor of a plan)
  7. Authorization (of the chosen plan) (122)

Finally, the patient consents to a procedure by deciding to do it (intent) and formally authorizing it (action), either verbally or in writing. According to Beauchamp and Childress, fulfilling these seven conditions is sufficient for informed consent, in accordance with respect for autonomy.

Even apart from those cases where respect for autonomy comes into conflict with the other three principles, it is sometimes unclear how best to promote it. For example, suppose a woman decides to get RU-486 (mifepristone) a day after having unprotected sex so that she can prevent a fertilized egg from implanting in her uterus. What should happen if the pharmacist opposes the drug because of their own deeply held religious convictions? The pharmacist's right to religious freedom conflicts with the woman's right to control her own body. It is also hard to respect the autonomy of an incapacitated patient if they did not make their medical preferences known in an advance directive. And medical decisions for minors become especially complex when there is disagreement among the doctor, one or both parents, and their underage child. How much control should children have over their own treatment, and what limits are there to what parents should be able to decide for their children? In places where abortion is legal, at what age should a young woman be able to consent to the procedure without informing her parents? Obviously, the principle of respect for autonomy raises a lot of vexing questions, many of which we explore in later chapters. For now, it suffices to show that moral reasoning about medical treatment begins from the presumption that patients should get to decide what happens to them.

## Principle 2: Nonmaleficence

The next three principles—nonmaleficence, beneficence, and justice—have to do with the provision of valued outcomes and their distribution. The principle of **nonmaleficence** enjoins us to avoid harming people, and the principle of beneficence obligates us to promote others' well-being, with harm and well-being defined broadly to include a range of devalued and valued states. They are **consequentialist** principles in the sense that what makes an action right or wrong is the consequences for the people who are affected by it.

There are many forms of consequentialist ethics, depending on the end that ought to be promoted: pleasure, happiness, rights, virtue, perfection, capabilities, or even beauty and truth. Beauchamp and Childress do not specify a particular end, talking instead in terms of furthering people's interests, which may involve all these things (and more) (2019, 158). The most prominent form of consequentialism is John Stuart Mill's **utilitarianism**, which is the view that we ought to maximize happiness, in both the short and long terms, for everyone who is affected by our actions (the principle of utility).

Initially, it may seem strange that Beauchamp and Childress distinguish nonmaleficence and beneficence, since they seem to be versions of the same principle. Surely, not harming someone is one way to help them, and helping someone is incidentally not to harm them. However, the duty not to harm someone is a separate obligation—indeed, it often carries more moral weight than the duty to help or make better. To take an extreme example, a doctor should not dissect an otherwise healthy person and distribute their organs to five people in need of transplants

(Foot 1967). Saving five lives at the expense of one life maximizes benefits, but it does so by deliberately harming someone, which is one reason why this is obviously wrong. More concretely, subjecting a patient to dialysis when they have multi-organ failure and the treatment only serves to prolong their suffering violates the principle of nonmaleficence, even if it benefits the patient in a narrow sense of cleaning their blood. Ross notes that nonmaleficence is "a duty of a more stringent character" than beneficence; harming someone is worse than simply not helping them (2002, 21). That is why people often say, roughly paraphrasing the Hippocratic Oath, that a physician's foremost obligation is *primum non nocere*, "first, do no harm." Beauchamp and Childress, however, do not necessarily prioritize nonmaleficence over the other three principles, saying that "the weights of these moral principles vary in different circumstances" (2019, 157).

The principle of nonmaleficence imposes a negative duty on us—that is, a duty to refrain from inflicting harm—not an obligation to promote the good. Beauchamp and Childress define harm as "a thwarting, defeating, or setting back of some party's interests" (2019, 158). They note that one can be wronged without being harmed—for example, if a doctor discloses my private medical information to someone who does not know me, care about the information, or remember it—and one can be harmed without being wronged—for example, when someone suffers because of medically recommended, promising chemotherapy treatments that turn out to be ineffective. There are broader and narrower conceptions of harm, everything from death to discomfort to mere offense. Beauchamp and Childress do not see the need to be more specific, choosing instead to focus on obvious cases of harm in the context of medicine, such as pain, disability, and death (159).

The principle of nonmaleficence is especially relevant in establishing clinicians' foundational obligations to patients. For example, clinicians ought to give due care to their patients so they are not subjected to unreasonable risks. Clinicians are negligent if they do not act as a "reasonable and prudent person" would, whether they are acting recklessly or merely carelessly (Beauchamp and Childress 2019, 159–61).

The obligation to "do no harm" is not always clear, however, and it raises many questions that medical practitioners and philosophers have struggled to address. For example, what are the conditions under which a clinician, who is normally obligated to treat a patient in need, could justifiably deny someone treatment? What state would a patient have to be in for a treatment to be considered futile? Is whole-brain death, the loss of higher brain functions, or low quality of life sufficient to make all treatment futile? Who determines a person's quality of life when they cannot speak for themselves? When do the burdens or risks of treatment outweigh the benefits? If we have a good reason to withhold treatment from a patient, does that also justify withdrawing treatment that they are already receiving, or is withdrawing treatment worse than withholding treatment? Is "ordinary care," providing the resources that anyone (healthy or unhealthy) needs to live, different in principle from "extraordinary care," such as surgical interventions and dialysis? Is letting a patient die (passive euthanasia) morally equivalent to killing them (active euthanasia)? And when a terminally ill patient asks a physician to legally prescribe them secobarbital to cause their own death (medical aid in dying), is the doctor harming the patient in fulfilling that request—agreeing that their life is not worth living, cutting off other treatment options prematurely, not pressing the benefits of **palliative care** (managing symptoms, especially pain, and helping them cope with side effects)—or is the doctor preventing harm by allowing the patient to avoid further suffering and loss of dignity?

## Principle 3: Beneficence

If you ask medical professionals why they went into the field, most of them will probably say that they wanted to help people. This is the impulse behind the principle of **beneficence**: we have a general obligation to improve other people's lives. This theme runs through the history of ethics: the Buddha bases ethical conduct (*sila*) on compassion (*karuna*) for all living things, Confucius says that we should extend to others the humaneness (*jen*) that we feel for our family, Francis Hutcheson says that our common moral sense only approves of actions that are motivated by disinterested benevolence, Mill says that we ought to maximize happiness, Kant says that fully respecting others involves furthering the ends they set for themselves, and Ross lists beneficence as one of his seven prima facie duties.

Beauchamp and Childress specify two concepts within the broader principle of beneficence: **positive beneficence**, which enjoins us to provide benefits to others, and **utility**, which has us weigh the risks, benefits, and costs in order to maximize the good (2019, 217). Both are positive duties in that they require us to act for the betterment of others, unlike the negative duty of nonmaleficence. Acting beneficently may involve preventing potential harm from occurring (e.g., making sure a patient's vaccinations are up to date), removing an existing harm (e.g., treating a person's illness), or promoting the good in general (e.g., leading a vaccination awareness campaign in one's community).

Kant calls beneficence an imperfect duty, meaning that there is some latitude in how we discharge it (1996a, 4:423–24). A physician who promotes vaccines is not obviously better or worse than one who gets patients into treatment for drug addiction. Both are acting rightly in trying to improve the health of individuals and communities. Other philosophers have argued that there is a method for identifying the best option among the alternatives. For example, Mill argues that we should act impartially—not privileging one person over another—and seek to maximize the amount of happiness, regardless of its distribution. Ross claims that we take on special obligations to some people that allow us to privilege them in our moral calculations. For example, a doctor should not cancel an appointment with an established patient who is sick just because a stranger is sicker. Beauchamp and Childress illuminate this by distinguishing **specific beneficence** and **general beneficence**: the former depends on special relationships (with children, friends, and patients, for example), and the latter is directed at anyone who can benefit from our actions (2019, 219–21).

Philosophers disagree about how demanding the duty of beneficence is, especially because it often requires self-sacrifice, using my own time, effort, or money. Utilitarianism is committed to the idea that we should promote happiness to the point of **marginal utility**, which is the point when any additional self-sacrifice would cause more harm for me than good that is produced for others. As Peter Singer famously notes, most Americans have a long way to go before they reach that point. They have a long way to go before they reach even a more moderate position: "we should prevent bad occurrences unless, to do so, we had to sacrifice something morally significant" (Singer 1972, 241). Getting coffee at Starbucks every morning is morally insignificant, especially compared to the good that money could do for the poor, both in our own country and abroad.

Beauchamp and Childress propose something that looks like Singer's moderate position. On their view, person X is obligated to or has a duty of rescue toward person Y if and only if the following conditions hold:

1. Y is at risk of significant loss of or damage to life, health, or some other basic interest.
2. X's action is necessary (singly or in concert with others) to prevent this loss or damage.
3. X's action (singly or in concert with others) will probably prevent this loss or damage.
4. X's action would not present significant risks, costs, or burdens to X.
5. The benefit that Y can be expected to gain outweighs any harms, costs, or burdens that X is likely to incur. (2019, 222)

There is a lot here that needs to be specified, such as what counts as a "basic interest." If someone is barely surviving in a state of extreme poverty, are their basic interests being met—they are surviving, after all—such that I can continue going to Starbucks? How can my action be necessary when so many other people could contribute instead? This raises coordination and free rider problems. Beauchamp and Childress talk in terms of "significance" and setting "reasonable thresholds" for when something is significant (222). Is this subjective—"I *really* like Starbucks coffee in the morning"—or is there a more objective standard along the lines of Singer's "moral significance"? The third and fifth conditions are about anticipating the effects of our actions. This raises questions about what we can reasonably anticipate, how far ignorance of the circumstances serves as an excusing condition, and our obligation to develop epistemic virtues so that we can properly assess outcomes.

The last condition, weighing the positive effects on Y's well-being against the costs to X, also raises complex questions. In public health especially, we need to know how best to distribute our limited medical resources in order to produce the most good. Two of the most common tools to do this are **cost-benefit analysis (CBA)** and **cost-effectiveness analysis (CEA)** (Beauchamp and Childress 2019, 251–56). One advantage of CBA is that it converts all costs and benefits into the same unit of measurement: economic value. This allows us to compare the value of different public programs, such as whether it is better to invest in healthcare, public education, food assistance programs, or low-income housing. Performing a CBA requires us first to put a value on human life. Drawing on behavioral economics, analysts often talk about willingness to pay, which, in the context of healthcare, is how much people would pay to reduce the risk of death. For example, a patient with a headache could get a brain scan to make sure it is not caused by a tumor. It is extremely unlikely that it is caused by a tumor, and a brain MRI (magnetic resonance imaging) costs on average between $1,600 and $8,400 in the U.S. If you had to pay that cost yourself, would you get a brain scan for a simple headache? Most people would say no. By comparison, a colonoscopy costs between $1,250 and $4,800 in the U.S., and it lowers the chance of death due to colorectal cancer by 88 percent. Therefore, while many private insurance programs in the U.S. and Medicare refuse to reimburse for that MRI scan, they typically cover a screening colonoscopy since the latter produces more benefit for the cost.

One advantage of CEA is that it can compare nonmonetary benefits and burdens, such as lives saved or lost, without having to assign monetary value to them. This allows us to compare similar things with similar outcomes, such as whether to continue using a current treatment or adopt a different one. A common unit of measure for cost-effectiveness analyses is **quality-adjusted life years (QALYs)**. A QALY includes both quantity of life (in terms of life years) and quality of life (in terms of how good one's health is). One year of life in perfect health is 1 QALY (1 year of life × 1 utility = 1 QALY). Of course, it is difficult to assign actual numbers to different conditions. Polling people's attitudes would give us only a snapshot at a particular time. Young, able-bodied athletes may see death as preferable to a life with diminished mobility, only to realize that they can live full lives when they are older and have arthritic knees. But even rough estimates of well-being are useful. For example, numerous studies show that people with COVID-19 vaccines and boosters are slightly less likely to get infected and significantly less likely to die from the coronavirus than those who are unvaccinated. Most side effects are minor and temporary (e.g., injection site pain and fatigue), and long-term risks (e.g., blood clotting) are extremely rare (Centers for Disease Control and Prevention 2024). At the national level, if no Americans had been vaccinated against COVID, it would have cost $34 billion in direct medical expenses in the first year of the pandemic (represented by nearly 6.3 million hospital days and over 283,000 deaths) and an additional $32 billion in the labor sector due to lost productivity. Widespread vaccination could have reduced these costs by 80 percent or more; actual vaccination patterns ended up reducing medical costs by 60 percent and productivity losses by 53 percent. The researchers concluded that if we are willing to pay $100,000 per QALY, vaccination was cost-effective in 66 percent of simulations (Padula et al. 2021). As a matter of public policy, then, it is cost-effective for individuals to get vaccinated for COVID, and it is cost-effective for governments to reduce vaccine resistance among the unvaccinated.

There are some problems with both CBA and CEA. For example, cost-effectiveness analyses can support discrimination against people with disabilities (Brock 2009). According to CEA, if two people, one with disabilities and one without, both need the same life-saving intervention, it is better to give it to the nondisabled person because their health-related quality of life will be higher. Cost-benefit analyses also focus too much on people's preferences rather than beliefs about what is right or best for the community as a whole. We should not gauge preferences to determine whether we should protect the environment, teach math in schools, enter a war, or find a criminal defendant guilty (Sagoff 2008). Similarly, there are values to consider besides preferences when we make important health-related decisions—for example, if someone has a right to care or if we ought to correct an injustice. The latter concern is one motivation behind Beauchamp and Childress's fourth principle because how goods are distributed (justice) is as important as how much good is produced (beneficence).

## Principle 4: Justice

The fourth principle, justice, emphasizes that people exist not as isolated individuals but in social relationships that carry moral weight. It reminds us that promoting a valued end, such as happiness, is not right if the goods are unjustly distributed. It matters who and how much someone is benefited, and the reasons they receive those benefits, in comparison to others.

Philosophers have been trying to define justice since Plato's *Republic*. The most influential recent attempt to establish a theory of justice, and one that has had an outsized impact on medical ethics, is the philosophy of John Rawls. In *A Theory of Justice,* Rawls says that a society is just when everyone in that society, the best and the worst off, would agree that it is just. To determine which society everyone would freely agree to, Rawls devises a hypothetical situation called the **original position**. In the original position, we should imagine ourselves as choosing from behind a **veil of ignorance**: you do not know your physical and intellectual abilities, including whether you are disabled; you do not know your age, race, gender, or religion; you do not know whether you are rich or poor; and you do not know the particular goals that you have, whether you want to be an artist, accountant, or mechanic. In short, all your "natural assets and abilities" are unknown to you (Rawls 1999, 118). This gives society a fair starting point, which is why Rawls's position is called **justice as fairness**.

If you did not know who you are, what you believe, or what you value, Rawls thinks that you would want two things: the freedom to pursue whatever it is you value and the means to do it. You would want what Rawls calls **primary goods**, including natural goods such as health and intelligence, and social goods such as rights and liberties, income and wealth, and the social bases of self-respect. These are the basic things that everyone needs to develop their capacities and try to live a good life.

To ensure that we have these primary goods, Rawls thinks that all of us would adopt two basic principles of justice: the liberty principle and the distribution principle.

1. **Liberty principle**: "Each person is to have an equal right to the most extensive basic liberty compatible with a similar liberty for others" (Rawls 1999, 53).

Every person has a right to pursue what they conceive of as good, provided that this does not interfere with the right of others to pursue their goods. This is respect for autonomy, limited by the harm principle. However, freedom does not mean much if one does not have the resources to do what one wants to do, so Rawls thinks that we would also adopt a second principle:

2. **Distribution principle**: "Social and economic inequalities are to be arranged so that they are both (a) reasonably expected to be to everyone's advantage, and (b) attached to positions and offices open to all" (53).

The second part (b) prohibits discrimination. If you did not know your race, gender, or other characteristics, you would not want to be prohibited from living what you think of as a good life. The first part (a) says that, in the original position, we would accept inequalities as long as the least well-off were better off than they would be under a system of equality.

If, from behind the veil of ignorance, you did not know whether you would be rich or poor, your initial inclination would probably be to give everyone the same amount and kinds of primary goods. Otherwise, you may end up destitute while others live in luxury, which would hamper your ability to live a good life. However, consider the following three options (Table 1), with $d_{1-3}$ being the three social arrangements (or decisions) you could choose and $c_{1-3}$ being the three social situations (or circumstances) where you could end up. The numbers indicate primary goods, such as health and wealth, with lower numbers being a worse quality of life and higher numbers being a better quality of life.

|  |  | Circumstances | | |
|---|---|---|---|---|
|  |  | $c_1$ | $c_2$ | $c_3$ |
| Decisions | $d_1$ | -5 | -5 | 40 |
|  | $d_2$ | 5 | 5 | 5 |
|  | $d_3$ | 6 | 8 | 10 |

Table 1. Possible distributions of primary goods.

With these options, and not knowing which circumstance you would end up in, Rawls thinks that all of us would choose $d_3$. We would not choose $d_1$ because we would not freely consent to a situation where we might be completely deprived of our primary goods (if we end up in $c_1$ or $c_2$). And we would not choose $d_2$ because we would be better off under $d_3$ even if we were the least well-off ($c_1$). This is a version of the **maximin principle**, where we make the worst outcome as good as it can be: in Rawls's account, we want to maximize the well-being of those with the minimum ("maximin"). A just scheme is one in which natural inequalities (e.g., different natural abilities) and social inequalities (e.g., the different socioeconomic classes into which people are born) damage people's prospects as little as possible. When they do hinder people, we must compensate them for their disadvantages (a rule of redress).

Three theories of justice that are especially relevant to medical ethics—what Beauchamp and Childress call **egalitarian theory, capability theory,** and **well-being theory** (2019, 274–75, 277–80)—all have roots in Rawls's justice as fairness. Norman Daniels (1985, 2007) claims that because everyone deserves fair equality of opportunity and health is a primary good, everyone deserves a basic level of healthcare. Amartya Sen (1980, 1999) and Martha Nussbaum (2003, 2013) claim that people need certain capabilities to have the actual opportunity to live well; we are obligated to provide healthcare so everyone has a chance to flourish. Madison Powers and Ruth Faden (2006, 2019) claim that societies must promote overall well-being by providing healthcare and addressing systemic inequalities that negatively impact people's health.

Beauchamp and Childress pose several questions that arise when applying a theory of justice. Even if there is a right to healthcare, what sort of public system should be in place to provide that care: socialized medicine, a nonprofit multi-payer system, a government-regulated system of private insurers, or a completely free market? How much healthcare are people entitled to? When there are limited resources, how do we balance this right against other rights, such as the right to education? How do we allocate healthcare—by need, by likelihood of patient benefit, by social utility, or by something else? Do people forfeit the right to care when their poor health is a result of their own bad decisions, be they unhealthy, risky, or immoral? If healthcare is a human right, is a state only obligated to provide for its own citizens (statist or nationalist theories), or must it also support noncitizens in the country and in other countries (global or cosmopolitan theories)? Answering these questions goes beyond the clinical space to a consideration of the proper role of government.

## Ethics, Professional Codes, and the Law

Sometimes, it seems like following the standards of one's profession is sufficient to discharge one's moral duties. However, Beauchamp and Childress claim that such codes are often grounded in traditional expectations rather than the common morality, and they are designed to serve organizational or corporate goals, such as reinforcing members' identification with the profession or reassuring potential clients that they are trustworthy, rather than guiding professionals to do the right thing. Acting ethically involves cultivating judgments that may be contested by other reasonable and well-meaning moral agents—by patients, other clinicians, and ethics committee members. Professional codes should thus be subjected to moral scrutiny to determine whether what they enjoin us to do is "coherent, defensible, and comprehensive within their domain" (Beauchamp and Childress 2019, 8).

Beauchamp and Childress have a more sanguine view of the law and other public policies, which they think do or should reflect our moral commitments: "Moral analysis is part of good policy formation," so "legal decisions often express communal moral norms" (2019, 9). They say that moral principles are only one element of policy formation, alongside such factors as efficiency, economic feasibility, and political procedure. The complexity of the law thus reveals the limitations of moral theory "because abstract norms do not contain enough specific information to provide direct and discerning guidance" (10). Ethicists should be modest in their claims so as not to assume that moral judgments about individual acts entail the same judgments regarding laws or policies, since the government has to consider things such as "the symbolic value of law" and the costs of enforcement (10). For example, euthanasia may be the best option for an individual patient, but it may be appropriate for the government to prohibit it legally because of the risk of abuse (10). According to Beauchamp and Childress, the law may even teach us to be better people, revealing the falsity of our own moral assumptions: "Legal decisions often . . . stimulate ethical reflection that over time alters those [moral] norms" (9).

The relationship between ethics and the law is a matter of longstanding debate, an accounting of which would take us beyond the scope of this book. Here it suffices to say that philosophers of law disagree about whether the law is or should be defined by ethical norms. To take only two examples: natural law theorists believe that human law should express the natural/moral law in our particular social circumstances, such that the law advances the ends of humanity and promotes the good; while legal positivists believe that the validity of law depends on whether it was formed by the right political institutions. On the former view, we should disobey the law (that is, engage in civil disobedience) when human law diverges from the higher, moral law; on the latter view, any obligation to obey the law is the result of social pressure to maintain the community and its benefits, and such an obligation is not absolute.

All of this is to say that the morality of the law is an open question, as is what to do when our moral values conflict with the law. Beauchamp and Childress do not address either issue, but it is something that clinicians need to confront. For example, several states in the U.S. have abortion bans in place with vaguely written exemptions when it is necessary to save the lives of pregnant women. Fearing prosecution, many doctors refuse to discuss abortion, or they send women to neighboring states when they seek abortions or experience complications due to miscarriage. Those who cannot travel are forced to suffer until their medical conditions are immediately life-threatening before doctors will terminate their pregnancies. Challenges to these laws are making their way through the courts. In the meantime, what should doctors do? Should respect for the four principles override their obligation to the law (if there is such an obligation)? Should they protect their licenses even at the expense of patients' well-being? It is well and good for Beauchamp and Childress to talk about how moral norms inform the law, but we also need to ask what clinicians should do when the law is wrong and it cannot be changed or is being debated.

## Sample Applications

In most clinical situations, there is no conflict among the four principles, and the right thing to do is obvious: the clinician recommends a treatment to the patient, explaining the reasons for their opinion along with the benefits and risks; the patient asks questions and chooses the treatment because it will address their health concern; and the patient has no financial impediment to receiving the treatment because they are insured and can afford it. That respects patient autonomy—a clinician does not have to be completely neutral on a course of action but has to inform the patient and solicit their consent—it improves the patient's well-being without substantial risk of harm, and the patient is treated equitably regardless of their race, class, or gender. Even when a conflict seems to arise—a patient refuses a recommended treatment—it may be because the patient values something over extended life. For example, a stage 4 cancer patient may forego aggressive treatment if they would prefer a shorter life (with pain management) to a few extra months with severe side effects from chemotherapy. And if a patient cannot afford a desired, recommended, and necessary treatment, there is no moral dilemma. It may be the community's moral failure and a strategic problem for the healthcare system—namely, to find out how to cover it.

Often the principles all point to the same conclusion. Imagine a patient (Patient A) with severe cystic fibrosis who will die without a lung transplant. Patient A wants to live, and a successful transplant has a good chance of extending their life and giving them a better quality of life. Performing a transplant would thus carry out Patient A's wishes (respect for autonomy) and improve their condition (beneficence). Suppose there is an available organ from a deceased person (Person B) who was a willing organ donor, and that organ is only a match for Patient A. In that case, Person B's choice is being honored (respect for autonomy), no one is being harmed to retrieve the organ (nonmaleficence), and no other patient needs it and can use it (justice). Although there is a risk of harm with any transplant, not doing the transplant poses a greater risk. The four principles would all dictate that we perform the operation.

In cases of actual moral conflict or disagreement, we must consider how the four principles are applicable, deliberate about their relative weights, and achieve reflective equilibrium. There are ways to tweak the above scenario that would put the different principles into conflict:

- The deceased Person B, whose lung is a perfect match for Patient A, did not agree to be an organ donor. Taking it against the person's will would benefit Patient A but not respect the autonomy of Person B. Should we take it anyway? And did Person B simply not express consent, or did they explicitly refuse? How would that affect our judgment of what it means to respect their autonomy?

- Patient A is fifteen years old and does not want the transplant, but their parents want them to get it. How much control should Patient A have over their own treatment? Should we ignore the minor patient's wishes so that we can do what the parents think is best for their child?

- Person B is alive and in a chronic vegetative state with little to no chance of recovery. Should we remove their feeding tube and allow them to die so we can save Patient A? This would cause intentional harm to Person B in order to benefit Patient A. How much weight should we assign to the principle of nonmaleficence, given Person B's condition?

- Patients A, C, D, E, and F all need lung transplants, and Person B is a match for all of them. There is a limited availability of organs. What principle of justice should we use to decide who gets it? Should we consider age, how close someone is to dying (need-based criterion), how long someone has been on the national transplant waiting list (first-come, first-served), the amount of benefit (life expectancy after the transplant), or other factors?

- Patient A wants the transplant, but they have comorbidities that mean they will likely only live another month, even if they survive the operation. Patient A is uninsured and unable to pay for the procedure, so the cost will be borne by the already struggling healthcare system. Is it worth the risk and expense?

It is difficult to answer these questions. However, principlism gives us the tools to focus on the morally relevant features and weigh different values against one another. Respecting patient autonomy tends to take precedence in these deliberations, so harvesting a person's organs without their consent is a nonstarter. There is increasing legal recognition that mature minors have the capacity for autonomous decision-making. Physicians have traditionally privileged nonmaleficence over beneficence—first, do no harm—meaning that, as long as a patient is alive, we should not kill them to use their organs for the sake of others. Questions of allocation are more complicated.

## Moral Character

In addition to the four principles they are most known for, Beauchamp and Childress also address two other foundational issues—moral character and moral status—that clarify who best acts on these principles and to whom we have moral obligations. Following Aristotle's account of virtue, Beauchamp and Childress's account of **moral character** focuses on who we are rather than what we do, right being instead of right action. For example, clinicians who are motivated by compassion for their patients are morally better than clinicians who act solely out of duty, without any sense of personal concern. Beauchamp and Childress identify five "focal virtues" that healthcare professionals ought to have:

1. Compassion: wants to understand others' feelings and has sympathy for them
2. Discernment: makes judgments based on relevant facts and values, and acts appropriately
3. Trustworthiness: inspires confidence in others that one has the right motives
4. Integrity: professes and acts on one's moral convictions
5. Conscientiousness: does what is right because it is right (2019, 38–45)

As Beauchamp and Childress say, these ideals of character are widely valued and ought to be promoted. In addition to training in moral reasoning, which is part of the standard curriculum in many medical schools, physicians and other clinicians should develop these virtues. Learning the four principles is not enough; clinicians need character traits that facilitate good judgment in using the principles effectively.

Although developing these virtues is important, we need to be mindful of how they emerge in the clinical space, where overemphasizing them can have negative effects. Having these virtues means that clinicians will act to further their patients' well-being. However, actual clinicians know that they stand at the intersection of sometimes conflicting demands from multiple stakeholders, including insurance companies, government regulators, and the hospitals or clinics that employ them (and their productivity metrics). When forced to make decisions that are not optimal for their patients, clinicians may feel that their attempts to be virtuous are thwarted by external conditions over which they have no control, such as available resources and bureaucratic demands. Over time, experiencing such moral distress causes frustration, cynicism, and guilt. By seeing how virtues are and are not allowed to express themselves in existing healthcare environments, we can begin to confront moral distress as a systemic issue rather than as individual instances of professional burnout. Theories of moral reasoning tend to focus on an individual agent deliberating about options in the abstract. But we should also be aware of the material conditions under which decisions are made and the fact that multiple individuals (such as a healthcare team) are often involved.

## Moral Status

In response to widespread doubts that we could reach consensus on a common morality, Beauchamp and Childress offer an explanation of moral diversity, both changing moral positions over time and pluralistic views held at the same time. They attribute different moral views to changing positions on **moral status**, not changing principles. That is, the universal, common morality does not change; its scope changes because of who is allowed into the moral community (2019, 447). For example, the abolition of slavery in the U.S. did not reflect the fact that we only then recognized the value of autonomy; rather, we only then began to expand the moral community to include Black people. Because membership in the moral community is not settled, it leaves open the question of who deserves justice or whose situations ought to be improved by our acts of beneficence.

The issue of moral status often arises in medical contexts since healthcare professionals deal with human beings at the margins of life and death: embryos and fetuses, anencephalic babies, patients in persistent vegetative states, and so on. Clinicians also treat people with developing or diminished capacity, such as pediatric patients, people with cognitive disabilities, patients with psychiatric disorders or addictions, and elderly patients suffering from dementia. Beauchamp and Childress talk about "degrees," "a continuum," and "levels" of moral status because the properties that people have can vary, which makes people more or less morally considerable (2019, 84).

Beauchamp and Childress describe five theories of moral status, which are differentiated by the properties that identify someone as morally considerable: (1) human properties, (2) cognitive properties, (3) moral agency, (4) sentience, and (5) relationships (2019, 67–80). Just as Beauchamp and Childress draw on traditional moral theories to develop their four principles, they draw on the five properties to develop possible guidelines regarding moral status "to clarify the nature, basis, and moral significance of these guidelines" (85). These guidelines capture different moral intuitions about whom to include in the moral community.

Their first two guidelines specify criteria put forward in the first and fourth theories, the criteria of (1) human properties and (4) **sentience** (the capacity to feel pleasure and pain):

> Guideline 1. All human beings who are sentient or have the biological potential for sentience have some level of moral status; all human beings

who are not sentient and have no biological potential for sentience have no moral status. (Beauchamp and Childress 2019, 85)

One problem with this view is that it is unclear why sentience and the "biological potential" for sentience would bestow equivalent moral status. As Judith Jarvis Thomson says, we should not treat an acorn as if it were an oak tree (1971, 47–48). Recognizing this, Beauchamp and Childress put forward a *"competitive"* guideline that captures this intuition:

> Guideline 2. All human beings who are sentient have some level of moral status; all human beings who are not sentient, including those with only a potential for sentience, have no moral status. (2019, 85)

This removes the potentiality component, but it retains the automatic moral elevation of some sentient beings for distinctively nonmoral traits: genetic similarity, or membership in the human species. But why is this morally relevant? Mary Anne Warren (1973) says that equating humans and persons rests on a category mistake: the former is a genetic or biological category, and the latter is an evaluative category that places someone in the moral community.

Beauchamp and Childress remove the appeal to human properties in their third guideline and focus instead on (4) sentience and (2) cognitive properties:

> Guideline 3. All sentient beings have some level of moral status; the level is elevated in accordance with the level of sentience and the level of cognitive complexity. (2019, 86)

In accordance with utilitarianism, here Beauchamp and Childress say that the ability to feel pleasure and pain makes something morally considerable, and things that are more conscious deserve more moral consideration. It is one reason why great apes deserve stronger protections than rats when it comes to animal experimentation (86). However, cognitive capacity is simply slipped in at the end—a not uncontroversial move. We tend not to think that children or the developmentally disabled have less right to moral consideration than fully functioning adults (Singer 2023, 8). The same question arises with their fourth guideline, which adds (3) moral agency:

> Guideline 4. All human beings capable of moral agency have equal basic rights; all sentient human beings and nonhuman animals not capable of moral agency have a diminished set of rights. (Beauchamp and Childress 2019, 86)

Beauchamp and Childress themselves recognize that this guideline entails the "controversial" conclusion that humans who lack moral agency have reduced moral status (87). They add the species criterion because, for many people, moral agency is only had by human beings, and it is an either-or proposition. Marc Bekoff and Jessica Pierce (2009) have challenged both assumptions by finding gradations of moral agency in nonhuman animals. Singer (2023) rejects the idea that someone ought to be privileged simply because of their species. He says that this is no more justifiable than favoring someone because of their race or gender. Speciesism is a prejudice, just like racism or sexism.

Beauchamp and Childress's fifth guideline returns to sentience, focuses on nonhuman animals, and specifies its application to research:

> Guideline 5. All sentient laboratory animals have a level of moral status that affords them some protections against being caused pain, distress, or suffering; as the likelihood or the magnitude of potential pain, distress, or suffering increases, the level of moral status increases and protections must be increased accordingly. (2019, 87)

Beauchamp and Childress say that this guideline incorporates both (4) sentience and (5) relationships since animals in laboratories are presumed to benefit human communities. Humans take on obligations of reciprocity and nonmaleficence when they establish relations with animals (87). We owe something to animals in labs (and presumably pets in our homes, to say nothing of the animals we raise for food) that we do not owe to animals in the wild.

Beauchamp and Childress acknowledge that the guidelines are inconsistent with one another and give us different moral conclusions—say, about whether an embryo, prior to achieving sentience, is morally considerable (2019, 84–85). When there are disagreements about who or what is morally considerable, the guidelines do not provide a method of adjudication. Beauchamp and Childress hope that such "guidelines can be progressively specified to the point of practicability," but they do not provide assurance that they can be (88). They stress the "importance" of addressing moral status—indeed, Raanan Gillon (1994) has made moral status a key part of his own "four principles plus scope" version of principlism. But Beauchamp and Childress also recognize the "limits" of existing theories (2019, 88). Many intractable moral and political issues hinge on this question of who belongs within the moral community, so it is unsurprising that philosophers continue to debate how to resolve that question in our practical decision-making. At least the five guidelines provide a vocabulary for articulating what grounds moral considerability so that discussions about medical decisions and policies can capture deep-seated moral intuitions, not only about what should happen but about the assumptions around moral status that underlie those judgments.

## Objections to Principlism

Decades after it was initially proposed, principlism remains the dominant approach in medical ethics, and for good reason. Beauchamp and Childress provide objective standards to focus complex ethical debates. Those standards are a compelling distillation of themes that recur throughout the history of ethics, including two principles (nonmaleficence and beneficence) that have roots in the Hippocratic Oath. The method of ethical analysis mimics what happens in the clinical space, such that practitioners can "work up" an ethical problem in much the same way that they diagnose an ailment and decide on a treatment. Perhaps because of its relative dominance in medical ethics, principlism has been the target of many objections.

### 1. Methodological concerns

Some people worry that patient autonomy has been overemphasized in recent years, but this is hardly Beauchamp and Childress's fault. Although they list autonomy first, they insist it does not automatically take priority over the other principles. Others object that principlism is not action-guiding since it provides only a framework for moral reasoning and lacks "explicit decision rules" that would allow us to come to a definitive conclusion in any given case (Holm 1995, 336). However, Beauchamp (2003) says that context-specific norms should be developed based on the four principles so that we can apply them in particular cases. And every moral theory depends on judgment. Even the "categorical imperative procedure" that has been attributed to Kant needs maxims as input, and there is a longstanding debate about how to formulate them correctly. It is doubtful that an algorithm would truly capture the essence of moral reasoning anyway. Still others contend that Beauchamp and Childress's framework is too much like a checklist, to be applied mechanically rather than through a shared process of reason-giving. That objection misunderstands the principles' status as prima facie obligations that need to be weighed against one another (Beauchamp and Childress 2019, esp. 15–16). The whole point is to guide discussion so that we can achieve reflective equilibrium rather than some quasi-mathematical derivation. However, even if we grant this point, Robert Veatch (1995) claims that without an explicit method of resolving conflicts among principles, Beauchamp and Childress's "constrained balancing" suffers from the same defect as Ross's intuitionism. What looks like moral reasoning cloaks an appeal to preconceived prejudices. Since someone cannot justify favoring one principle over another, they must fall back on their deeply felt (and ultimately unjustified) personal values.

## *2. Ethics of care objection*

Some philosophers have challenged Beauchamp and Childress's appeal to principles, claiming that they overlook the important role of feeling. Feminist ethicists in particular have criticized traditional moral theories for being too concerned with abstract principles instead of the relationships between people that generate our moral obligations to one another. Traditional ethical theories such as utilitarianism and Kantianism conceive of the prototypical moral agent as an autonomous individual, specifically a rational adult, who applies abstract principles to other unmarked, abstract individuals with whom he—it is usually male—engages in contractual relationships. A founder of care ethics, Carol Gilligan (1982), calls this the justice approach. Although care ethicists do not abandon principles entirely, they think something important has been left out. **Care ethics** focuses on our personal differences, our emotional reactions, and our obligations to specific people—a mother's relationship with her children, a teacher's relationship with his students, or a doctor's relationship with her patients. The word "care" is not only about what we do for others but how we feel about others, which is why relationships are morally significant.

Unlike the justice approach, which appeals to universal laws, the care approach does not demand that we suspend our special relationships when we make moral decisions. We ought to have an emotional commitment to particular people, not simply an abstract moral obligation to all rational beings or all sentient beings, but to our particular loved ones and those who depend on us (Collins 2017).

*3. Moral imperialism objection*

Another objection to principlism is that it purports to present universal ethical principles even though it is deeply infused with Western conceptions of individual rights and duties. In this sense, the dominance of the approach represents a kind of **moral imperialism**. This claim has three parts to it: first, that the four principles are not part of a common morality across all cultures or even across different religious and ethnic traditions within a culture; second, that there is no universal understanding of what those principles mean; and third, that even when there is agreement on principles, they are prioritized so variably in different cultures that it hardly constitutes a common morality. Unlike the objection from the standpoint of feminist ethics, this is mostly a factual issue: Is every reasonable person implicitly or explicitly committed to the four principles, and in the way that Beauchamp and Childress understand them?

The challenges to the supposedly universal scope of Beauchamp and Childress's common morality come from many quarters. For example, a wide-ranging study of European bioethics identified four values at the core of ethical decision-making across European countries: autonomy, dignity, integrity, and vulnerability. These four values are codified in the so-called Barcelona Declaration, which calls for them to inform policies devised by the European Commission (Kemp and Rendtorff 2000). Only one of those values—autonomy—is shared with principlism. There is also variation between Western and Asian values. Ruiping Fan (1997) has said that the Western conception of autonomy emphasizes individual independence, both in forming a personal, subjective conception of the good and in deciding for oneself, while East Asian cultures emphasize dependence on the family and the community as well as an objective conception of the good. Angeles Alora and Josephine Lumitao (2001) say that Western bioethicists focus on individuals, principles, concepts, and intellectual discourse, while Filipino bioethicists focus on social units (especially the family), moral virtues, embodiment, and the phenomenology of lived experience.

Even when the four principles seem to appear in non-Western traditions, they often mean different things. A recent study in South Africa found that biomedical researchers tend to understand autonomy through a communitarian rather than a libertarian, rights-based lens. In this cultural context, family members and the larger community are involved in the consent process. The concept of relational autonomy is not easily reduced to an individual agreeing to a contract (Akpa-Inyang and Chima 2021). Similarly, Anna Westra, Dick Willems, and Bert Smit (2009) say that Muslims do not have the same conceptions of autonomy and nonmaleficence. For Muslims, respect for autonomy does not mean that there should be informed consent, leading to an individual choice on the part of the patient. Rather, Muslim patients are bound to God and their imam, and they are only allowed to make decisions that are right, or are deemed to be right based on their religious leader's interpretation of the Qur'an. In some cases, this supports paternalistic beneficence as the best way to respect the patient. Furthermore, Muslims believe that human life has unconditional value, so withdrawing treatment that may prolong life would amount to harm. By contrast, Beauchamp and Childress talk about whether continuing treatment is "desirable" and say that we "need to balance benefits and burdens to determine overall effectiveness" (2019, 163). Using the same principle, then, they would come to different conclusions regarding treatments that may be futile or otherwise damaging.

Even when people profess the same principles and mean the same things by them, they may weigh them differently because of their different cultural backgrounds. For example, during the AIDS crisis in Africa, Western drug companies running clinical trials focused on study design, informed consent, and fair selection of research subjects, thus overlooking the burdens that were disproportionately felt by poor African women and children (Ryan 2004). Arguably, an overemphasis on autonomy and a one-dimensional conception of justice failed to prevent additional harm or to confront patterns of injustice that could have been partially addressed by preferentially recruiting test subjects from among those most affected by the disease. There is variation in how people order the four principles even within the United States itself. A study of a Navajo community by Joseph Carrese and Lorna Rhodes (1995) found that they rejected the notion of open and honest communication of "bad news" to severely ill patients. Since, on this view, thought and language can shape reality, expressing "positive thoughts" is one way to help patients. A beneficent concern for Navajo patients' well-being is more important than respecting patient autonomy by being transparent about their (perhaps bleak) prospects. Finally, based on case studies, Miguel Bedolla (1995) says that Mexican-Americans routinely privilege beneficence over autonomy. Søren Holm (1995) concludes that principlism is not a truly common morality but an "American common morality" that privileges autonomy and leads to the "underdevelopment" of any positive obligations to promote beneficence and justice for all people.

Although these are factual claims about cultural variation, critics of principlism draw a moral conclusion from them: bioethics should not neglect the social and cultural dimensions of moral experience, including religious, ethnic, gender-based, and ideological dimensions. As alternatives, they tout more pluralistic forms of bioethics. Although they risk a moral relativism that Beauchamp and Childress are trying to avoid, critics often propose ethical frameworks that are attuned to the specific value commitments of patients, families, and clinicians. Whether or not this is a damning criticism of principlism, clinicians should attend to the diverse religious and ethnic traditions in their community and be aware of how cultural differences affect patients' engagement with medicine.

## Alternatives to Principlism

Alternatives to principlism purport to describe clinical deliberations more accurately, to be based in actual cases, and to be more useful as guides to action. The most promising alternatives include the **appeal to common morality**, casuistry or case-based reasoning, and narrative ethics. On the first view, Bernard Gert, Charles Culver, and K. Danner Clouser (2006) conceive of morality as an informal, public system of rules, ideals, virtues, morally relevant features, and procedures for determining which rule to follow and when. Importantly, morality is public in the sense that all rational agents understand what it requires, allows, and forbids, and that they ought to follow it impartially. Moral theory discovers the common morality and tries to describe and justify it. The goal of morality is to lessen evil or harm, and Gert, Culver, and Clouser identify ten rules that forbid actions that directly cause harm (e.g., do not kill), forbid actions that eventually cause harm (e.g., do not deceive), or require actions that avoid harm (e.g., obey the law).

**Casuistry** or **case-based reasoning** begins from the bottom up with actual clinical practice, instead of applying principles to particular cases. Moral reasoning starts with paradigm cases of right action and then proceeds by analogy, looking at how new cases converge and diverge from the paradigms. For example, Albert Jonsen, Mark Siegler, and William Winslade (2021) propose the Four Box Method that collects and sorts the relevant facts about a particular case: medical indications, patient preferences, quality of life, and contextual features.

Grounded in religious ethics and literary theory, the **narrative approach** identifies priorities and assigns meaning to values in the context of an individual's or community's stories about themselves. Truth and values are constructed through a process of individual and shared meaning-making. The stories patients tell about themselves explain why they value what they do and what ultimately motivates them—their personal identity and their conception of what makes their life worthwhile—which informs their ethical deliberations (Montello 2014).

These alternatives are all, in their own ways, trying to ground ethical theory in ethical practice and to give clinicians, patients, and ethics committees clearer moral guidance. On these views, principlism lacks decision rules that would give us definitive answers to our moral questions, leaving us only with moral considerations that are ambiguous, have variable weight in different circumstances, and often lead us in different directions.

Although these approaches are presented as alternatives to principlism, the values of autonomy, nonmaleficence, beneficence, and justice are crucial in all of them. For example, the specific questions in the case-based approach may be aligned with the four principles, even though they start from a focus on clinical practice. Jonsen, Siegler, and Winslade recommend that clinicians consider whether "the patient [has] been informed of benefits and risks, understood this information, and given consent," which respects autonomy; identify "the goals of treatment" to evaluate whether it supports the patient's well-being; and acknowledge any "problems of allocation of scarce health resources that might affect clinical decisions," which speaks to the principle of justice (2021, 9). Thus, the Four Box Method is not purely casuistical. It prompts us to identify the salient facts or factors in a specific clinical context as a way of organizing and clarifying our moral reasoning. These alternatives provide different methods of moral reasoning, but they often draw on the same intuitions that Beauchamp and Childress call the common morality.

## Conclusion: The Impact of Principlism

Although we must keep these critiques and alternatives in mind—and Beauchamp and Childress attempt to incorporate some of them into principlism—we should not lose sight of what *Principles of Biomedical Ethics* has done for contemporary bioethical debates. Beauchamp and Childress have drawn on several major Western moral traditions to formulate common principles that clinicians, ethics committees, and academics can use in practice. The four principles are applicable across different healthcare systems and in the clinical, public health, and research settings. Their framework is sensitive to the legal and regulatory environment, especially in North America and Europe, such that the moral conclusions reached are consistent with what is legally required. Above all, principlism is useful for clarifying our reasoning and identifying the sources of moral disagreements, both interpersonally and cross-culturally. Although we should acknowledge its limitations, it has been and remains an extremely powerful tool in medical ethics.

## REFERENCES

Akpa-Inyang, Francis, and Sylvester C. Chima. 2021. "South African Traditional Values and Beliefs Regarding Informed Consent and Limitations of the Principle of Respect for Autonomy in African Communities: A Cross-Cultural Qualitative Study." *BMC Medical Ethics* 22: article no. 111. doi:10.1186/s12910-021-00678-4.

Alora, Angeles Tan, and Josephine M. Lumitao. 2001. "An Introduction to an Authentically Non-Western Bioethics." In *Beyond a Western Bioethics: Voices from the Developing World*, edited by Angeles Tan Alora and Josephine M. Lumitao, 3–19. Washington, DC: Georgetown University Press.

Beauchamp, T. L. 2003. "Methods and Principles in Biomedical Ethics." *Journal of Medical Ethics* 29, no. 5 (October): 269–74. doi:10.1136/jme.29.5.269.

Beauchamp, Tom L., and James F. Childress. 2019. *Principles of Biomedical Ethics*. 8th ed. New York: Oxford University Press.

Bedolla, Miguel A. 1995. "The Principles of Medical Ethics and Their Application to Mexican-American Elderly Patients." *Clinics in Geriatric Medicine* 11, no. 1 (February): 131–37. doi:10.1016/S0749-0690(18)30313-6.

Bekoff, Marc, and Jessica Pierce. 2009. *Wild Justice: The Moral Lives of Animals*. Chicago: University of Chicago Press.

Brock, Dan W. 2009. "Cost-Effectiveness and Disability Discrimination." *Economics and Philosophy* 25, no. 1 (March): 27–47. doi:10.1017/S0266267108002265.

Carrese, Joseph A., and Lorna A. Rhodes. 1995. "Western Bioethics on the Navajo Reservation: Benefit or Harm?" *JAMA: Journal of the American Medical Association* 274, no. 10 (September 13): 826–29. doi:10.1001/jama.1995.03530100066036.

Centers for Disease Control and Prevention. 2024. "Selected Adverse Events Reported after COVID-19 Vaccination." Last modified October 30, 2024. https://www.cdc.gov/coronavirus/2019-ncov/vaccines/safety/adverse-events.html.

Collins, Stephanie. 2017. "Care Ethics: The Four Key Claims." In *Moral Reasoning: A Text and Reader on Ethics and Contemporary Moral Issues*, edited by David Morrow, 192–204. New York: Oxford University Press.

Daniels, Norman. 1985. *Just Health Care*. Cambridge: Cambridge University Press. doi:10.1017/CBO9780511624971.

———. 2007. *Just Health: Meeting Health Needs Fairly*. Cambridge: Cambridge University Press. doi:10.1017/CBO9780511809514.

Fan, Ruiping. 1997. "Self-Determination vs. Family Determination: Two Incommensurable Principles of Autonomy." *Bioethics* 11, nos. 3–4 (July): 309–22. doi:10.1111/1467-8519.00070.

Foot, Philippa. 1967. "The Problem of Abortion and the Doctrine of the Double Effect." *Oxford Review* 5: 5–15.

Gert, Bernard, Charles M. Culver, and K. Danner Clouser. 2006. *Bioethics: A Systematic Approach*. 2nd ed. Oxford: Oxford University Press. doi:10.1093/0195159063.001.0001.

Gilligan, Carol. 1982. *In a Different Voice: Psychological Theory and Women's Development*. Cambridge, MA: Harvard University Press.

Gillon, Raanan, ed. 1994. *Principles of Health Care Ethics*. Chichester, UK: Wiley.

Holm, Søren. 1995. "Not Just Autonomy—the Principles of American Biomedical Ethics." *Journal of Medical Ethics* 21, no. 6 (December): 332–38. doi:10.1136/jme.21.6.332.

Jonsen, Albert R., Mark Siegler, and William J. Winslade. 2021. *Clinical Ethics: A Practical Approach to Ethical Decisions in Clinical Medicine*. 9th ed. New York: McGraw Hill.

Kant, Immanuel. 1996a. *Groundwork of the Metaphysics of Morals*. In *Practical Philosophy*, translated and edited by Mary J. Gregor, 41–108. Cambridge:

Cambridge University Press. As is customary in Kant scholarship, references to Kant's writings throughout the book give the volume and page number(s) of the Royal Prussian Academy edition (*Kants gesammelte Schriften*), which are included in the margins of the translations.

———. 1996b. *The Metaphysics of Morals*. In *Practical Philosophy*, translated and edited by Mary J. Gregor, 363–602. Cambridge: Cambridge University Press.

Kemp, Peter, and Jacob Dahl Rendtorff. 2000. *Basic Ethical Principles in European Bioethics and Biolaw*. 2 vols. Barcelona and Copenhagen: Institut Borja de Bioetica and Centre for Ethics and Law.

Montello, Martha, ed. 2014. "Narrative Ethics: The Role of Stories in Bioethics." Special issue, *Hastings Center Report* 44, no. S1 (January–February). https://www.thehastingscenter.org/publications-resources/special-reports-2/narrative-ethics-the-role-of-stories-in-bioethics/.

Nussbaum, Martha C. 2003. "Capabilities as Fundamental Entitlements: Sen and Global Justice." *Feminist Economics* 9, nos. 2–3: 33–59. doi:10.1080/1354570022000077926.

———. 2013. *Creating Capabilities: The Human Development Approach*. Cambridge, MA: Belknap.

Padula, William V., Shreena Malaviya, Natalie M. Reid, Benjamin G. Cohen, Francine Chingcuanco, Jeromie Ballreich, Jonothan Tierce, and G. Caleb Alexander. 2021. "Economic Value of Vaccines to Address the COVID-19 Pandemic: A U.S. Cost-Effectiveness and Budget Impact Analysis." *Journal of Medical Economics* 24, no. 1: 1060–69. doi:10.1080/13696998.2021.1965732.

Powers, Madison, and Ruth Faden. 2006. *Social Justice: The Moral Foundations of Public Health and Health Policy*. Oxford: Oxford University Press. doi:10.1093/oso/9780195375138.001.0001.

———. 2019. *Structural Injustice: Power, Advantage, and Human Rights*. Oxford: Oxford University Press. doi:10.1093/oso/9780190053987.001.0001.

Rawls, John. 1999. *A Theory of Justice*. Rev. ed. Cambridge, MA: Belknap.

Ross, W. D. 2002. *The Right and the Good*. Edited by Philip Stratton-Lake. Oxford: Clarendon.

Ryan, Maura A. 2004. "Beyond a Western Bioethics?" *Theological Studies* 65, no. 1 (March): 158–77. doi:10.1177/004056390406500105.

Sagoff, Mark. 2008. *The Economy of the Earth: Philosophy, Law, and the Environment*. 2nd ed. Cambridge: Cambridge University Press. doi:10.1017/CBO9780511817472.

Sen, Amartya. 1980. "Equality of What?" In *Tanner Lectures on Human Values*, edited by Sterling M. McMurrin, 195–220. Cambridge: Cambridge University Press.

———. 1999. *Development as Freedom*. Oxford: Oxford University Press.

Singer, Peter. 1972. "Famine, Affluence, and Morality." *Philosophy & Public Affairs* 1, no. 3 (Spring): 229–43. https://www.jstor.org/stable/2265052.

———. 2023. *Animal Liberation Now*. New York: Harper Perennial.

Thomson, Judith Jarvis. 1971. "A Defense of Abortion." *Philosophy & Public Affairs* 1, no. 1 (Autumn): 47–66. https://www.jstor.org/stable/2265091.

Veatch, Robert M. 1995. "Resolving Conflict among Principles: Ranking, Balancing, and Specifying." *Kennedy Institute of Ethics Journal* 5, no. 3 (September): 199–218. doi:10.1353/ken.0.0138.

Warren, Mary Anne. 1973. "On the Moral and Legal Status of Abortion." *Monist* 57, no. 1 (January): 43–61. doi:10.5840/monist197357133.

Westra, Anna E., Dick L. Willems, and Bert J. Smit. 2009. "Communicating with Muslim Parents: 'The Four Principles' Are Not as Culturally Neutral as Suggested." *European Journal of Pediatrics* 168, no. 11 (November): 1383–87. doi:10.1007/s00431-009-0970-8.

## FURTHER READING

Arras, John. 2017. *Methods in Ethics: The Way We Reason Now*. Oxford: Oxford University Press. doi:10.1093/acprof:oso/9780190665982.001.0001.

> A systematic, critical discussion of the main philosophical methods in bioethics over the last sixty years. Arras devotes separate chapters to Beauchamp and Childress's principlism, Gert's defense of common morality, the new casuistry, narrative ethics, pragmatism, the "internal morality" of clinical practice, and reflective equilibrium.

Beauchamp, Tom L. 2010. *Standing on Principles: Collected Essays*. Oxford: Oxford University Press.

> Contains fifteen previously published essays that modify or defend different aspects of the principlist approach. The book has three sections: a historical survey of the rise of principlism in the 1970s, with an emphasis on the Belmont Report; practical applications of principlism to such issues as informed consent and hastened death; and thoughts on the importance of theory in applied ethics and the role of the common morality.

Clouser, K. Danner, and Loretta M. Kopelman, eds. 1990. "Philosophical Critique of Bioethics." Special issue, *Journal of Medicine and Philosophy* 15, no. 2 (April). doi:10.1093/jmp/15.2.121.

> Six articles that criticize principlism by James Gustafson, Robert Holmes, Baruch Brody, Ronald Green, Loretta Kopelman, and K. Danner Clouser and Bernard Gert. For example, Brody claims that respect for autonomy, nonmaleficence, beneficence, and justice are "mid-level" principles

that must be justified theoretically by some more basic ethical principle. Clauser and Gert claim that because the principles are not derived from some common root, conflicts between them are irresolvable.

DeMarco, J. P. 2005. "Principlism and Moral Dilemmas: A New Principle." *Journal of Medical Ethics* 31, no. 2 (February): 101–5. doi:10.1136/jme.2004.007856.

Argues that Beauchamp and Childress's four principles lead to irresolvable dilemmas. DeMarco then offers a fifth principle, the mutuality principle, according to which basic moral values should mutually enhance one another. He tests the fifth principle by considering the hypothetical case involving parents who are Jehovah's Witnesses refusing a blood transfusion for their child.

Dubose, Edwin R., Ronald P. Hamel, and Laurence J. O'Connell, eds. 1994. *Matter of Principles? Ferment in U.S. Bioethics*. Valley Forge, PA: Trinity Press International.

Conference proceedings with essays focusing on cross-cultural critiques of principlism and five proposed alternatives (phenomenology, hermeneutics, narrative ethics, casuistry, and virtue ethics). The book sets the discussion in the context of bioethics in the 1990s and includes an afterword that promotes the value of religion and theology in bioethics.

Hodges, Kevin E., and Daniel P. Sulmasy. 2013. "Moral Status, Justice, and the Common Morality: Challenges for the Principlist Account of Moral Change." *Kennedy Institute of Ethics Journal* 23, no. 3 (September): 275–96. doi:10.1353/ken.2013.0011.

Examines how the universal common morality works in tandem with conceptions of moral status to account for variability in morals over time. Hodges and Sulmasy say that no adequate account of their relationship can be given to support a robust principle of justice.

Huxtable, Richard. 2013. "For and against the Four Principles of Biomedical Ethics." *Clinical Ethics* 8, nos. 2–3: 39–43. doi:10.1177/1477750913486245.

Briefly surveys four of the major objections to principlism—that it is imperialist, inapplicable, inconsistent, and inadequate—as well as responses to those objections. The article is primarily addressed to healthcare professionals and students. Huxtable claims that, despite some concerns about principlism, the four principles focus practitioners on morally salient features of clinical practice and serve as a useful starting point for deliberation.

Page, Katie. 2012. "The Four Principles: Can They Be Measured and Do They Predict Ethical Decision Making?" *BMC Medical Ethics* 13: article no. 10. doi:10.1186/1472-6939-13-10.

Empirical study of how prevalent the four medical ethical principles (plus truth telling and confidentiality) are in our actual decision-making process. Page finds that, although people profess a commitment to these principles (nonmaleficence especially), they tend not to actually use them in their moral reasoning.

Savulescu, J., ed. 2003. "Festschrift in Honour of Raanan Gillon." Special issue, *Journal of Medical Ethics* 29, no. 5 (October).

Celebrates Raanan Gillon's work by testing his assertion that the four principles approach can be applied interculturally to analyze ethical problems in medicine. Contributors, including Beauchamp, focus on four hypothetical scenarios: the Jehovah's Witness case, the child of a Jehovah's Witness case, selling kidneys for transplantation, and genetic manipulation to produce germline transmissible genetic enhancement. The authors thus demonstrate how to apply principlism as well as alternatives such as communitarianism, virtue ethics, and casuistry.

Veatch, Robert M., ed. 2003. "Is There a Common Morality?" Special issue, *Kennedy Institute of Ethics Journal* 13, no. 3 (September).

Collects three papers that challenge the notion of a common morality, along with a response by Beauchamp. Leigh Turner claims that empirical, cross-cultural observations do not support the idea that there are shared moral norms. David DeGrazia claims that striving for consensus hampers ideas that challenge unjustified moral beliefs. And Jeffrey Brand-Ballard claims that we confront a dilemma: attempting to bring general norms and considered judgments into reflective equilibrium covers over their inconsistency, but acceding to pluralism leaves us without concrete moral guidance.

# CHAPTER 2
# Collective Responsibility in Medicine

**Key topics in this chapter:**

- Two ways of justifying collective responsibility, applied to healthcare settings
- The prevalence of medical errors and the concept of just culture as an attempt to address them
- A case study illustrating the intersection of individual responsibility on the part of the clinician and collective responsibility on the part of the healthcare institution

## Introduction

The modern clinical environment is extremely complex. Primarily for economic reasons, most doctors have given up private practice and are now employed by hospitals and clinics, and most independent hospitals and clinics have been absorbed by larger healthcare systems. In this context, doctors are not patients' only point of contact, and patients may not have longstanding relationships with individual primary care clinicians. Often, teams that may include attending physicians, nurse practitioners, physician assistants, registered nurses, nurse assistants, clinical pharmacists, and medical scribes, among others, collectively provide care for patients. Their actions are governed by the standards of professional organizations, policies of their employers, regulations of government agencies, and state and federal laws. Any clinician's actions intersect with the actions of others; the effects of those actions are not attributable only to the individual. In such an environment, it makes sense to talk about collective responsibility in addition to personal responsibility and to call attention to the diffusion of responsibility throughout the organization and beyond. In other words, medical ethics is relevant not only to individual clinicians but also to the organization as a whole, its constituent departments, administrators, and board of directors/trustees. In this chapter, we will focus on medical errors to illustrate this idea. Holding organizations such as hospitals and clinics responsible for errors, in addition to individual practitioners, will show the need for process improvements that fulfill our collective duty to respect autonomy, prevent harm, improve well-being, and promote justice.

## The Concept of Collective Responsibility

Much of the work on collective responsibility has been done by business ethicists, who focus on how we can attribute responsibility to artificial entities such as corporations. In this context, **collective responsibility** has to do with who is to blame for moral failures and the attribution of moral responsibility to groups of agents, rather than what it often means in nonphilosophical contexts: that everyone ought to work together to make things better (e.g., "we have a collective responsibility to address the opioid crisis"). This more technical concept of corporate agency has generated two kinds of explanations: (1) some theorists claim that the decision-making process of organizations is enough like individual moral agency to warrant the attribution of blame; and (2) others claim that moral decision-making is diffused through the organization as a whole due to its bureaucratic structure, such that no individuals can be held responsible for what the corporation does. Both approaches affirm that corporations can be held responsible. However, they justify that claim differently: the former by drawing an analogy between the individual moral agent and the corporation, and the latter by focusing on individual agents within the corporation and their reduced personal accountability.

Peter French (1979) represents the first approach. Traditionally, what defines an individual moral agent is the adoption of some aim, an evaluation of whether that aim ought to be pursued, and the attempt to achieve it. For example, Immanuel Kant defines humanity as the ability to set ends rather than acting purely on instinct or because of external forces (1996b, 6:387, 392). He says that to be fully rational, an agent must do what is right (act reasonably by following the categorical imperative) and will the means to the end they have adopted (act rationally by following the hypothetical imperative) (1996a, 4:413–16; Rawls 1989, 88). French claims that a corporation is a distinct moral agent because it does what moral agents do (see also Goodpaster and Matthews 1982). It adopts a strategic plan and accomplishes its goals by means of its employees. In other words, the whole is more than the sum of its parts: the corporation's actions cannot be attributed to any individual or set of individuals because they are acting on behalf of the organization, and those individuals may not have personally adopted the organization's broader goals when they accomplish the specific tasks that, collectively, further its aims. The actions of employees are guided by what French calls the corporate internal decision (CID) structure. According to French, "the CID Structure accomplishes a subordination and synthesis of the intentions and acts of various biological persons into a corporate decision" (1979, 212). Individual workers carry out the goals of the company, as defined by the CID. The CID structure gives the organization a direction even when all the employees and executives have changed. Something persists, and that something is the corporation. Its functioning as an agent, beyond the individual wills of the people who participate in it, means that it can be held responsible for its actions. In one article, French (1982) claims that the medical profession itself is an "aggregate collectivity," meaning that each individual clinician, as part of that collective, is partly responsible for the state of healthcare and has a general obligation to help when needed. In this chapter, however, we are focused on healthcare organizations such as hospitals and clinics, which have clearer CID structures, rather than the profession as a whole.

Business ethicists have attributed collective responsibility to what are arguably looser structures than what is present in healthcare. Individual employees in non-healthcare fields further the strategic plans of their organizations, as do hospital employees. But with the possible exception of aviation, whose high-reliability strategies the healthcare industry tries to emulate, no industry is as focused as healthcare on standard practices that guide the actions of its workers (see Kapur et al. 2016).

1. There are clinical practice standards for healthcare professionals and different standards for different positions. For example, there are medical boards that license and review physicians of different specialties, each with their own expectations.

2. There are standards specific to given tasks. For example, the continued use of patient restraints must be reassessed and documented at regular, designated intervals.

3. There are formal standards and informal guidelines that are specific to individual organizations. For example, each hospital has expectations around monitoring patients who are given high-alert medications.

These restrictions are administered by a number of bodies: laws and regulations are enforced by federal and state governments (via regulatory agencies), professional standards are imposed by licensing agencies and accrediting organizations such as the Joint Commission, and performance and ethical expectations are monitored by professional organizations and employers. Payors also decide whether to reimburse healthcare organizations based on whether their own rules are followed. For example, in the U.S., the Centers for Medicare and Medicaid Services (CMS) has strict conditions that organizations must meet in order to participate in the Medicare and Medicaid programs, and they are surveyed regularly to confirm compliance. There is very little that clinicians do that is not governed by some kind of codified expectations. And within a healthcare organization, its governing body adopts a strategic plan that is operationalized through its Quality Assurance and Performance Improvement (QAPI) plan. The QAPI plan lists projects that are assigned to project leaders and carried out by different departments. Thus, French's claims about individual decisions being absorbed into a collective action are exemplified in the modern clinical setting (see also De George 1982).

David Luban, Alan Strudler, and David Wasserman (1992) typify the second approach to corporate responsibility. They claim that the bureaucratic structure of many businesses means that individuals have little awareness of the whole process, so blaming any one person for environmental damage, dangerous products, or harmful working conditions is often impossible. If a rank-and-file employee cannot be expected to know everything about how their contribution fits into what the corporation as a whole is doing, and if the executives do not know exactly what their subordinates are doing, then no identifiable individual can be held responsible for wrong actions by the corporation. In other words, the corporate structure erodes personal moral responsibility and diffuses it throughout the organization.

Although the lack of knowledge is probably not applicable to healthcare practitioners—treatments for individual patients are charted and discussed with the care team (in huddles)—there is something akin to a bureaucratic structure that makes the actions of any one clinician significant only in a larger context. In the case of healthcare systems, there is a general commitment to preventing and reducing patient harm (nonmaleficence) and improving patient health outcomes (beneficence) that can only be accomplished within a system that promotes it. For example, a patient who undergoes total knee replacement surgery requires an entire surgical team composed of (at least) an orthopedic surgeon, an anesthesiologist or certified registered nurse anesthetist (CRNA), an operating room nurse, and a surgical technologist. The anesthesiologist or CRNA does a preoperative assessment to identify needs and risk factors, and they monitor the patient after surgery. The patient is then evaluated and their pain managed by doctors, nurses, physician assistants, and nurse practitioners in the hospital (perhaps in the intensive care unit), and the patient undergoes rehabilitation with physical therapists. The health outcomes of the procedure depend on all these people. There are also housekeepers who clean the operating room, sterile processing technicians who prepare the surgical supplies, whoever schedules the surgery and selects the team members, and even the governing body that credentials the clinicians.

With regard to medical errors specifically, a team-based approach has been the industry standard at least since 1995, when MedTeams, a U.S. Department of Defense research project, reviewed risk management cases in a Rhode Island emergency department and found that 43 percent of medical errors were due to problems with team coordination. They concluded that better training in team behavior would have mitigated or prevented 79 percent of the identified errors. In response, they developed an Emergency Team Coordination course that trained clinicians on people's roles and responsibilities, communication, and cross-monitoring, resulting in a 58 percent reduction in observable errors (Leedom and Simon 1995; Morey et al. 2022). Other studies followed. The Institute of Medicine published a report in 2000, *To Err Is Human*, in which they found that medical errors cause up to 98,000 deaths annually in the U.S. (Kohn, Corrigan, and Donaldson 2000; see also Leape 1994). A more recent review of the scientific literature on medical error showed that more than 250,000 Americans die each year from **adverse medical events** (the umbrella category for medical errors, defined as unintended, negative effects of medical treatment), making it the third leading cause of death (Makary and Daniel 2016). The World Health Organization has called for a reduction in medical errors worldwide, and the Joint Commission disseminates national patient safety goals annually to address these problems.

In the U.S., the evidence- and team-based approach to improving health outcomes was legally codified with the Patient Safety and Quality Improvement Act of 2005, which established a voluntary reporting system to collect safety data and resolve quality issues. It created what has come to be known as **just culture** (as opposed to a blame-and-shame culture), which is the industry standard. The idea behind just culture is that medical errors are primarily the result of system failures rather than individual lapses. Healthcare decisions are so complex that mistakes are inevitable. The point of just culture is to minimize mistakes by having clinicians report them and then subject them to root cause analyses so that similar mistakes can be prevented in the future. To improve outcomes, there is an emphasis on transparency, where adverse and near-miss events are reported and talked about. To encourage such reporting, clinicians are not punished for good-faith errors (that is, those not caused by malicious intent, negligence, or gross incompetence), and reporters are protected from retaliation.

The goal is to lessen avoidable harm and improve overall outcomes for patients by implementing system-wide policies that guide the actions of clinicians. The field known as **human factors engineering** uses what we know about people—their cognitive processes, behavior, capabilities, and limitations—and applies it to redesigning equipment, workspaces, and devices with the goal of minimizing human error (see Leape 1994). Weaker solutions include individual instruction and training; stronger solutions are system-oriented and introduce forcing functions that focus attention to complete a task, thus preventing undesirable actions. For example, many years ago, concentrated potassium was removed from patient floor stock in general hospital wards, which prevented it from being given intravenously too rapidly or in an undiluted form—something that had led to patient deaths. Pharmacy computers can be programmed so as not to fill an order unless allergy information is entered. Syringes and IV medication bags can be labeled with barcodes that must match a patient's ID band. The goal is to lessen the inevitable errors that clinicians make by rendering them impossible or at least less likely. The responsibility for doing this—everything from employee training to product design to system design—rests with the organization rather than the individual clinician.

## Case Study: RaDonda Vaught and VMC

None of this is to say that clinicians should be given immunity for gross negligence or willful misconduct. Responsibility for violating established policies or not providing the legal standard of care for one's patients may fall on the individual person, usually the attending of record (the clinician ultimately responsible for a patient's care). However, given the healthcare industry's commitment to just culture, there is a high standard for administrative sanctions imposed on individuals and an even higher standard for legal culpability.

A high-profile case of medical error involving a nurse named RaDonda Vaught exemplifies the intersection of personal and collective responsibility. On December 24, 2017, Charlene Murphey (age seventy-five) was admitted for a subdural hematoma (bleeding between the brain and the skull) to Vanderbilt University Medical Center (VMC) in Tennessee. Two days later, Murphey was scheduled for a positron emission tomography (PET) scan, so she was prescribed two milligrams of Versed—the brand name for midazolam, a sedative—to blunt the claustrophobic effects of being in the scanner. Vaught, a floating "Help All" nurse for VMC's Neurological Intensive Care Unit, volunteered to retrieve and administer the medication.

Vaught typed "VE" (for Versed) into an Automatic Dispensing Machine (ADM), and it found no hits. So, Vaught used a computerized override to obtain the drug. Distracted by a conversation with a newly hired trainee under her supervision, Vaught typed in "VE" again and chose the first result that appeared: vecuronium, a powerful paralyzing agent. Vaught then ignored five warnings or pop-ups when overriding the system:

1. The following message appeared: "Override medications should only be accompanied by STAT orders or when the clinical status of a patient would be significantly compromised by the delay that would result from pharmacist review." Murphey's case did not meet urgent or emergent criteria.

2. A pop-up screen asked for a reason for the override. The message "PARALYZING AGENT" was at the top of the screen. Vaught had to select a reason for the override and then confirm the override.

3. The screen returned to the selected medication, where another "PARALYZING AGENT" message appeared.

4. Once the medication was selected, another pop-up screen appeared with the message "PARALYZING AGENT" and the following warnings: "Causes Respiratory Arrest" and "Patient Must Be Ventilated." Vaught had to press a button to move on to the next screen.

5. The ADM requested a quantity amount, and the screen once again contained the warning "PARALYZING AGENT" as well as a yellow "ALERT" caution sign.

This series of warnings was designed to make it less likely that a paralyzing agent such as vecuronium would be accidentally given to a patient. In this case, Vaught was distracted, and, as we will see, overriding such messages had become commonplace at VMC. Vaught also ignored other red flags between the time of the override and when she administered the medication:

6. Vecuronium comes in a powder form, as opposed to a liquid form like Versed. Vaught had to add a diluent to the bottle and shake it to reconstitute the medication, a process not needed for Versed.

7. The instruction label of the medication identified the contents as "Vecuronium" along with the message "PARALYZING AGENT." Vaught had to read the instructions to know that the medication needed to be reconstituted.

In the radiology department, Vaught did not have access to barcode verification, which would have compared the medication being administered with what was ordered; second nurse verification, which would have had someone double check the drug, dose, and patient; or electronic health records (EHRs), where she could have checked the order herself. Vaught administered the drug to Murphey at an unspecified time.

Vaught exited the room, leaving Murphey unattended. Had Murphey been monitored by a nurse, the signs of the medication's paralytic effects could have been detected, medication to counteract vecuronium administered, and resuscitation efforts begun. Murphey was later found pulseless and unresponsive. She was intubated, and after chest compressions, her heart restarted. Fifteen to thirty minutes later, after being informed of Murphey's condition and her error, Vaught reported to the Educator's Office and admitted to giving Murphey the wrong medication. Vaught then filled out a report in Veritas, the hospital's reporting system.

According to a physician's documentation, a scan of Murphey's brain on December 27 revealed "progression towards but not complete brain death . . . very low likelihood of neurological recovery." Murphey was removed from mechanical ventilation and died ten minutes later. Dr. Eli Zimmerman then falsified Murphey's death certificate, neglecting to document the fatal paralytic agent that had been administered and marking the manner of death as "natural," the result of a brain bleed. VMC also failed to report Murphey's actual cause of death to the Tennessee Department of Health, as required by law. Vaught was fired on January 3, 2018, because, according to the termination letter, "you did not validate the five rights of medication administration [right patient, right drug, right time, right dose, right route], per policy, which is part of your responsibility and within your scope of practice as a Registered Nurse."

Nothing happened after that until Murphey's wrongful death was anonymously reported to the Tennessee State Department of Health on October 3, 2018. The DOH investigated Vaught but decided not to pursue disciplinary action, claiming that Vaught's case "did not constitute a violation of the statutes and/or rules governing the profession." The Centers for Medicare and Medicaid Services then investigated VMC. They found numerous system deficiencies and individual failures relating to Murphey's death, and they ruled that VMC would be expelled from the Medicare program unless it produced a satisfactory plan of correction. VMC later submitted a 330-page plan of correction to CMS, pledging to:

1. monitor critically ill patients during transport;
2. monitor patients who have received medications that cause respiratory depression;
3. expand administration policies to require more documentation;
4. require that paralyzing agents be signed off by two nurses before and after administration; furthermore, paralyzing agents can only be retrieved from the ADM by searching "para," as opposed to the drug name itself.

In early December 2018, Vaught was interviewed by the Tennessee Bureau of Investigation, to whom she admitted that she was distracted while overriding the ADM, that she should have called the pharmacy instead of using the override function, and that she should have recognized the differences between Versed and vecuronium. In February 2019, Vaught was indicted by a Nashville grand jury on charges of reckless homicide and abuse of an impaired adult. In September 2019, the Tennessee Department of Health reversed its earlier decision and charged Vaught with unprofessional conduct, abandoning and neglecting a patient who required care, and failing to maintain accurate patient records. The Nursing Board revoked Vaught's nursing license in July 2021 and fined her $3,000.

On March 25, 2022, a trial jury found her guilty of criminally negligent homicide (a lesser charge) and abuse of an impaired adult. The judge gave Vaught a light sentence: three years of supervised probation under judicial diversion, with the record expunged on completion of the sentence. In May 2023, Vaught formally requested that her nursing license be reinstated, claiming she did not receive due process from the Tennessee Board of Nursing. Her appeal was denied in November 2023. For his falsification of the death certificate, Dr. Zimmerman apparently did not suffer any legal or professional consequences.

## Diffusion of Responsibility in the Vaught Case

In this case, there were both individual errors and system errors. Vaught's mistakes are obvious: ignoring the many warnings when dispensing, preparing, and administering the drug; not comparing the drug she had to the drug that was ordered; and not monitoring the patient after giving her the medication. Given Vaught's many avoidable errors, it was not unusual for VMC to have fired her or for the Nursing Board to have revoked her license. What Vaught did was egregiously wrong, and reporting the error does not absolve her. However, the criminal charges against Vaught were unusual, and they were met with almost universal alarm among clinicians. Thousands of medical errors resulting in adverse outcomes, including death, take place every year, and they are usually (except in cases of intentional harm) relegated to administrative enforcement and civil litigation. Penalties can be imposed on both the individual clinician (e.g., licensure actions) and the organization (e.g., damages awarded to a patient in a medical malpractice lawsuit). Vaught and VMC both were morally obligated to act differently and avoid patient harm, given not only her own mistakes but the prevalence of system errors that made Vaught's mistakes possible.

The diffusion of responsibility described by Luban, Strudler, and Wasserman (1992) is evident throughout the Vaught case. Using a team-based approach to quality, as is customary in healthcare, can help to identify structural safeguards that were lacking and that contributed to Murphey's death, including:

1. The use of the override function was common practice at VMC in the fall of 2017 because of integration issues between the ADM and the EHR system. Indeed, Murphey herself had previously

received, during the same hospital visit, at least twenty medication doses based on override orders (Lambert and Schiff 2022). The phenomenon of overriding alerts is prevalent enough across the U.S. that it has a name: alert fatigue (Singh et al. 2013). The point of alerts is to call attention to possible risks, but if there are too many for clinicians to process in order to get their work done, skipping past the alerts becomes habitual. In this case, the dangerous override could have been prevented in many ways, such as allowing overrides only when medications are required in emergent circumstances, waiting for pharmacist review of medication orders, or having a prompt requiring documentation of a witness when removing especially dangerous drugs (such as paralyzing agents) via override. VMC also did not have a committee regularly review and approve all medications for which overrides are permitted, clinical locations where they are allowed, and practitioner types who can use the override function.

2. The warnings were not sufficient to prevent such a mistake. The Institute for Safe Medication Practices (ISMP) (2019) commented on the Vaught case:

> whether the nurse made an error in judgment when deciding to obtain the medication via override is not the issue; the real issue in this case is that there were no effective systems in place to prevent or detect the accidental selection, removal, and administration of a neuromuscular blocker that had been obtained via override.

Such an accidental selection was made more likely by the fact that the ADM was not configured to search automatically by both brand and generic names, and it did not require clinicians to type in at least five letters to retrieve search results. The ISMP (2016) had published a set of safe practices for paralytic agents in June 2016 that VMC had not implemented. According to ISMP (2022), the 2016 guidelines "provided recommendations for addressing risks that likely would have avoided this error."

3. The radiology area where the error occurred had no barcode scanners to verify the medication prior to administering it (Institute for Safe Medication Practices and the Just Culture Company 2022).

4. VMC had no policy or procedure for monitoring patients following the administration of high-alert medications.

If we take just culture seriously, VMC missed opportunities to correct these problems in advance, such as addressing the frequent overrides to obtain medication. In a no-fault environment, someone should have said something earlier to bring about a policy change. The plan of correction that VMC itself submitted to CMS included changes that would correct the first, second, and fourth problems. Although it was forced on them, the plan of correction was the result of an evidence- and team-based approach to avoiding medical errors, which depends on clinicians duly reporting good-faith errors (as Vaught did).

As we have discovered over the past twenty-five years of research into patient safety, punishing clinicians for mistakes that are not grossly negligent has an overall adverse effect on health outcomes. Indeed, fear of consequences is the most common reason clinicians give for underreporting medical errors (Aljabari and Kadhim 2021). An important part of just culture is the nonpunitive response to errors, a turn away from a blame-and-shame culture so that individual clinicians feel comfortable reporting them. When errors are reported, root cause analyses can be conducted and system changes can be instituted to make such mistakes less likely in the future. As French (1979) shows us, an individual clinician's actions take on moral significance only in the context of a broader, institutional goal—in this case, the improvement of quality and patient safety. That goal is realized by modifying standard practices that produce errors or creating standard practices where none exist in order to prevent them.

In the Vaught case, the heads of the American Nurses Association and the Tennessee Nurses Association sent a letter to the presiding judge prior to Vaught's sentencing, warning of "the residual impact on nurses and other healthcare professionals feeling safe to report errors" (Grant, Cole, and Lawson 2022). The guiding principles behind just culture in healthcare are fundamentally opposed to the principles underlying the criminal law. In the context of criminal law, reporting a mistake is an admission of guilt. If clinicians know they may be prosecuted, they will be reluctant to incriminate themselves. This conflict revealed itself in the Vaught case. Vaught immediately reported her mistake and remained cooperative throughout the investigation because that is an expectation of just culture—and then she was charged with and convicted of a crime.

VMC covered up the mistake and did not generate a plan of correction until CMS demanded it.

## Conclusion: The Collective Responsibility to Reduce Harm

The choices of individual clinicians are not isolated actions but points in a complex process of healthcare delivery. This is not to say, of course, that individuals cannot be held morally and legally responsible for gross negligence or intentional harm. But the conditions under which healthcare professionals work both mitigates individual responsibility and spreads the blame to the larger organization. The policies and practices that could have prevented Murphey's death would have been carried out by several departments, including the neuro ICU, radiology, pharmacy, information technology, and medical staff services. Although only an individual nurse was blamed, she acted within a network of systems. With stronger safety controls, her mistakes may not have had such grave consequences. VMC had all the elements of moral agency, including a corporate internal decision structure. Insofar as commonly accepted practices were unsafe, staff training was deficient, or technology was not appropriately programmed to minimize harm, the organization as a whole was partly responsible for Murphey's death.

As illustrated by the Vaught case, responsibility for harm usually rests not only on the individual clinician—Vaught herself is clearly at fault—but also on the larger organization. VMC can be blamed for harm because both individuals and collective entities have moral obligations. Unless clinicians are acting recklessly or maliciously, they act under technological, physical, and social conditions that guide their behavior. Moral duties to patients and the public thus not only constrain clinicians in their specific decisions but also apply to the organization as a whole and its constituent parts. Boards of trustees should credential only qualified clinicians, hospital administrators should compensate based on quality metrics and not just productivity metrics, safety and quality improvement committees should encourage reporting of errors, ethics committees should help clinicians and families of patients to weigh conflicting prima facie duties, and so on. Together they can formulate policies and design systems that respect autonomy, reduce harm, improve health, and promote justice.

## REFERENCES

Aljabari, Salim, and Zuhal Kadhim. 2021. "Common Barriers to Reporting Medical Errors." *Scientific World Journal* 2021. doi:10.1155/2021/6494889.

De George, Richard T. 1982. "The Moral Responsibility of the Hospital." *Journal of Medicine and Philosophy* 7, no. 1 (February): 87–100. doi:10.1093/jmp/7.1.87.

French, Peter A. 1979. "The Corporation as a Moral Person." *American Philosophical Quarterly* 16, no. 3 (July): 207–15. https://www.jstor.org/stable/20009760.

———. 1982. "Collective Responsibility and the Practice of Medicine." *Journal of Medicine and Philosophy* 7, no. 1 (February): 65–86. doi:10.1093/jmp/7.1.65.

Goodpaster, Kenneth, and John B. Matthews. 1982. "Can a Corporation Have a Conscience?" *Harvard Business Review* 60, no. 1 (January–February): 132–41. https://hbr.org/1982/01/can-a-corporation-have-a-conscience.

Grant, Ernest J., Loressa Cole, and Kirk W. Lawson. 2022. Letter to Judge Jennifer L. Smith. May 5. https://www.nursingworld.org/~49a0c0/globalassets/practiceandpolicy/ethics/vaught-judge-letter-05092022.pdf.

Institute for Safe Medication Practices. 2016. "Paralyzed by Mistakes—Reassess the Safety of Neuromuscular Blockers in Your Facility." June 16. https://www.psqh.com/analysis/paralyzed-by-mistakes-reassess-the-safety-of-neuromuscular-blockers-in-your-facility/.

———. 2019. "Another Round of the Blame Game: A Paralyzing Criminal Indictment That Recklessly 'Overrides' Just Culture." February 14. https://www.ismp.org/resources/another-round-blame-game-paralyzing-criminal-indictment-recklessly-overrides-just-culture.

———. 2022. "ISMP Speaks Out against Criminalization of Medication Errors." April 7. https://home.ecri.org/blogs/ismp-news/ismp-speaks-out-against-criminalization-of-medication-errors.

Institute for Safe Medication Practices and the Just Culture Company. 2022. "Lessons Learned about Human Fallibility, System Design, and Justice in the Aftermath of a Fatal Medication Error." Webinar. May 6. https://home.ecri.org/blogs/ismp-on-demand-events/lessons-learned-about-human-fallibility-system-design-and-justice-in-the-aftermath-of-a-fatal-medication-error.

Kant, Immanuel. 1996a. *Groundwork of the Metaphysics of Morals*. In *Practical Philosophy*, translated and edited by Mary J. Gregor, 41–108. Cambridge: Cambridge University Press.

———. 1996b. *The Metaphysics of Morals*. In *Practical Philosophy*, translated and edited by Mary J. Gregor, 363–602. Cambridge: Cambridge University Press.

Kapur, Narinder, Anam Parand, Tayana Soukup, Tom Reader, and Nick Sevdalis. 2016. "Aviation and Healthcare: A Comparative Review with Implications for Patient Safety." *JRSM Open* 7, no. 1 (January). doi:10.1177/2054270415616548.

Kohn, Linda T., Janet M. Corrigan, and Molla S. Donaldson, eds. 2000. *To Err Is Human: Building a Safer Health System*. Washington, DC: National Academy Press.

Lambert, Bruce L., and Gordon D. Schiff. 2022. "RaDonda Vaught, Medication Safety, and the Profession of Pharmacy: Steps to Improve Safety and Ensure Justice." *Journal of the American College of Clinical Pharmacy* 5, no. 9 (September): 981–87. doi:10.1002/jac5.1676Ci.

Leape, Lucian L. 1994. "Error in Medicine." *JAMA: Journal of the American Medical Association* 272, no. 23 (December 21): 1851–57. doi:10.1001/jama.1994.03520230061039.

Leedom, Dennis K., and Robert Simon. 1995. "Improving Team Coordination: A Case for Behavior-Based Training." *Military Psychology* 7, no. 2: 109–22. doi:10.1207/s15327876mp0702_5.

Luban, David, Alan Strudler, and David Wasserman. 1992. "Moral Responsibility in the Age of Bureaucracy." *Michigan Law Review* 90, no. 8 (August): 2348–92. doi:10.2307/1289575.

Makary, Martin A., and Michael Daniel. 2016. "Medical Error—the Third Leading Cause of Death in the US." *BMJ* 353: i2139. doi:10.1136/bmj.i2139.

Morey, John C., Robert Simon, Gregory D. Jay, Robert L. Wears, Mary Salisbury, Kimberly A. Dukes, and Scott D. Berns. 2002. "Error Reduction and Performance Improvement in the Emergency Department through Teamwork Training: Evaluation Results of the MedTeams Project." *Health Services Research* 37, no. 6 (December): 1553–81. doi:10.1111/1475-6773.01104.

Rawls, John. 1989. "Themes in Kant's Moral Philosophy." In *Kant's Transcendental Deductions: The Three 'Critiques' and the 'Opus postumum,'* edited by Eckart Förster, 81–113. Stanford: Stanford University Press. doi:10.1515/9781503621619-009.

Singh, Hardeep, Christiane Spitzmueller, Nancy J. Petersen, Mona K. Sawhney, and Dean F. Sittig. 2013. "Information Overload and Missed Test Results in Electronic Health Record-Based Settings." *JAMA Internal Medicine* 173, no. 8 (April 22): 702–4. doi:10.1001/2013.jamainternmed.61.

## FURTHER READING

Blegen, Mary A., Thomas Vaughn, Ginette Pepper, Carol Vojir, Karen Stratton, Michal Boyd, and Gail Armstrong. 2004. "Patient and Staff Safety: Voluntary Reporting." *American Journal of Medical Quality* 19, no. 2 (March–April): 67–74. doi:10.1177/106286060401900204.

An investigation of reporting rates for medication administration errors, patient falls, and occupational injuries (accidental needlesticks, exposure to bodily fluids, and back injuries). The researchers found that patient and staff safety occurrences are underreported. Reporting rates depended especially on the perception of quality management processes on the unit, and specifically whether the information would be used to improve patient safety; personal fears, such as worries that colleagues would think less of them; and concerns about the administrative response, such as blaming the individual rather than system errors.

Burlison, Jonathan, Rebecca R. Quillivan, Lisa M. Kath, Yinmei Zhou, Sam C. Courtney, Cheng Cheng, and James M. Hoffman. 2020. "A Multilevel Analysis of U.S. Hospital Patient Safety Culture Relationships with Perceptions of Voluntary Event Reporting." *Journal of Patient Safety* 16, no. 3 (September): 187–93. doi:10.1097/PTS.0000000000000336.

Studies the organizational and cultural factors that affect frequency of incident reports. The study concludes that three factors are most crucial for encouraging voluntary reporting of safety events: meaningful feedback and communication about the event, communication about how systems and processes are changed as a result, and support for safety from hospital leadership.

Carayon, Pascale, and Abigail R. Wooldridge. 2019. "Improving Patient Safety in the Patient Journey: Contributions from Human Factors Engineering." In *Women in Industrial and Systems Engineering: Key Advances and Perspectives on Emerging Topics*, edited by Alice E. Smith, 275–99. Dordrecht: Springer. doi:10.1007/978-3-030-11866-2_12.

Using a systems approach, the authors address patient safety by examining the environments of and transitions between different care settings. They illustrate their methodology with two examples: medication management and care coordination for elderly patients with chronic conditions.

Gawron, Valerie J., Colin G. Drury, Rollin J. Fairbanks, and Roseanne C. Berger. 2006. "Medical Error and Human Factors Engineering: Where Are We Now?" *American Journal of Medical Quality* 21, no. 1 (January–February): 57–67. doi:10.1177/1062860605283932.

Provides an overview of human factors engineering, focusing on human and system errors. The authors then discuss how to collect and analyze error data to reduce medical mistakes and improve health outcomes.

Iglehart, John K., ed. 2014. "Exploring Alternatives to Malpractice Litigation." Special issue, *Health Affairs* 33, no. 1 (January). https://www.healthaffairs.org/toc/hlthaff/33/1.

Collects federally funded research papers on evidence-based patient safety and medical liability demonstrations as alternatives to malpractice lawsuits. Articles cover the successes and challenges of communication-and-resolution programs, how to involve patients and families in medical error events, and how healthcare reform and tort reform may be pursued simultaneously.

Joint Commission. n.d. *Standards*. Accessed January 15, 2025. https://www.jointcommission.org/standards/.

The Joint Commission is the main accrediting body for healthcare organizations in the U.S., and accreditation is a condition of licensure for Medicaid and Medicare reimbursements from the federal and state governments. This site includes links to current national safety goals for hospitals, ambulatory healthcare, assisted living communities, laboratory services, and so on.

Jukola, Saana, and Mariacarla Gadebusch Bondio. 2023. "Not in Their Hands Only: Hospital Hygiene, Evidence and Collective Moral Responsibility." *Medicine, Health Care and Philosophy* 26, no. 1 (March): 37–48. doi:10.1007/s11019-022-10120-0.

Claims that we typically attribute responsibility for hospital-acquired infections wrongly to individual clinicians alone. Instead, by means of their policies and employment conditions, hospitals are both causally and ethically responsible. Therefore, the organization as a whole is obligated to develop effective infection controls.

Muyskens, James. 1981. "Collective Responsibility and the Nursing Profession." In *Biomedical Ethics*, edited by Thomas A. Mappes and Jane S. Zembaty, 102–8. New York: McGraw-Hill.

Argues that nurses are failing to meet reasonable expectations for professional conduct because they are overworked and understaffed. This is not the fault of individual nurses but the profession as a whole, which Muyskens considers a collective entity.

Pellegrino, Edmund D., ed. 1982. "Collective Responsibility in Health Care." Special issue, *Journal of Medicine and Philosophy* 7, no. 1 (February). https://academic.oup.com/jmp/issue/7/1.

A collection of one editorial and eight articles, including the contributions by French and De George referenced above, that address the issue of shared moral responsibility. Articles consider not only how the organization as a whole can be morally responsible but also how a clinician's responsibility as part of the organization may conflict with their personal and professional responsibilities.

Rubin, Susan B., and Laurie Zoloth, eds. 2000. *Margin of Error: The Ethics of Mistakes in the Practice of Medicine.* Hagerstown, MD: University Publishing Group.

> A collection of twenty-one essays around the theme of medical error. In part one, on conceptual issues, contributors use methods of literary interpretation and sociocultural analysis to expose our moral positions on error, and they evaluate the strengths and weaknesses of different moral frameworks. Part two covers errors in medical practice, including a chapter by Virginia Sharpe on the accountability of individuals and healthcare teams and a proposal for a no-fault system to encourage reporting. Part three addresses the underexamined issue of errors in ethics consultation, including how to develop a standard to understand and evaluate such errors.

# CHAPTER 3
# Paternalism and Patient Autonomy

**Key topics in this chapter:**
- Why paternalism dominated medicine for so long, and recent critiques of its foundational assumptions
- The historical shift from paternalism to patient autonomy and informed consent
- The difference between liberty and autonomy, and how that contrast generates alternative models of the clinician-patient relationship
- How autonomy only makes sense in the context of a person's social, economic, cultural, and political life

## Introduction

Many issues in medical ethics are situational: not everyone has to decide whether to get an abortion or to request medical aid in dying. But the relationship between patients and healthcare workers is universal. Everyone regularly encounters medical professionals, be they physicians (medical doctors and doctors of osteopathic medicine), advanced practice clinicians (physician assistants and nurse practitioners), or nurses (licensed practical nurses, registered nurses, clinical nurse specialists, and advanced practice nurses)—known collectively as **clinicians** or practitioners. This language was developed as an alternative to "providers," which frames the medical encounter in economic, consumerist terms (Mangione, Mandell, and Post 2021; Scarff 2021). Although some professional organizations and physicians object to the generic term "clinicians" because it does not recognize different levels of expertise, we use it regularly in this book because patients encounter a range of healthcare professionals, and the ethical issues apply generally.

Because health is an important part of the good life and decisions around health are personal, the clinician-patient relationship raises important ethical questions. Philosophers and physicians have tried to define obligations to patients as long as medicine has been a profession. Although it is commonly accepted that clinicians ought to preserve patients' health, reduce their suffering, and respect their autonomy, how to accomplish those ends is more contested, and dilemmas may arise when they are pursued simultaneously.

## Medical Paternalism

People go to doctors and other clinicians when they need diagnoses and courses of treatment for illnesses, injuries, and other medical conditions, or to prevent future illnesses and injuries. Many factors contribute to the inherent power differential between patients and healthcare professionals. The patient needs care and is therefore physically and often emotionally vulnerable. Patients depend on clinicians for their specialized knowledge about what is ailing them and what to do about it. And clinicians are gatekeepers to treatment insofar as patients' insurance only covers tests and specialists if clinicians deem them necessary, and insofar as patients have access to many drugs only if clinicians prescribe them. These conditions, along with the respected social status that medical professionals tend to have, combine to form a structure of legitimized authority for clinicians and corresponding deference on the part of patients. This power dynamic naturally lends itself to medical paternalism.

The contemporary emphasis on patient autonomy is relatively recent, arising partly in response to the medical abuse of experimental subjects and patients in Nazi Germany and during the post-war period. Before then, the history of European medicine had prioritized beneficence and nonmaleficence. The ancient **Hippocratic Oath** treats medicine as esoteric knowledge to be safeguarded by those educated in its proper use: "I will impart a knowledge of the art to my own sons, and those of my teachers, and to students bound by this contract and having sworn this Oath to the law of medicine, but to no others" ("Hippocratic Oath" 2002). Given the proximity between "medication" and "poison" (both are translations of the Greek word *pharmakon*), professional physicians pledge not to share their knowledge of how to heal, which is also knowledge of how to harm, with nonprofessionals, and they are bound by the Oath to protect the well-being of their patients: they should not administer "a lethal drug," "give a woman a pessary to cause an abortion," or "use the knife [to perform surgery]" ("Hippocratic Oath" 2002; see also Kass 1989). In addition, physicians promise to maintain the confidentiality of their patients and patients' families, and not to take advantage of their position as trusted caregivers: "Into whatever homes I go, I will enter them for the benefit of the sick, avoiding any voluntary act of impropriety or corruption, including the seduction of women or men" ("Hippocratic Oath" 2002).

The perilous knowledge of medicine puts physicians in a privileged role, and elements of the Oath reflect anxieties about how that knowledge might be misused. The contemporary availability of detailed medical information, including websites that invite the public to diagnose their own symptoms, would horrify Hippocrates (or whoever wrote the texts attributed to him). He argues that physicians should not share all the information that they have about a patient's condition with the patient themselves:

> Perform [medical tasks] calmly and adroitly, concealing most things from the patient while you are attending to him. Give necessary orders with cheerfulness and serenity, turning his attention away from what is being done to him; sometimes reprove sharply and emphatically, and sometimes comfort with solicitude and attention, revealing nothing of that patient's future or present condition. (Hippocrates 1923, 297, 299)

Information itself becomes medicine to be carefully administered, an intervention in the patient's attitude and behavior that the physician must control. For Hippocrates, a patient needs to know how to change their diet, for instance, but becoming aware of risks and possible outcomes could create unnecessary anxiety and undermine the processes of healing. As an example of how long this tradition of paternalism extended, physicians were, until recent decades, trained not to use the word "cancer" in discussions with patients but instead to use euphemisms such as "growths" or "neoplasms." In current practice, the use of technical jargon in patient interactions has a similar effect of withholding information (or its significance) from patients who are less medically literate.

On the **paternalistic model**, physicians—and it was traditionally physicians rather than other clinicians—are responsible for medical decision-making and for getting patients to comply with those decisions. The patient's role is to obey medical authority and trust that physicians will prioritize their well-being. The argument for paternalism springs from the intuition that physicians and other healthcare professionals have the expertise to prevent, diagnose, or treat pathology. Their highly specialized training gives them the authority to make the best possible medical decisions on behalf of the patient: how to evaluate a person's health, diagnose the problem, identify the treatment options, and select the treatment with the best chance of curing them and restoring their health. We might contrast this role with that of nurses, who traditionally focus on patients' comfort and ordinary care, with the effect that nurses tend to have more responsive dialogue with patients rather than making medical decisions for them.

In general, paternalism is the practice of some authority figures choosing what is best for others instead of letting them decide for themselves, as adults do for children. In a medical context, the physician takes on the role of a beneficent parent—or specifically, a father (*pater* in Latin), which, given cultural norms around that role, might suggest the problems associated with paternalism—by assuming that patients are unable to make appropriate decisions for themselves. When parents decide what their children eat, how they are educated, and when they go to bed, the assumption is that children do not know what is best, so those who know better will decide for them. Parents may effectively force a young child into getting vaccinations because it is in their long-term best interests, regardless of the child's current desire not to be jabbed by a needle.

Adults may make the wrong choices for themselves as well, and philosophers have long debated when or to what extent a person's self-regarding actions ought to be limited. Joel Feinberg (1986) distinguishes two varieties of paternalism. Under **hard paternalism**, a healthcare professional imposes a decision on a patient for their own good even when they are capable of deciding for themselves. Under **soft paternalism**, a patient is stopped from hurting themselves (e.g., refusing life-sustaining treatment following a car accident) until it is clear that they are making autonomous, fully informed decisions. Soft paternalism is generally accepted because it is only a temporary measure, when someone is in a state of distress. Hard paternalism is more difficult to justify. John Stuart Mill argues that we should only intervene to prevent harm to others, not for someone's own good (the **harm principle**) (1978, 9), while Sarah Conly argues that we should coerce people when they are confused about how to achieve the ultimate ends that they themselves have chosen (**coercive paternalism**) (2013, 43). The defense of hard paternalism follows Conly's line of argument, assuming that a person's professed ends may not be the ends to which they are actually committed.

In some cases, we as a community have decided that everyone, including otherwise competent adults, should be protected against the consequences of their own bad decisions. For example, the government acts paternalistically when it requires people to wear seatbelts in cars or helmets on motorcycles, when it sets aside a portion of people's earnings for their retirement (Social Security), or when it mandates that individuals purchase health insurance (Affordable Care Act). The typical justification of hard paternalism draws on the fact that many people do not make fully rational decisions, so the authority figure is doing for them what they would do if they were thinking rightly. A biker who grumbles about not feeling the wind in his hair will be grateful after he survives an accident with his skull intact. Thus, even apart from the cost to others (e.g., the financial burden of long-term care), the justification for limiting people's choices is that they may only understand the full risks of not getting a measles vaccine, not saving for retirement, or not wearing a helmet after they have already caused themselves irreparable harm. As a parallel to government paternalism, clinicians have the responsibility to correct what a patient thinks they want when it does not align with their "true preferences or values"—their long-term welfare, which may be obscured from them at the moment that they make their choice (Goldman 1980, 177).

Alan Goldman (1980) says that medical paternalism is based on two main assumptions. First, the doctor knows best how to make a person healthy, how to minimize pain, or how to treat a patient's condition most successfully. Second, the patient wants to be healthy, wants to minimize pain, or wants the best treatment. The patient wants to live, and that is their highest priority. The argument for paternalism, then, is very simple: the patient wants to be healthy (or as healthy as possible) above all else, and the doctor knows better than they do how to support their health, so the doctor should make decisions for the patient.

In this sense, paternalism protects the person's freedom by making sure that they do not harm themselves, and it safeguards the person's continued life and health, which is a condition for the possibility of all other projects. Paternalism may take the overt form of the clinician only presenting one treatment option, or it may take on more subtle forms, such as concealing the severity of a diagnosis or nudging a patient into a particular choice by emphasizing the benefits of one treatment and the risks of alternatives. In any of these scenarios, the patient is guided into consenting to a treatment without fully understanding their own medical situation and the options available to them.

One assumption is that the patient may make the wrong decision because they are scared or ignorant of at least some of the facts. This is the important point: a patient may *think* they know what they want, just as a child may think they do not want a vaccination shot. However, what children *really* want is not to be sick, so parents make them get the shot. The patient may think they want one treatment, but if that is not the best treatment, then what they really want is the treatment the doctor chooses. Of course, doctors usually try to explain the intricacies of diagnoses as well as the risks and benefits of possible treatments, but they cannot simplify the complexities of symptomatology, human biology, and pharmacology enough for the average patient to understand. Doctors thus have to oversimplify (e.g., "don't consume so many fatty foods" ignores the distinction between trans fats, saturated fats, and unsaturated fats), use metaphors and analogies (e.g., "using hormone blockers to prevent the spread of breast cancer is like breaking off a key in a lock"), and withhold information that they consider unnecessary (e.g., describing only the standard, preferred treatment and its side effects and not presenting other options). Patients seldom have a problem with this and may attempt to shortcut full-fledged explanations by posing a common question: "If you were in my position, doctor, what would you do?" By making decisions for the patient, the doctor is actually supporting the patient's freedom, unclouded by ignorance and fear.

## The Value of Autonomy

Despite the justifications for paternalism, there are risks associated with it: abuses and overreaches of authority, and misunderstanding what is in the patient's best interests. With regard to the first danger, the history of medicine provides innumerable examples. Well-meaning physicians sometimes overestimate their ability to diagnose and treat pathology, and other physicians take advantage of their authority to abuse patients for their own self-interest. The Hippocratic Oath does not substantively protect patients from negligence or corruption when all decision-making authority is placed in the hands of medical professionals who are overseen only by others who have received similar training and with whom they share professional bonds.

The second objection to paternalism is more philosophically interesting because it recognizes that the patient is a whole person rather than merely a set of biological systems. We can assume that a doctor has a better sense than the patient does of what the best course of treatment is. Even a mediocre doctor is likely to know more than the patient, whose information is based on what the doctor says anyway (or based on unreliable internet research). But clinicians are not experts in what their patients want, and indeed they often misidentify patients' values (Street and Haidet 2011). In *Cobbs v. Grant* (8 Cal. 3d 229 [1972]), the California Supreme Court distinguished the clinician's medical expertise from the "nonmedical judgment" that weighs the risks "against the individual subjective fears and hopes of the patient" (243). Each patient has purposes and ends of their own, which are sometimes only clear to the patient themselves, and other things they value may outweigh their continued health and existence. Goldman paraphrases Albert Camus in claiming that "anything worth living for is worth dying for. To realize or preserve those values that give meaning to life is worth the risk of life itself" (1980, 180). Self-determination means choosing not only how to protect one's life but what one wants to live for, and it is up to each individual to decide what is reasonable to risk to pursue their goals.

Healthcare professionals may be trained to fight against death as a kind of enemy and to treat a patient's health and continued life as the highest priority. But for many people, life does not have inherent value but instrumental value: it is good *for* something. And if that something is no longer possible, then there is no reason to live as long as we possibly can or to preserve our health at all costs. For example:

- None of us has a perfectly healthy lifestyle. Any decision to forego the optimal amount and kind of exercise or to eat less than nutritionally ideal food involves trade-offs between quantity and quality of life. On the other hand, a patient may be willing to risk their health by climbing a mountain or running daily despite aging knees because these activities are personally fulfilling to them (Veatch 2000).

- A patient diagnosed with terminal cancer, who has undergone multiple, unsuccessful rounds of chemotherapy, may decline further treatment in order to spend their remaining time, energy, and attention with their family and friends, or devoted to completing an intellectual or creative project. They may also take advantage of medical aid in dying, choosing a shorter life over a longer one so that they can have a sense of control at the end of life.

- A Jehovah's Witness may refuse a life-saving blood transfusion (e.g., in case of a life-threatening hemorrhage) because of the biblical prohibition on consuming blood. The person thinks that it is more important to die holding fast to their religious convictions than to continue living by doing the wrong thing.

People not only value different things; patients, not doctors, are also the best authority on what they value. So, patients need to decide for themselves. If a doctor chooses for a patient, the doctor may be misidentifying what the patient would choose if the patient were thinking rationally. The doctor would be imposing on the patient either the doctor's own values or their misinterpretation of the patient's values. Despite their best intentions, the treatment would not be helping the patient to achieve their ends.

Of Tom Beauchamp and James Childress's four principles—respect for autonomy, nonmaleficence, beneficence, and justice—autonomy carries by far the most weight in practice (Wolpe 1998). Based on its two Greek roots (*auto-* and *nomos*), the term **autonomy** literally means "giving the law to oneself," being self-governing or self-determining. In Kantian terms, to be autonomous is to give purposes or ends to oneself, as opposed to the condition of **heteronomy**, which is to have one's purposes fixed by natural laws, instincts, or the will of others (Kant 1996, 4:432–33, 440–41). Autonomy in the medical field is typically understood to be the self-determination of patients or research subjects, although occasionally, it refers to the autonomy of physicians, pharmacists, or other clinicians. Basically, respecting autonomy means allowing a patient to control what happens with their own body, provided that, in the clinician's judgment, such treatments are not medically unnecessary, carry too much risk given potential benefits, or are futile. The core of a commitment to autonomy means that a patient should be able to decide which available medical option is best and should have the right to refuse treatment altogether. To decide on behalf of another person is to treat them as incompetent and thus to deny them moral agency, even if one's intent is to protect their well-being. This relatively recent emphasis on autonomy is one reason why many medical students no longer take the ancient Hippocratic Oath. Often, they recite versions that promise to "accept each [patient] in a nonjudgmental manner, appreciating the validity and worth of different value systems and according to each person a full measure of human dignity" (Penn State College of Medicine, n.d.).

The principle of respect for autonomy is a principle of separation, a recognition that other people's judgments may not mirror one's own. Since values and the ordering of values can shift over time, depending on external or internal conditions, the patient is in the best position to make medical decisions that align with their interests. The physician risks using their own values to surreptitiously guide their judgment of what is best for the patient. Because of the asymmetrical authority placed in the physician and often-curtailed communication with the patient, these misapprehensions often go unchecked.

Autonomy has not only instrumental value—the doctor may misidentify the patient's priorities—but also inherent value. Even if the clinician is a beneficent caregiver who accurately mirrors the decisions that the patient would make for themselves, claiming decision-making power over a patient removes a key element of their personhood by regarding them as a passive object to be managed. There is a moral and existential loss for the patient in not being treated as an autonomous being—in not having access to all the information about one's medical condition, prognosis, and treatment options that a physician does, and in not making the decision about how and whether to treat a pathology. Honoring a patient's autonomy is a way of recognizing their alterity, the fact that they are not a generic human organism with predictable interests but a singular being whose identity and values are ultimately self-defined and may be spontaneously redefined. The doctor and the patient are moral equals. The former has no right to control the latter, even in the interest of helping them.

We could read the contemporary emphasis on autonomy in both clinical practice and medical research as an extension of ideas in the Hippocratic Oath. This ethical code alerts us to how the authority of physicians could be abused in their deeply personal but asymmetrical interactions with patients—hence the prohibitions on violating confidentiality and on sexual relationships with anyone in the homes of patients. Parallel to their knowledge of medicines that may also function as poisons, physicians must not take advantage of their specialized skills to harm patients. And one way to mistreat people is to infantilize them, rob them of agency, and reduce them to passive objects whose own articulations of values can be disregarded in favor of the medical authority's judgment. Prioritizing the patient's autonomy thus guards against a register of corruption and abuse of authority risked by the paternalistic approach.

## Informed Consent

Because of the dehumanizing medical abuses of the twentieth century, respecting autonomy is a core commitment of the Nuremberg Code and the Belmont Report, governing experimentation with human subjects, and the American Medical Association's (AMA) Principles of Medical Ethics, concerning clinical care. The Nuremberg Code begins:

> The voluntary consent of the human subject is absolutely essential. This means that the person involved should have legal capacity to give consent; should be situated as to be able to exercise free power of choice, without the intervention of any element of force, fraud, deceit, duress, over-reaching, or other ulterior form of constraint or coercion; and should have sufficient knowledge and comprehension of the elements of the subject matter involved as to enable him to make an understanding and enlightened decision. ("Permissible Medical Experiments," n.d., 181)

The first ethical principle of the Belmont Report is respect for persons, which includes the ideas that "individuals should be treated as autonomous agents" and "persons with diminished autonomy are entitled to protection" (National Commission 1979, 4). The Report specifies:

> to respect autonomy is to give weight to autonomous persons' considered opinions and choices while refraining from obstructing their actions unless they are clearly detrimental to others. To show a lack of respect for an autonomous agent is to repudiate that person's considered judgments, to deny an individual the freedom to act on those considered judgments, or to withhold information necessary to make a considered judgment, when there are no compelling reasons to do so. (National Commission 1979, 5)

The AMA Principles of Medical Ethics (2001) begin with the injunction to "provid[e] competent medical care, with compassion and respect for human dignity and rights." In other words, contemporary medical ethics demands a commitment to respect individuals' self-determination by protecting people from external coercion. On this reading, autonomy is synonymous with **negative liberty**, the freedom to make choices without constraint by others, limited only by the obligation not to harm others or infringe on their rights. This focus has come to define healthcare in the contemporary United States, perhaps because it aligns with a consumer model of medicine, in which patients can choose treatments and "providers" (as long as patients can afford them), and healthcare professionals are specialized technicians able to provide those services.

In the U.S., the courts have, in many landmark decisions, asserted the value of patient autonomy, defined its scope, and established legal protections, usually by requiring informed consent for any medical procedure. In *Schloendorff v. Society of New York Hospital* (105 N.E. 92 [N.Y. 1914]), the New York Court of Appeals acknowledged autonomous medical decision-making as a basic right: "Every human being of adult years and sound mind has a right to determine what shall be done with his own body" (129–30). The U.S. Supreme Court asserted that "this notion of bodily integrity has been embodied in the requirement that informed consent is generally required for medical treatment," which it says is found in the common law and justified by the Due Process Clause of the Fourteenth Amendment (*Cruzan v. Director, Missouri Department of Health*, 497 U.S. 261 [1990], at 269). For a patient to freely consent, the physician must provide "all information relevant to a meaningful decisional process" (*Cobbs v. Grant*, 8 Cal. 3d 229 [1972], at 242). *Canterbury v. Spence* (464 F.2d 772 [D.C. Cir. 1972]) established an "objective" test for the "adequate disclosure" of alternatives and risks: "The physician is under an obligation to communicate specific information to the patient when the exigencies of reasonable care call for it" (781); adequate disclosure is understood "in terms of what a prudent person in the patient's position would have decided if suitably informed of all perils bearing significance" (791). Finally, to freely consent to have procedures done, patients must not be coerced or subject to undue influence, and they must be of "sound mind," with the mental capacity to understand doctors' recommended courses of action, including any side effects or long-term consequences, and to make important medical decisions (*Schloendorff v. Society of New York Hospital*, 129).

The emphasis on informed consent as a counter to paternalism has produced the **informative model** of the clinician-patient relationship, in which the clinician offers objective information about the patient's condition and treatment options, the patient chooses one, and the clinician uses their technical expertise to enact that decision (for example, performing surgery). On this view, the doctor acts like a car mechanic. The patient does not understand what is wrong or what the possible treatments are, so the doctor gives the patient this information. And the patient does not have the technical expertise to carry out the chosen treatment on themselves, so the doctor does what the patient wants done. The doctor does not interfere in the decision and remains neutral regarding the options: "Here are three possible repairs. Here are the costs of each one. What do you want me to do?" Robert Veatch calls this the engineering model of the clinician-patient relationship (1972; 1991, 11–12), and Terrence Ackerman refers to it as the legalistic model, in which the physician "need be only an honest and good technician, providing relevant information and dispensing professionally competent care" (1982, 14). Medical school becomes a glorified trade school.

Although informed consent is the legal standard in the United States and is applied in both clinical and experimental settings, some theorists believe that informed consent is not much of an improvement over paternalism. First, getting informed consent usually means offering a patient a document delineating a treatment's risks and benefits, reading or summarizing it for the patient, and then having them sign it to demonstrate their understanding. There is often little attempt to ascertain whether the patient fully comprehends what they have heard or read, or whether they are simply acquiescing to the physician's authority. Onora O'Neill reminds us that the informed consent "ritual" is limited in two ways: to whom it applies (excluding people with limited or diminished cognitive abilities, and people in the midst of medical emergencies) and how well it captures whether someone is approaching a decision autonomously (2003, 4–5). What informed consent procedures can do, as a minimum standard, is ensure "that a patient (research subject, tissue donor) has not been deceived or coerced" (5). But fully respecting a patient's autonomy goes beyond obtaining their voluntary agreement to a medical procedure at a point in time. Consent is an ongoing process that must be continually documented in the electronic health record.

A second concern with informed consent is that the clinician is still determining what is in the patient's best interests. The doctor proposes what they take to be the best course of treatment, and most of the time, the patient simply defers to the doctor's technical expertise. This presupposes that the clinician knows which trade-offs the patient would make and how the proposed treatment will impact the patient's larger social circle (including their family), job performance, and other obligations (Veatch 1995).

Finally, Jay Katz (1984) argues that the objective standard of reasonableness established in *Canterbury v. Spence* places too much authority in the clinician. What counts as "reasonable care" is mostly a matter of medical judgment. And not every patient is a "prudent person." Clinicians end up guessing what needs to be disclosed and imposing their own value preferences onto their patients. Thus, according to Katz, informed consent only seems to support patient self-determination, leaving clinicians as the ultimate decision-makers.

Even if the previous concerns could be addressed and the informative model worked as described, it would have some broader negative implications. Specifically, allowing patients unfettered control over their own treatment decisions often leads to unnecessary procedures. If a patient demands a surgery or drug that randomized, controlled trials show not to be beneficial, doctors should comply, on this model. In positioning the patient as a consumer, the informative model only addresses individual liberty rather than issues of justice. This drives up the cost of healthcare. Not only are there financial incentives for clinicians to move forward with unnecessary interventions, and not only are clinicians often driven by rare or irrelevant counterexamples that are present to mind (the availability heuristic), but many clinicians want to reduce patient anxiety or are worried about being sued if their patients' health later declines (Epstein 2017). Spending money on an unnecessary repair to one's car only costs the car owner, but widespread overtreatment in medicine increases overall healthcare costs—$75.7 billion to $101.2 billion annually in the U.S. (Shrank, Rogstad, and Parekh 2019)—and subjects patients to potential harms (such as the risk of infection during surgery or drug side effects).

## Liberty versus Autonomy

A richer sense of freedom emerges as a secondary theme in discussions of autonomy in the Nuremberg Code and the Belmont Report: a person may have diminished autonomy because of internal constraints on their ability to make free choices. Internal constraints may be tangible, such as being an infant or being currently in shock, or they may be more subtle, such as psychological pressure to conform to social norms or grappling with debilitating anxiety or pain. Edmund Pellegrino argues that people often make medical decisions in a condition of "wounded humanity"—when they are injured, sick, fearful, or discouraged (1979, 44). Healthcare practitioners should therefore recognize that the ideal of the Western philosophical tradition—the adult, sovereign individual—is not the default patient. Treating patients as if threats to autonomy are exclusively external misses less obvious ways that decision-making can be unfree.

A stronger attention to autonomy, in contrast to liberty, arises out of the Kantian tradition. For Immanuel Kant, autonomy means that a person is not simply doing whatever they want, based on their immediate desires or impulses, but acting authentically to realize their own projects. An end becomes one's own in the full sense only when the person has rationally chosen it (Kant 1996, 4:431–33). On this view, a drug addict is not acting autonomously. They want whatever drug they are addicted to, but they are not rationally and freely choosing to take that drug. Therefore, someone interested in promoting autonomy is not going to let the person remain in the grip of their addiction; instead, they will fight for the addict to gain control over themselves. This is not simply a calculation about the well-being of the person—that their overall health and quality of life will be diminished—but a concern about how their freedom is diminished through the internal constraint of addiction.

Another way of making sense of internal constraints on autonomy is to use Harry Frankfurt's (1998) taxonomy of first- and second-order desires (see also Dworkin 1970). I may have impulses to overindulge in alcohol after a stressful day or to avoid seeing a doctor about a worrisome symptom, which are **first-order desires**. But I also have the capacity to critically reflect on those impulses and override them with **second-order desires**—what I want to want—which express my longer-term projects or deeper values—in this case, to promote my overall health, mobility, and mood. Second-order desires are desires to have certain kinds of desires, which (under ideal conditions) direct my behavior. Autonomy, then, involves acting in ways that do not cause friction or alienation between my first- and second-order desires, or that align my first-order desires with my second-order desires. On this model, freedom is not simply the ability to act without interference but to act in accordance with one's authentic values—autonomy rather than liberty.

The informative model does not have a way to distinguish between truly free decisions and those that are the products of internal constraints. Particularly in the midst of illness or injury, patients often experience a loss of control over their lives and a sense of helplessness. To assist patients in choosing autonomously rather than reactively, clinicians must create the conditions under which patients can regain a sense of control through rational reflection, and that requires more than nonintervention (Ackerman 1982, 16). Certain elements of paternalism support patient autonomy precisely because their autonomy may be impaired or diminished.

Ackerman discusses four kinds of constraints on a patient's ability to choose: physical, cognitive, psychological, and social constraints. **Physical constraints** are illnesses or injuries that keep a person from doing what they want: "Illness 'interposes' the body or mind between the patient and reality, obstructing attempts to act upon cherished plans" (Ackerman 1982, 15). Someone recently diagnosed with amyotrophic lateral sclerosis (ALS) will need to adjust their expectations to a newly diminished range of muscular control, shift more of their time and energy to managing symptoms, and make use of supportive equipment. Physical constraints may also be invisible, such as diseases that cause chronic pain. They diminish autonomy not by interfering with the decision-making process itself (decisional autonomy) but with the patient's ability to act on a decision (executional autonomy). This is the least controversial form of constraint in medical ethics: clinicians do what they can to heal, prevent, or manage illness or injury so that people can do what they want.

**Cognitive constraints** are less straightforward, but addressing them sits squarely within the informative model. These are limitations on the information the patient can access or on the patient's understanding of that information. If a patient is only given one treatment option when there are in fact four effective treatments, or if they are given information in language that they cannot understand, either due to lack of fluency or inability to grasp technical jargon, the resulting choice is mere obedience to authority. Healthcare professionals support patients' freedom by communicating in a language in which patients are fluent, presenting all relevant information, taking time to answer questions, and checking in to see if patients understand (Katz 1984, 130–64). A more nuanced understanding of autonomy takes seriously Hippocrates' caution about sharing information. Ackerman argues that physicians have to "tell the truth in a way, at a time, and in whatever increments are necessary to allow patients to effectively use the information" (1982, 17).

Respecting the liberty of each patient requires attention to overcoming these two kinds of constraints. However, Ackerman describes two other kinds of constraints that more subtly undermine autonomy and thus require physicians to cultivate more complex approaches to resolve them. **Psychological constraints** are forces that keep patients from deliberating clearly, such as depression, denial, or fear. These constraints interfere with the decision-making process itself—understanding one's current situation, weighing risks and benefits of various treatments, reflecting on what future best aligns with one's primary values—and arise as internal hindrances to autonomy. Emotional responses, such as denial, or psychological illnesses, such as depression, distort one's perceptions and subsequent choices in ways that are largely unobservable, since there is no external source of coercion. Clinicians should attend to verbal cues or body language that suggests that patients are making decisions clouded by psychological constraints.

Lastly, patient autonomy may be diminished by **social constraints**, such as pressure from family members or cultural norms. This form of constraint may be particularly intense for those who are most dependent on others for their care or are vulnerable to the withdrawal of social support: children, people with disabilities, the elderly, and people from marginalized communities. Social norms may not be explicitly articulated and instead operate in an internalized way: for instance, the expectation that men should "tough out" physical injuries or that children should not talk (or think) about sexuality. One element of social constraint may be patients' ingrained ideas about the clinician-patient relationship. If patients are socially trained to defer to clinicians, they may resist actively engaging in the decision-making process. That is, paternalism itself becomes habituated, at which point it functions not as an external constraint on autonomy but as an internal one. To address social constraints, clinicians may need to extend their cultural awareness and have conversations with family members or other caregivers.

The attention to different forms of internal constraint explains why states with legal medical aid in dying do not allow terminally ill patients to consent to it when they are clinically depressed (psychological constraint) and why it is illegal for people to coerce or exert "undue influence" on patients to make the request (social constraint). Attending to these kinds of constraints requires more than the clear transmission of information and competent provision of medical services. It demands that the clinician reflect on whether the patient's decision-making process is hampered by intangible, internal sources of coercion and then do their best to help the patient act in accordance with their own considered values. To highlight the need for conversation that clarifies a patient's values, this approach is sometimes called the **interpretive model** (Emanuel and Emanuel 1992, 2221–22).

The canon of Western philosophy tends to privilege autonomy as the central characteristic of rational persons (historically assumed to be adult, white, nondisabled males), but medicine is an arena in which we should recognize a spectrum of autonomy. Young children, people suffering from dementia, people with severe cognitive disabilities, people experiencing physical or psychological trauma, or people grappling with addiction may experience diminished or compromised autonomy that still deserves to be respected. The treatment of others, such as infants or comatose individuals, may be guided by the recognition of their ability to gain or regain autonomous decision-making.

## Deliberation and Practical Reasoning

Ezekiel Emanuel and Linda Emanuel (1992) go beyond Ackerman to claim that the doctor should, in some cases, even challenge the patient's own stated values. They reject paternalism for the same reason Goldman does: the patient may prioritize some things over health and prolonged life. They reject the informative model because it does not give us the kind of healthcare professional that we want: a good practitioner should not only be a good technician but should also have genuine concern for patients, an ability to understand their feelings, empathy for their diminished sense of self-control, and a desire to help them make the best medical decisions. As Beauchamp and Childress say, caring is "fundamental" to the relationship between clinicians and patients, and compassion is one of the "focal virtues" (2019, 35–36, 38–39; see also Chen and Tsai 2021). The informative model also assumes that patients know exactly what they want and that what they want is not going to change—in other words, each patient has a set hierarchy of values, and those values are clear or may be made clear to the patient. On the interpretive model, doctors should help patients discover what they really want, but what they want may be unsettled or contradictory. Emanuel and Emanuel (1992) instead propose the **deliberative model**: although the patient is allowed to decide based on their own deeply held values, the doctor can challenge what the patient claims to want and can even try to persuade them to take a certain action. This is a version of what Douglas Walton (1985) calls the practical reasoning model, where the clinician and the patient engage one another in a dialogic process of bilateral communication and feedback, questions and answers, negotiation and compromise (see also Quill and Brody 1996; Charles, Gafni, and Whelan 1997, 1999). Studies show that patients prefer a shared decision-making process over either consumerism (the informative model) or paternalism (Murray et al. 2007; see also Chewning et al. 2012; Noteboom et al. 2021).

Someone who smokes and eats fast food all day may be satisfied with their current state of health because they do not feel sick all the time. The clinician should try to convince them that these are the wrong choices in the long term, given the patient's love for their family and desire to experience important milestones with them. According to Emanuel and Emanuel (1992), this actually supports the patient's freedom insofar as it does not indulge their unreflective desires. By discussing things with the patient, the doctor helps them affirm their autonomy by considering whether their current values are the right ones or whether their professed values are consistent.

Some ethicists have challenged the idea that there is one correct model of the clinician-patient relationship by claiming that it is out of step with the complexity of clinical practice. First, not all patients have the same ability to make autonomous decisions, identify their own health-related values, and understand medical information. Because of this range of capacity, Aakash Agarwal and Beth Murinson (2012) propose a more variable approach that would identify the appropriate model of clinician-patient interaction specific to each individual. A second challenge comes from Greg Clarke, Robert Hall, and Greg Rosencrance (2004), who claim that proposed models of the clinician-patient relationship wrongly assume that the typical encounter involves an individual patient and an individual physician making decisions in isolation. In reality, patients consult family and friends, and they often defer to people they think have a better understanding of the relevant facts. This depends in part on cultural variation; some cultures tend to value individual autonomy and free choice, while others tend to see individuals as embedded in larger family units (Blackhall et al. 2001). The correct way to relate to patients changes from patient to patient and sometimes from moment to moment, depending on the nature of the medical decision. Thus, Clarke, Hall, and Rosencrance (2004) recommend that practitioners establish a constructive relationship with a patient by clearly identifying the members of the healthcare team and their roles, and then asking how the patient wants the clinical interactions to be conducted: "Who does the patient want to be present for support and advice when treatment decisions are discussed with the physician," and how much information do they want to get (e.g., lots of detail or just the key points)? And "different care decisions should be treated differently" since the clinician cannot always anticipate what will be important to a patient in various circumstances (18). This resistance to prioritizing one model reflects a case-based (casuistic) method, which is more emblematic of a practitioner's approach to medical ethics, as opposed to a theoretical commitment to abstract principles on which specific cases would be decided.

## Relational Autonomy

Conversations between clinicians and patients are set against familial, cultural, and other social backgrounds that can empower or disempower subjects in a range of registers. The expanded scope of **relational autonomy** focuses on social disparities such as class, race, gender, and sexuality, to take into account how people may operate under unfairly restricted options or with limited recognition of their status as autonomous agents (see Meyers 1989; Sherwin 1998; Kukla 2005). A woman living in Texas who seeks an abortion may be told by doctors that she has only one option: to carry the pregnancy to term, unless her own life is in immediate danger. If she has no resources to travel out of state for an abortion, her medical options have shrunk to one. She experiences coercion due to legal constraints on her bodily autonomy as well as social pressures that define femininity through maternity and punish violations of that norm. An inability to pay for treatment, or (as in this example) an inability to pay for access to treatment (transportation, childcare, time away from work) significantly limits patients' ability to make and act on decisions that align with their priorities.

Relational autonomy thus takes into account how patients' choices are constrained by forms of social injustice. It challenges a consumerist model in which people come into medical decision-making as equal buyers and sellers in the free market. For example, although some philosophers propose a commercial market for transplantable organs and tissues—the increased supply would better meet the demand—a focus on relational autonomy recognizes that a decision to donate might involve subtle (or not so subtle) forms of coercion. A person who might otherwise not afford to buy groceries or pay their heating bill may decide to sell a kidney or bone marrow, but these medically significant decisions attest to the forces undermining that person's ability to govern their own life. Participating in the selling of one's own organs or tissues may also erode a person's sense of themselves as an agent by framing their body as a commodity.

Relational autonomy emphasizes the "ongoing interpersonal, social, and institutional scaffolding" necessary for individual self-determination (Mackenzie 2015, 285). Our status as autonomous agents must be recognized by individual others and the institutions in which we operate, in a continuous and iterative manner. The traditional Western philosophical view separates autonomous beings (subjects) from determined things (objects). Relational autonomy adds a focus on how we acquire the status of agents and the gradations of autonomy. The development of autonomy begins in childhood, with adults who foster not only a gradually increasing sense of independence in decision-making but also the ability to name and reflect on our own values (Mackenzie 2015, 286). Those abilities then are either further supported by our relations with others or diminished by our interpersonal, cultural, and institutional environments. That is, respecting relational autonomy entails taking into account the wider systems in which patient decisions are embedded.

## Conclusion: The Power and Limits of Autonomy

Despite the differences among the specific models, there are commonly accepted principles that govern all clinician-patient relationships. Apart from legally required testing (such as paternity tests), medical procedures cannot be forced on fully conscious, rational persons against their will.

## Conclusion: The Power and Limits of Autonomy

The right to forgo treatment or have treatment discontinued at any time, including medical nutrition and hydration, even against medical advice, is widely recognized and legally protected by judicial precedent (American Medical Association, n.d., 1.1.3; *Cruzan v. Director, Missouri Department of Health*, 497 U.S. 261 [1990]). Conversely, patients who are young children, impaired by drugs or alcohol, mentally disabled, or suffering from dementia are not allowed to make unilateral medical decisions for themselves. Usually, competent adult guardians, such as parents and medical proxies, are entrusted with authorizing treatment on their behalf.

Even when a patient knows what they want and clinicians are willing to carry it out—that is, when both patient and clinician autonomy are respected—patients may request procedures that are medically unnecessary and go beyond overtreatment. These cases represent the limit cases of autonomy: Should every request for treatment made by a rational adult be honored? For example, philosophers have debated whether doctors should perform surgeries on so-called amputee wannabes who request to have otherwise healthy limbs amputated so they can align their actual body with their ideal body image. Like those with Body Identity Integrity Disorder, wannabes need not be delusional and may be as responsive to reasons as the rest of us, so they seem to be as capable of consenting to their transformation as people are to other forms of extreme body modification (such as tongue splitting and eye piercing). Still, the debate is usually framed as a question of whether such patients are making autonomous, informed decisions. Tim Bayne and Neil Levy (2005) claim that if a wannabe is not psychologically impaired, conceives of the amputation as a psychological good, and has an informed and stable desire for the surgery, then physicians ought to respect that desire and carry it out. On the other side, Sabine Müller (2009) claims that such a decision is not autonomous because, although the patient desires the amputation, they do not identify or endorse that desire (that is, they have a first-order desire for amputation but a second-order desire that the first-order desire not be effective); and Peter Brian Barry (2012) claims that, although such a decision is autonomous, a wannabe is not fully informed about the phenomenal facts concerning amputation (what it is like to be an amputee), so they cannot meaningfully consent to it. As such debates reveal, the meaning of patient autonomy and how best to promote it remain deeply contested issues in medical ethics. How we respond to this type of case may reveal what we think the role of the physician is: to provide services as long as patients clearly identify their core values, are informed about the outcomes, and can pay for them, or to contest patients' stated desires and refuse to perform medically unnecessary procedures?

Finally, some medical ethicists question the dominance of autonomy as a principle. For instance, there are situations in which the well-being of patients would have to be compromised to secure their participation in decision-making. A patient who has experienced a life-threatening accident and is deeply sedated could only be asked about treatment options by being brought out of sedation and thus subjected to significant pain. If the patient has not left an advance directive that covers this medical situation, then respecting their right to decide entails sacrificing the principle of beneficence. The legal requirements and dominant moral expectations that demand this ritual of informed consent can violate the duty to care. Patient autonomy may also be overridden for their own benefit (e.g., restraining a patient with suicidal ideation) or the benefit of others (e.g., isolating a patient with measles).

Despite these foundational debates, autonomy has pride of place in contemporary clinical ethics. Respect for autonomy answers the central question of what medicine is for by avoiding any predictable, generic answer. The practice of medicine, as much as is feasible, takes its value and goals from the singular decisions of the unique individuals who are patients, organ donors, and research subjects.

## REFERENCES

Ackerman, Terrence F. 1982. "Why Doctors Should Intervene." *Hastings Center Report* 12, no. 4 (August): 14–17. doi:10.2307/3560762.

Agarwal, Aakash Kumar, and Beth Brianna Murinson. 2012. "New Dimensions in Patient-Physician Interaction: Values, Autonomy, and Medical Information in the Patient-Centered Clinical Encounter." *Rambam Maimonides Medical Journal* 3, no. 3 (July): e0017. doi:10.5041/RMMJ.10085.

American Medical Association. 2001. "AMA Principles of Medical Ethics." June. https://code-medical-ethics.ama-assn.org/principles.

———. n.d. "Code of Medical Ethics." Accessed January 15, 2025. https://code-medical-ethics.ama-assn.org/.

Barry, Peter Brian. 2012. "The Ethics of Voluntary Amputation." *Public Affairs Quarterly* 26, no. 1 (January): 1–18. https://www.jstor.org/stable/41698212.

Bayne, Tim, and Neil Levy. 2005. "Amputees by Choice: Body Integrity Identity Disorder and the Ethics of Amputation." *Journal of Applied Philosophy* 22, no. 1 (March): 75–86. doi:10.1111/j.1468-5930.2005.00293.x.
Beauchamp, Tom L., and James F. Childress. 2019. *Principles of Biomedical Ethics.* 8th ed. New York: Oxford University Press.
Blackhall, Leslie J., Gelya Frank, Sheila Murphy, and Vicki Michel. 2001. "Bioethics in a Different Tongue: The Case of Truth-Telling." *Journal of Urban Health* 78, no. 1 (March): 59–71. doi:10.1093/jurban/78.1.59.
Charles, Cathy, Amiram Gafni, and Tim Whelan. 1997. "Shared Decision-Making in the Medical Encounter: What Does It Mean? (or It Takes at Least Two to Tango)." *Social Science & Medicine* 44, no. 5 (March): 681–92. doi:10.1016/s0277-9536(96)00221-3.
———. 1999. "Decision-Making in the Physician-Patient Encounter: Revisiting the Shared Treatment Decision-Making Model." *Social Science & Medicine* 49, no. 5 (September): 651–61. doi:10.1016/s0277-9536(99)00145-8.
Chen, Huei-Ya, and Wei-Ding Tsai. 2021. "Reflections on the Doctor-Patient Relationship in Medical Humanities from the Perspective of Care Ethics." In *Proceedings of 6th International Conference on Contemporary Education, Social Sciences and Humanities,* edited by Olga Chistyakova and Iana Roumbal, 299–307. Dordrecht: Atlantis. doi:10.2991/assehr.k.210902.046.
Chewning, Betty, Carma Bylund, Bupendra Shah, Neeraj K. Arora, Jennifer A. Gueguen, and Gregory Makoul. 2012. "Patient Preferences for Shared Decisions: A Systematic Review." *Patient Education and Counseling* 86, no. 1 (January): 9–18. doi:10.1016/j.pec.2011.02.004.
Clarke, Greg, Robert T. Hall, and Greg Rosencrance. 2004. "Physician-Patient Relations: No More Models." *American Journal of Bioethics* 4, no. 2 (Spring): W16–19. doi:10.1162/152651604323097934.
Conly, Sarah. 2013. *Against Autonomy: Justifying Coercive Paternalism.* Cambridge: Cambridge University Press. doi:10.1017/CBO9781139176101.
Dworkin, Gerald. 1970. "Acting Freely." *Noûs* 4, no. 4 (November): 367–83. doi:10.2307/2214680.
Emanuel, Ezekiel J., and Linda L. Emanuel. 1992. "Four Models of the Physician-Patient Relationship." *JAMA: Journal of the American Medical Association* 267, no. 16 (April 22–29): 2221–26. doi:10.1001/jama.1992.03480160079038.
Epstein, David. 2017. "When Evidence Says No, but Doctors Say Yes." *ProPublica.* February 22. https://www.propublica.org/article/when-evidence-says-no-but-doctors-say-yes.
Feinberg, Joel. 1986. *The Moral Limits of the Criminal Law.* Vol. 3, *Harm to Self.* Oxford: Oxford University Press. doi:10.1093/0195059239.001.0001.
Frankfurt, Harry G. 1998. *The Importance of What We Care About: Philosophical Essays.* Cambridge: Cambridge University Press. doi:10.1017/CBO9780511818172.

Goldman, Alan H. 1980. "Refutation of Medical Paternalism." In *The Moral Foundations of Professional Ethics*, 173–95. Totowa, NJ: Rowman & Littlefield.

Hippocrates. 1923. *Decorum*. In *Hippocrates*, vol. 2, translated by W. H. S. Jones, 267–301. Cambridge, MA: Harvard University Press.

"Hippocratic Oath." 2002. Translated by Michael North. National Library of Medicine, National Institutes of Health. https://www.nlm.nih.gov/hmd/greek/greek_oath.html.

Kant, Immanuel. 1996. *Groundwork of the Metaphysics of Morals*. In *Practical Philosophy*, translated and edited by Mary J. Gregor, 41–108. Cambridge: Cambridge University Press.

Kass, Leon R. 1989. "Neither for Love nor Money: Why Doctors Must Not Kill." *Public Interest* 94 (Winter): 25–46. https://www.proquest.com/magazines/neither-love-nor-money-why-doctors-must-not-kill/docview/1298107982/se-2.

Katz, Jay. 1984. *The Silent World of Doctor and Patient*. New York: Free Press.

Kukla, Rebecca. 2005. "Conscientious Autonomy: Displacing Decisions in Health Care." *Hastings Center Report* 35, no. 2 (March–April): 34–44. doi:10.2307/3527761.

Mackenzie, Catriona. 2015. "Autonomy." In *The Routledge Companion to Bioethics*, edited by John D. Arras, Elizabeth Fenton, and Quill R. Kukla, 277–90. New York: Routledge.

Mangione, Salvatore, Brian F. Mandell, and Stephen G. Post. 2021. "The Language Game: We Are Physicians, Not Providers." *American Journal of Medicine* 134, no. 12 (December): 1444–46. doi:10.1016/j.amjmed.2021.06.031.

Meyers, Diana. 1989. *Self, Society, and Personal Choice*. New York: Columbia University Press.

Mill, John Stuart. 1978. *On Liberty*. Edited by Elizabeth Rapaport. Indianapolis: Hackett.

Müller, Sabine. 2009. "Body Integrity Identity Disorder (BIID)—Is the Amputation of Healthy Limbs Ethically Justified?" *American Journal of Bioethics* 9, no. 1 (January): 36–43. doi:10.1080/15265160802588194.

Murray, Elizabeth, Lance Pollack, Martha White, and Bernard Lo. 2007. "Clinical Decision-Making: Patients' Preferences and Experiences." *Patient Education and Counseling* 65, no. 2 (February): 189–96. doi:10.1016/j.pec.2006.07.007.

National Commission for the Protection of Human Subjects of Biomedical and Behavioral Research. 1979. *The Belmont Report: Ethical Principles and Guidelines for the Protection of Human Subjects of Research*. Washington, DC: U.S. Department of Health and Human Services. https://www.hhs.gov/ohrp/regulations-and-policy/belmont-report/read-the-belmont-report/index.html.

Noteboom, Eveline A., Anne M. May, Elsken van der Wall, Niek J. de Wit, and Charles W. Helsper. 2021. "Patients' Preferred and Perceived Level of Involvement in Decision Making for Cancer Treatment: A Systematic Review." *Psychooncology* 30, no. 10 (October): 1663–79. doi:10.1002/pon.5750.

O'Neill, Onora. 2003. "Some Limits of Informed Consent." *Journal of Medical Ethics* 29, no. 1 (March): 4–7. doi:10.1136/jme.29.1.4.

Pellegrino, Edmund D. 1979. "Toward a Reconstruction of Medical Morality: The Primacy of the Act of Profession and the Fact of Illness." *Journal of Medicine and Philosophy* 4, no. 1 (March): 32–56. doi:10.1093/jmp/4.1.32.

Penn State College of Medicine. n.d. "Oath of Modern Hippocrates." Accessed January 15, 2025. https://students.med.psu.edu/md-students/oath/.

"Permissible Medical Experiments." n.d. In *Trials of War Criminals before the Nuremberg Military Tribunals under Control Council Law No. 10: Nuremberg, October 1946–April 1949*, vol. 2, 181–82. Washington, DC: U.S. Government Printing Office.

Quill, Timothy E., and Howard Brody. 1996. "Physician Recommendations and Patient Autonomy: Finding a Balance between Physician Power and Patient Choice." *Annals of Internal Medicine* 125, no. 9 (November 1): 763–69. doi:10.7326/0003-4819-125-9-199611010-00010.

Scarff, Jonathan R. 2021. "What's in a Name? The Problematic Term 'Provider.'" *Federal Practitioner* 38, no. 10 (October): 446–48. doi:10.12788/fp.0188.

Sherwin, Susan. 1998. "A Relational Approach to Autonomy in Health Care." In *The Politics of Women's Health: Exploring Agency and Autonomy*, edited by Susan Sherwin, 19–47. Philadelphia: Temple University Press.

Shrank, William H., Teresa L. Rogstad, and Natasha Parekh. 2019. "Waste in the US Health Care System: Estimated Costs and Potential for Savings." *JAMA: Journal of the American Medical Association* 322, no. 15 (October 15): 1501–9. doi:10.1001/jama.2019.13978.

Street, Richard L. Jr., and Paul Haidet. 2011. "How Well Do Doctors Know Their Patients? Factors Affecting Physician Understanding of Patients' Health Beliefs." *Journal of General Internal Medicine* 26, no. 1 (January): 21–27. doi:10.1007/s11606-010-1453-3.

Veatch, Robert M. 1972. "Models for Ethical Medicine in a Revolutionary Age: What Physician-Patient Roles Foster the Most Ethical Relationship?" *Hastings Center Report* 2, no. 3 (June): 5–7. doi:10.2307/3560825.

———. 1991. *The Patient as Partner*. Part 2, *The Patient-Physician Relation*. Bloomington: Indiana University Press.

———. 1995. "Abandoning Informed Consent." *Hastings Center Report* 25, no. 2 (March–April): 5–12. doi:10.2307/3562859.

———. 2000. "Doctor Does Not Know Best: Why in the New Century Physicians Must Stop Trying to Benefit Patients." *Journal of Medicine and Philosophy* 25, no. 6 (January): 701–21. doi:10.1076/jmep.25.6.701.6126.

Walton, Douglas N. 1985. *Physician-Patient Decision-Making: A Study in Medical Ethics*. Westport, CT: Greenwood.

Wolpe, Paul Root. 1998. "The Triumph of Autonomy in American Medical Ethics: A Sociological View." In *Bioethics and Society: Sociological Investigations of the Enterprise of Bioethics*, edited by Raymond DeVries and Janardan Subedi, 38–59. New York: Prentice Hall.

## Further Reading

Berg, Jessica W., Paul S. Appelbaum, Charles W. Lidz, and Lisa S. Parker. 2001. *Informed Consent: Legal Theory and Clinical Practice*. 2nd ed. New York: Oxford University Press. doi:10.1093/oso/9780195126778.001.0001.

> An interdisciplinary discussion of informed consent as it plays out in medical contexts, with a focus on practical guidelines for clinicians. The authors argue that informed consent should be understood as a continuous process rather than a distinct event, and they make recommendations to overcome some limitations of how informed consent is currently put into practice. Grounded in a study of the legal requirements of informed consent in the United States, they apply this doctrine to a range of situations, including patients who refuse treatment, end-of-life care, and medical experimentation.

Bergsma, Jurrit, and David C. Thomasma. 2000. *Autonomy and Clinical Medicine: Renewing the Health Professional Relation with the Patient*. Dordrecht: Kluwer. doi:10.1007/978-94-017-0821-0.

> Argues against traditional conceptions of autonomy (in terms of dignity and individualism) and puts forward an alternative, based in both psychology and philosophy, where autonomy is an aspect of personal identity that varies from person to person and changes according to one's state of health. In the clinician-patient relationship, two people are confronted with the patient's suffering. Autonomy is at the basis of coping strategies that the clinician and patient can use to bring about healing.

Cavanaugh, T. A. 2018. *Hippocrates' Oath and Asclepius' Snake: The Birth of the Medical Profession*. New York: Oxford University Press. doi:10.1093/med/9780190673673.001.0001.

> Examines the origins of Western medical ethics by considering the Hippocratic Oath in its cultural context. Cavanaugh discusses the Greek

attention to the doctor as a "wounder" and "healer," and he analyzes the role that the Oath plays in modern medicine, in relation to patient and professional autonomy.

Craigie, Jillian, and Lisa Bortolotti. 2015. "Rationality, Diagnosis, and Patient Autonomy in Psychiatry." In *The Oxford Handbook of Psychiatric Ethics*, edited by K. W. M. Fulford, C. W. van Staden, and John Z. Sadler, 387–404. New York: Oxford University Press. doi:10.1093/oxfordhb/9780198732365.013.28.
   Considers what patient autonomy means and how it should be supported by clinicians when a person has been diagnosed with a psychiatric illness. The concept of rationality has been central to the philosophical and legal understanding of autonomy, and mental health diagnoses are frequently invoked to justify overriding a person's autonomy in favor of beneficence. The authors critique the ethical implications of this approach.

Curlin, Farr, and Christopher Tollefsen. 2021. *The Way of Medicine: Ethics and the Healing Profession*. Notre Dame, IN: University of Notre Dame Press.
   Rejects what the authors call "the provider of services model" in favor of a historical tradition they seek to revive, "the Way of Medicine." On this view, medicine has an end—namely, health—to which all medical endeavors and the ethical virtues of clinicians ought to be directed. On Curlin and Tollefsen's view, the physician has the authority of expertise and decides the appropriate range of options based on their professional understanding of health. The patient must choose from those (limited) options because patient autonomy is only good if it is directed at the objective end of health.

Ells, Carolyn. 2001. "Lessons about Autonomy from the Experience of Disability." *Social Theory and Practice* 27, no. 4 (October): 599–615. https://www.jstor.org/stable/23559192.
   Considers the philosophical conception of self at work in dominant understandings of autonomy and argues that people with disabilities offer critical reflection on those assumptions. Ells claims that relational autonomy more accurately captures the experiences of people with chronic disabilities.

Gilbar, Roy, and José Miola. 2015. "One Size Fits All? On Patient Autonomy, Medical Decision-Making, and the Impact of Culture." *Medical Law Review* 23, no. 3 (Summer): 375–99. doi:10.1093/medlaw/fwu032.
   Discusses the traditional concept of autonomy in European philosophy and argues that the concept of relational autonomy may be more supportive of the self-determination of patients from non-Western cultural

backgrounds. The authors apply their view to legal decisions regarding healthcare in the United Kingdom.

Mallia, Pierre. 2013. *The Nature of the Doctor-Patient Relationship: Health Care Principles through the Phenomenology of Relationships with Patients*. Dordrecht: Springer. doi:10.1007/978-94-007-4939-9.

Explains and justifies Beauchamp and Childress's four principles—respect for autonomy, nonmaleficence, beneficence, and justice—by exploring the relationship between patient and physician. Mallia claims that the four principles are grounded in the phenomenology of the healthcare relationship and the historical tradition of medical thought. Linking these principles in the physician-patient relationship retains the focus on the patient and guards against medicine becoming a tool of government regulators and insurance companies.

Rothman, David J. 1991. *Strangers at the Bedside: A History of How Law and Bioethics Transformed Medical Decision Making*. New York: Routledge.

Chronicles a crucial period in American medical history, the decade following Henry Beecher's 1966 publication of "Ethics and Clinical Research," which criticized unethical experimentation practices, and how resulting shifts in the culture of medicine changed the dynamic of the clinician-patient relationship. Rothman considers the clinician's role in earlier historical periods and the more recent involvement of the legal system in medical decision-making. As the title suggests, Rothman argues that these changes have increasingly distanced physicians from their patients and turned medicine into a more bureaucratic and transactional enterprise.

Tauber, Alfred I. 2005. *Patient Autonomy and the Ethics of Responsibility*. Cambridge, MA: MIT Press.

A philosophical discussion of how patient autonomy has been historically framed by political concepts, and an argument to reframe autonomy in moral terms, with a stronger emphasis on beneficence and the ethics of care. Tauber argues that dominant conceptions of patient autonomy do not lead to the development of trust between patient and physician, and he makes practical recommendations for how such trust can be cultivated.

# CHAPTER 4
# Clinicians' Obligations to Patients and Themselves

**Key topics in this chapter:**

- Clinicians' professional expectations and ethical duties to be honest with patients, including disclosure of medical errors and when exceptions are warranted
- Different ways to justify maintaining patient confidentiality and when it can be breached
- The scope and limits of clinician autonomy, understood through the lens of conscientious refusal
- How the healthcare industry impacts clinician well-being, including the risk of moral distress

## Introduction

The previous chapter addressed a central issue in the clinician-patient relationship: how the autonomy of the person as patient should be respected, and how that goal interacts with the need to protect patients' well-being and with the professional authority of clinicians. This chapter focuses on moral questions that arise from the practitioners' perspective: What level of transparency fulfills their obligations to respect autonomy and act beneficently? Should all medical errors be disclosed? What are the limits of patient confidentiality? These issues concern the exchange of information among clinicians, patients, and (in some cases) a wider community.

Furthermore, how do we protect the autonomy and well-being of clinicians? What role should their personal judgments play in which treatments they offer patients? How should clinicians deal with the psychological weight of doing morally charged work, particularly when they are unable to act according to their own values and judgments? More specifically, respecting clinician autonomy means defining the scope of conscientious refusal, and promoting clinician well-being means addressing the problem of moral distress. Deliberation around these issues will typically happen among professionals and thus be less evident to patients, but they have a significant impact on treatment, privacy, and other aspects of the patient experience. In recent decades, legal and professional standards have established guidelines for confronting some of these challenges, but for others, more clarification and institutional change are needed.

## Truth-Telling, Autonomy, and Beneficence

Respecting a patient's autonomy means they must get accurate information about their medical condition, treatment options, and the risks associated with them. There are both deontological and consequentialist reasons for clinicians to be honest: being fully informed is a crucial part of autonomous self-determination, the patient has a right to be informed about their own medical condition, and deception may undermine the relationship of trust between clinician and patient. Although the **duty of transparency** is not in the Hippocratic Oath (and in fact Hippocrates suggests that medical information should be sparingly shared with the patient), clinicians are regularly told to be truthful with patients (and others) by their professional organizations. For example, the American Medical Association's Principles of Medical Ethics (2001) enjoin physicians to "be honest in all professional interactions." Tom Beauchamp and James Childress claim that when clinicians and patients enter into a relationship, they each implicitly promise to be honest with one another which, they say, gives the patient a right to truthful information (2019, 328).

As Beauchamp and Childress also note, veracity is only a prima facie obligation that may be overridden by other obligations, typically beneficence (2019, 328). For example, if a patient is in such a psychologically fragile state that a cancer diagnosis would lead to self-injurious behavior, the physician may not reveal the truth until a later time. A survey in 1961 found that almost 90 percent of physicians avoided telling patients about a terminal cancer diagnosis out of concern for how they would respond (Oken 1961). Even with the contemporary insistence on transparency, physicians may be hesitant to discuss bluntly with patients their chances of survival and quality of life following available treatments (Gawande 2014).

Especially in the medical context, however, the duty of transparency is not easily overridden. David Thomasma claims that all the reasons why the truth may be withheld—"recipient survival, community survival, and the ability to absorb the full impact of the truth at a particular time"—are "only temporary trump cards in any event . . . because respect for persons is a foundational value in all relationships" (1994, 377). To shelter a person from the reality of their medical situation is to deprive them of the agency to make decisions that align with their values and priorities.

The consequentialist argument against truth-telling is often weaker than it seems. Clinicians should not assume that a patient's ignorance about their condition will protect their well-being. The author of the 1961 study notes that concerns about patient harm were rarely substantiated; rather, the doctors were motivated by "emotion-laden *a priori* personal judgments" (Oken 1961, 86). In fact, an earlier survey showed that most cancer patients (89 percent) wanted to know their diagnoses (Kelly and Friesen 1950). The increased emphasis on patient autonomy in the 1970s led to a dramatic change in physicians' attitudes (Sokol 2006): in 1979, 98 percent of physicians reported that they informed cancer patients of terminal diagnoses (Novack et al. 1979).

Despite the general obligation to be truthful, there are exceptional cases where it is unclear whether beneficence or transparency is the more pressing prima facie duty. For example:

- A heavily sedated patient who is intubated and on mechanical ventilation is diagnosed with terminal cancer, with only a month to live. Should clinicians wake the patient so that, when she becomes fully aware, they can inform her about the condition, or should they only tell the patient's family, who would prefer that she not be informed and die peacefully?

- A patient has a life-threatening disease with only a 10 percent chance of successful treatment. The patient claims to understand this information but expresses an unreasonable level of confidence that the treatment will work. Should the clinician play along and emphasize the possibility of success or make sure that the patient fully grasps the seriousness of the prognosis?

- A frail, elderly patient is anxious about getting encephalitis from the COVID-19 vaccine. This side effect is extremely rare, and the risks of not being vaccinated are much worse, especially given the patient's age and health. Should the doctor lie to the patient and say that it is not a possible side effect?

In each of these cases—lies of both omission and commission—the patients are (or could be) cognitively capable, autonomous beings with a right to be informed about and understand their conditions and treatment options, and clinicians have a corresponding obligation to tell them the truth. In each case, telling the whole truth will likely lead to unnecessary distress—that is, psychological suffering that serves no purpose because it will not change their prognoses or their treatment decisions. It may even lead to quicker physical deterioration. Whether patient autonomy or beneficence is the overriding value in these and similar cases is a matter of moral judgment. Clinicians often consult with ethics committees to figure out what to do.

The weight of the different prima facie duties may also depend on a patient's acculturated expectations. There is cultural variation regarding the kinds of relationships that patients want with their clinicians and the information they hope to receive. For example, Leslie Blackhall et al. (2001) found that, while European Americans and Black Americans tend to privilege individual autonomy, Latinos and Korean Americans tend to view the self as part of a family unit. Although members of the former cultures tend to want full disclosure of their diagnoses and prognoses, members of the latter culture may see it "as an act of cruelty," "traumatic and demoralizing, sapping the patient of hope and the will to live" (69). In this study, only 48 percent of Latinos and 33 percent of Korean Americans agreed that a terminally ill patient should be told about their prognosis (61). In many countries outside of the United States, patients may also have different expectations. Greater support for nondisclosure of cancer diagnoses, especially for pediatric patients, is more common in countries such as Spain, Italy, Greece, Japan, China, and some Middle Eastern countries (see, respectively, Centeno-Cortés and Núñez-Olarte 1994; Surbone, Ritossa, and Spagnolo 2004; Mystakidou et al. 1996; Mayer et al. 2005; Wang et al. 2018; Rosenberg et al. 2017; see also Zahedi 2011). In developing countries, clinicians may also be reluctant to disclose cancer diagnoses because they lack access to quality cancer treatment and hospice care facilities (Kazdaglis et al. 2010).

In the U.S., standard clinical protocol is to ask patients whether they want all the relevant information or if it should instead be communicated to their proxies. The right to refuse medical interventions includes the right to decline to be informed fully about one's medical situation. This is a way to respect patient autonomy, promote well-being, and honor cultural differences around decision-making.

## Disclosure of Medical Errors

As part of the commitment to transparency, all the major medical associations say that clinicians ought to inform patients when they make mistakes that affect or may affect the course of treatment. For example, the British Medical Association says that doctors have "both a legal and ethical duty . . . to be honest about acknowledging mistakes in diagnosis or treatment" (2024, 17); the American College of Physicians says that clinicians should disclose errors if the information is "material to the patient's well-being" (Sulmasy and Bledsoe 2019); and the American Medical Association says that clinicians should inform patients about medical errors, including "possible" errors, even if they "will not alter the patient's medical treatment or therapeutic options" (n.d., 8.6). Regulators and accreditors, such as the Joint Commission in the U.S. and the General Medical Council in the U.K., also require disclosure. Although some jurisdictions mandate disclosure of unanticipated outcomes, including ten U.S. states, most of them enforce it with accreditation and professional discipline. Fatal hospital errors sometimes result in prosecution for manslaughter, as in the RaDonda Vaught case discussed in Chapter 2 (Merry 2009). Many more jurisdictions, including thirty-eight U.S. states, legally prohibit apologies from being used as evidence in medical liability/malpractice cases. This encourages clinicians to acknowledge patients' unfulfilled expectations and to discuss how treatments could have gone better.

Despite the professional and legal consensus on disclosing medical errors, surveys show that most clinicians are reluctant to do so. Thomas Gallagher et al. (2006) found that only 42 percent of physicians would explicitly acknowledge errors to patients, with the majority (56 percent) calling attention to the adverse event without identifying its cause. Lauris Kaldjian et al. (2007) found that, although almost all the physicians and trainees they surveyed recognized the obligation to disclose, less than half of them actually admitted major or minor errors to patients (see also Lamb et al. 2003; cf. Sweet and Bernat 1997). There are several possible reasons for this reluctance: confusion about what constitutes an error, concerns that disclosure will cause anxiety in patients and erode their trust in the practitioner or the profession, or fear that it will expose clinicians and their employers to lawsuits. Clinicians who admit mistakes may also lose their colleagues' respect and be burdened with bad reputations among patients (Wu et al. 1997, 772). In addition, there is a culture in medicine that discourages disclosure: physicians "manage" errors through denial (e.g., negating the concept of error by emphasizing the "inexact science" of medicine), discounting personal responsibility by shifting blame to others, and distancing themselves from the problem by stressing the inevitability of error (Mizrahi 1984).

None of these reasons for not disclosing stands up to ethical scrutiny, however. As Françoise Baylis (1997) says, we can distinguish avoidable medical errors from anticipated risks; patient anxiety and lack of confidence may be warranted rather than something to avoid; and the absence of explanations, not honesty about good-faith mistakes, is more likely to prompt litigation. Furthermore, self-interested motives, especially worries about one's own reputation, seldom carry much moral weight. The desire to avoid social opprobrium or to conform to cultural expectations may explain a person's reluctance to do the right thing, but it does not justify it.

Although medical ethicists disagree about when to disclose (immediately or when the patient is ready to hear it?), how much to tell (must one use the word "error" or "mistake"?), and the conditions under which disclosure is necessary (does it have to affect health outcomes?), almost all of them agree that clinicians are obligated to inform patients about medical errors and to apologize. Philosophers articulate this responsibility in terms of wider moral duties. Beauchamp and Childress see it as just another kind of bad news, and they claim that the obligation of veracity cannot be overridden by any of the supposed reasons for nondisclosure (2019, 334–36). Albert Wu et al. (1997) claim that disclosure is justified on both consequentialist and deontological grounds: knowledge of the mistake may facilitate proper treatment, thus helping the patient (beneficence) and preventing further harm to the patient and others in their situation (nonmaleficence); it may prevent anxiety by identifying the etiology of the problem (nonmaleficence); it allows the patient to make informed decisions about future care (respect for autonomy); and it may allow the patient to receive compensation to which they are entitled (justice). Martin Smith and Heidi

Forster (2000) say that, as one of the "professional virtues," "the virtue of truthfulness" is not only integral to the clinician-patient relationship but also "strengthens [clinicians'] inner selves." To promote that virtue, clinicians should practice "the routine disclosure of mistakes" (46). When a clinician notices a mistake by a colleague, they should encourage them to report it to their institution and disclose it to the patient. If their colleague refuses, the clinician may have an obligation to navigate the complex interpersonal dynamics and report it themselves (Gallagher et al. 2013).

## Confidentiality

In the service of building trust with patients, clinicians must freely share information with them but must not disseminate their private health information to others. This obligation is longstanding and widely recognized, not only ethically but also professionally and legally. The Hippocratic Oath (2002) includes a pledge of **confidentiality**: "Whatever I see or hear in the lives of my patients, whether in connection with my professional practice or not, which ought not to be spoken of outside, I will keep secret, as considering all such things to be private." This prohibition recognizes the intimate nature of medical communication and how much effective treatment depends on building trust with patients. Many contemporary professional codes of conduct include similar expectations. For example, the World Medical Association (2022) says that "the physician must respect the patient's privacy and confidentiality, even after the patient has died." The United Nations recognizes privacy and confidentiality as basic human rights in the Universal Declaration on Bioethics and Human Rights (Article 9). Many countries have established informational privacy in the healthcare setting as a legal right. In the United States, medical confidentiality is codified in the **Health Insurance Portability and Accountability Act (HIPAA)** (Pub. L. 104–191 [1996]) and is specified in the 2000 HIPAA Privacy Rule, which prohibits the misuse of individually identifiable health information, formalizes confidentiality practices and oversight, and requires healthcare organizations to notify patients about their privacy rights. In the United Kingdom, patient confidentiality is a matter of common law.

Like the disclosure of errors, the ethical obligation to protect patient privacy can be justified on both deontological and utilitarian grounds. There are several different duty-based approaches: the **right to privacy** includes the right to deny others access to one's personal information, respect for autonomy entails that clinicians should allow patients to decide how their information is used, and there is an implicit promise in a clinical setting not to disclose sensitive information without a patient's consent. Consequentialist arguments usually focus on how lack of confidentiality would erode the bond of trust between clinicians and patients, and how it would discourage people from getting the treatment they need. Clinicians cannot successfully diagnose and treat patients without accurate information, and patients whose information is not held in confidence would sometimes—when the ailment or its cause is socially condemned or personally embarrassing—be less likely to tell the truth or the whole truth. If sick people avoid seeking aid, their own health and the health of others (in the case of communicable diseases, for example) would be compromised. Furthermore, if sensitive information were leaked to the public, patients could be stigmatized—imagine a patient in a conservative community who confesses to homosexual desires in therapy—or discriminated against by their employers or potential employers—for example, if they tested positive for HIV. The long-term consequences of not respecting patient privacy, for both patients themselves and the public, would be worse than the consequences of maintaining confidentiality.

Clinician-patient confidentiality can be waived by patients. They can, for example, consent to have their information shared with another doctor to give a second opinion or provide treatment for what the first doctor diagnosed, as when an oncologist's cancer diagnosis is shared with an infusion center that will administer the chemotherapy. In signing a consent for care and treatment form, a patient agrees to have their medical information given to their insurance company. HIPAA allows healthcare professionals to share information with other practitioners at the clinic unless a patient explicitly requests otherwise—that is, patients are presumed to consent to have their information shared with the whole care team. Mark Siegler (1982) has said that this is broadly construed to include numerous people at the clinic: various physicians (primary physician, surgeon, etc.), house officers (surgical and ICU staff, etc.), nurses (on multiple shifts), pharmacists, nutritionists, chart reviewers (quality and risk management officers, financial officers, insurance auditors, etc.), and more (see also Beltran-Aroca et al. 2016). The desire for the best possible care, with a team of clinicians, is in tension with the patient's interest in maintaining confidentiality. Thus, Siegler says, "the confidentiality principle is compromised systematically in the course of routine medical care" (1982, 1518). Those who have responded to Siegler in the intervening years have mostly agreed with his conclusion, claiming that strict confidentiality is impossible and that patients should simply adjust their unrealistic expectations around privacy (e.g., Anesi 2012). If nothing else, clinicians and patients need "a new Hippocratic bargain" to clarify what is expected and what is possible in the age of electronic health records, which only compound the problem (Rothstein 2010; see also Foreman 2006).

In addition to the general erosion of confidentiality, the laws and professional expectations that enjoin clinicians to respect patient privacy also include exceptions even when patients do not consent. That is, none of them construe confidentiality as absolutely binding; it is a prima facie obligation. The conditions under which clinicians ought to break confidentiality were first set out in a landmark court case, *Tarasoff v. Regents of the University of California*, originally heard in 1974 (13 Cal. 3d 177, 529 P.2d 553, 118 Cal. Rptr. 129) and later reheard in 1976 (17 Cal. 3d 425, 551 P.2d 334, 131 Cal. Rptr. 14). A patient had confessed to his psychologist that he was going to kill Tatiana Tarasoff. Although the therapist informed the campus police and his superior, no one warned Tarasoff herself, whom the patient later killed. The question was whether the psychologist and the institution that employed him were partly responsible or, as the majority opinion put it, whether "Tatiana's death proximately resulted from defendants' negligent failure to warn Tatiana or others likely to apprise her of her danger" (433). The California Supreme Court "conclude[d] that the public policy favoring protection of the confidential character of patient-psychotherapist communications must yield to the extent to which disclosure is essential to avert danger to others. The protective privilege ends where the public peril begins" (443). Although the 1974 decision only established a legal **duty to warn** the threatened individual, the 1976 decision established a legal **duty to protect** them, the latter of which may entail not only warning the potential victim but also notifying the police, having the patient hospitalized, or taking other precautions. The assumption is that healthcare professionals have a moral obligation to protect the well-being of all people, not only their patients.

To override the duty to maintain confidentiality, there must be a foreseeable and imminent threat of serious harm, and the person or group at risk must be clearly identifiable. These conditions ensure that the value of the harm averted is greater than the harm caused by the sacrifice of confidentiality. In short, breaking confidentiality must be worth it. Common reasons to break confidentiality include protecting people from future wrongful activity by notifying third parties of threats (as in the *Tarasoff* case) or reporting to the police injuries resulting from child abuse, intimate partner violence, or elder abuse; preventing or detecting serious crimes by reporting violence-related injuries such as gunshot wounds; and promoting public health by reporting to the local health department communicable diseases such as tuberculosis, which may require isolation or quarantine, or sexually transmitted infections such as syphilis, whose detection may (depending on the state) result in partner notification and contact tracing by the health department.

As with any other prima facie duty, the obligation to maintain confidentiality does not simply disappear when it is overridden. In warning the potential victim, a patient's confidentiality must be respected as much as possible: as it says in the *Tarasoff* decision, a clinician must disclose the information "discreetly, and in a fashion that would preserve the privacy to the fullest extent compatible with the prevention of the threatened danger" (441). For example, a doctor must disclose a patient's tuberculosis diagnosis to the public health department, but they should not reveal unrelated physiological or psychiatric information that is not reportable and is unnecessary to protect public health.

Some U.S. states mandate a duty to protect or a duty to warn; some merely permit the breach of confidentiality, either by legislative statute or judicial precedent; and a few are silent on the issue both statutorily and in case law (Edwards 2010; National Conference of State Legislatures 2022). States also have different standards for when to breach confidentiality. In 1985, California enshrined the *Tarasoff* ruling in state law, although they narrowed its applicability to when "the patient has communicated to the psychotherapist a serious threat of physical violence against a reasonably identifiable victim or victims" (Cal. Civ. Code § 43.92[a]). By contrast, Washington state broadened the duty to protect beyond actual threats to identifiable victims. In *Volk v. DeMeerleer* (187 Wn. 2d 241 [Wash. 2016]), the Washington Supreme Court found that once a "special relationship" is established between a mental health professional and a patient, the clinician "'incur[s] a duty to take reasonable precautions to protect *anyone* who might foreseeably be endangered by' the patient's condition" (256; quoting *Petersen v. State*, 100 Wn. 2d 421 [Wash. 1983], at 428).

Although clinician-patient confidentiality is legally protected in many countries outside the U.S., there is no uniform standard. First, countries differ regarding the basis of the law, whether in domestic, common, or international human rights law. For example, Brazil has a statute similar to HIPAA called the General Data Protection Act (*Lei Geral de Proteção de Dados* [LGPD]) (2020). In the United Kingdom, no domestic legislation protects confidentiality; it is incorporated into their system through the Human Rights Act (1998), which applies the European Convention on Human Rights to U.K. residents (Perlin 2006). In India, there is no law governing patient confidentiality; the Indian Medical Council's ethics regulations (2002) include a privacy rule (7.14) that has been applied by the courts.

Countries also set out different conditions under which clinicians can or should breach their patients' confidentiality. In South Africa, for example, "personal information may be disclosed in the public interest where the benefits to an individual or to society of the disclosure outweigh the patient's interest in keeping the information confidential." They give as an example "third parties at grave personal risk, such as the spouse or partner of a patient who is HIV positive, who after counselling refuses to disclose his or her status to such spouse or partner" (Health Professions Council of South Africa 2021, 8.2.4.1). In Vietnam, medical professionals are fined if they do not report patients with drug addictions to the local health authorities (Decree 46-CP, 1992). And in New Zealand, clinicians may (but do not have to) disclose private health information to a police officer if it is "required ... for the purposes of exercising or performing any of that person's powers, duties or functions," even if the officer does not have enough evidence for a warrant (Health Act 1956, sec. 22C). Different countries balance privacy against public health and safety in different ways.

## Conscientious Refusal

Although medical ethicists tend to focus on how and how much to support patient autonomy, clinicians also have a right to self-determination that may impact their professional obligations. In addition to what Edmund Pellegrino calls physician autonomy (moral status because of expert knowledge) and professional autonomy (membership in a moral community with collective obligations to society), clinicians have personal autonomy to follow their consciences (1994, 51–53; see also American Medical Association, n.d., 1.1.7). As an expression of personal values, some clinicians may decide not to perform procedures to which they have moral objections. The law usually accommodates **conscientious refusal** (also called conscientious objection) in order to respect clinicians' freedom to exercise their religious views or maintain their moral integrity. For example, all death with dignity laws say that healthcare professionals may decline to assist terminally ill patients in dying. The Oregon statute says that "no health care provider shall be under any duty, whether by contract, by statute or by any other legal requirement to participate in the provision to a qualified patient of medication to end his or her life in a humane and dignified manner" (ORS 127.885 § 4.01[4]). Conscientious refusals are especially common with abortion procedures. Washington state's Reproductive Privacy Act, which requires any state-funded medical facility that provides maternity care also to offer "substantially equivalent" abortion services, allows individual clinicians to opt out as long as the institution as a whole can accommodate patient demand (RCW 9.02.100, 9.02.160 [1991]).

As several philosophers note, however, we need to balance clinicians' rights and patients' rights (Pellegrino 1994; Wicclair 2011; Childress 2020, 127–52). Society has restricted access to healthcare through the licensure process; for example, patients cannot buy prescription drugs on the open market. This means clinicians who refuse to assist patients may be using their professional power, which society has granted them, to impose their personal views on people who cannot otherwise receive care. The problem with conscientious refusal is that it may deprive patients of timely access to desired and legal medical services. Various state laws govern conscientious refusal. For example, even if a pharmacist has a moral or religious objection to filling a prescription for emergency contraception, some states require them to dispense it (and any other legally prescribed drugs), citing the duty of care. Other states require them to refer the prescription to another pharmacist or to advise the patient on where they can obtain the medication. Recently, some states have legally allowed pharmacists simply to refuse to fill the prescription, with no obligation to inform the patient about how to obtain the medication otherwise (Achey and Robertson 2022). In rural areas or other communities that face shortages of healthcare professionals (including pharmacists), conscientious refusal may play an outsized role in controlling access to treatment. Christian Fiala and Joyce Arthur (2017) argue against the right to refuse treatment on religious grounds because it conflicts with the right to healthcare and patient autonomy. Conscientious refusal in reproductive healthcare should be legally prohibited because it is not evidence-based medicine, and it puts someone's unjustified, personal convictions ahead of their professional obligations (see also Savulescu 2006). Alongside these legal questions, clinicians' moral obligations are a matter of scholarly debate: Are they obligated to fulfill their professional obligations to provide the service, or would any participation (such as referral to another clinician) make them complicit in an act that they have judged to be wrong (Eberl 2019; Reis-Dennis and Brummett 2022)?

A point of contemporary cultural conflict is whether clinicians can conscientiously refuse to treat adult transgender patients, either to assist in gender reassignment or to provide routine medical care, or if such refusal is inherently discriminatory because it targets a class of people rather than a specific procedure (Dinelli 2022). On the latter view, it would compound the structural barriers (e.g., lack of insurance coverage for transgender-related services), anticipation barriers (e.g., avoiding doctors for fear of mistreatment), and other interpersonal barriers (e.g., lack of clinician sensitivity) to transgender patients receiving adequate care (Warner and Mehta 2021). Legally protecting clinicians' refusal to treat transgender patients amounts to "legislation of discrimination . . . under the guise of religious and moral conscience" (James, Lioi, and Yang 2022). Aaron Ancell and Walter Sinnott-Armstrong (2017) defend a middle position. Although cases of invidiously discriminatory conscientious objection are morally wrong, they claim that we can both legally allow clinicians to exercise their freedom of conscience and protect patients' right against undue burdens if clinicians and their employers publicize the patient population they refuse to serve, direct affected patients to clinicians who will serve them, and cover the costs, either by hiring clinicians who will treat them or by paying the additional expenses of going elsewhere, including the difference in the clinic bill, time, and transportation.

## Moral Distress, Moral Injury, and Burnout

Clinicians deal with morally charged issues that affect individual patients, and their work is structured by policies, institutions, and laws they do not control. Their attempt to navigate this terrain, all while staying true to their own values, impacts clinician well-being. What if the situation of being a clinician in the healthcare industry is, perhaps inevitably, psychologically and morally harmful?

Clinicians face many unique challenges. First, although the demand for services has grown dramatically as people live longer, the supply of physicians has decreased. Over seventy-four million people in the U.S. live in places where access to a primary care physician is scarce, which could only be addressed with an additional 12,973 doctors ("Primary Care" 2024). By 2036, the U.S. is projected to have between 13,500 and 86,000 fewer physicians than it needs (Association of American Medical Colleges 2024). By 2030, the U.S. will also have 63,720 fewer full-time registered nurses than it needs (National Center for Health Workforce Analysis 2022). Staffing shortages lead to excessive work hours and caseloads for clinicians, as well as increased time on call (on nights and weekends). Clinicians also have less control over the kind of work they do. While doctors themselves used to decide how much time they spent with patients, the questions they asked, and the treatments they used, their work is now highly regimented by hospitals and clinics. Their employers have expectations around quality measures, patient satisfaction scores, and productivity, usually measured in relative value units (RVUs). Insurance companies require prior authorization for many treatments, allowing them to assess the appropriateness of clinicians' decisions using so-called utilization reviews (to control costs). Government regulations impose administrative burdens, mostly around documentation and reporting, including EHR meaningful use requirements. On average, primary care physicians spend approximately a quarter of their workday entering data into the EHR, including not only visit notes, diagnoses, and orders, but also information needed for billing, quality measurements, and compliance (Arndt et al. 2017). This emphasis on clerical work distracts from patient care. Finally, clinicians are regularly responding to people in physical and psychological distress, some of which can be alleviated, but some of which can be addressed only partially and imperfectly. Given the moral dimension of these roles and a medical culture that tends to acknowledge the vulnerability of patients but not practitioners, clinicians may struggle to process the psychological intensity of caring for people (Gazelle, Liebschutz, and Riess 2015).

These countervailing pressures often leave clinicians with an impossible choice: either to care for their patients with the amount of time and effort that they think is appropriate, or to satisfy the demands of their employer, the insurance companies, and the government, sometimes at the expense of their own well-being. When practitioners cannot act in alignment with their values due to these pressures—when they act wrongly, fail to prevent a wrong, or witness wrongdoing by others—they experience **moral distress** (Jameton 1984). According to Denise Dudzinski (2016), several factors make distress a distinctively moral emotion: a heightened sense of moral responsibility, concern for patient well-being, feelings of powerlessness, blame for preventable wrong or harm, and conflicting professional and ethical obligations. One physician explains moral distress as a misalignment between personal and organizational priorities: "We're being put in conflict with what our original calling was. . . . We want to heal people and be available—but systems are at odds with that. We constantly hit roadblocks honoring our values" (Doggett 2023). Although moral distress is situational, experiencing it persistently may lead to **moral injury**, a term that originated in military psychology (Litz et al. 2009). Moral injury results from the erosion of a person's integrity or "the enduring psychological, spiritual, behavioral, social, and emotional harm inflicted on an individual's conscience" (Weisleder 2023, 262).

Sometimes moral distress and injury are misinterpreted as **burnout**, characterized as "a long-term stress reaction" to overwork that includes "emotional exhaustion," "depersonalization" (a lack of empathy, or a tendency to view patients and colleagues as objects), and a "feeling of decreased personal achievement" (American Medical Association 2023). However, moral distress and injury are systemic problems rather than individual deficiencies, and although distress can lead to burnout, they are not the same phenomenon (Dean, Talbot, and Dean 2019). Collectively, moral distress, moral injury, and professional burnout lead to lower patient satisfaction and worse health outcomes (Panagioti et al. 2018), contribute to the overuse of resources and higher costs (Kushnir et al. 2014; Han et al. 2019), and exacerbate the shortage of primary care physicians, thus hindering the achievement of healthier communities and placing more of a burden on other clinicians (Willard-Grace et al. 2019). Because of this, some people add to the Triple Aim of healthcare—improving the patient experience, improving population health, and reducing per capita costs—a fourth component: improving the work life of healthcare professionals.

Addressing these problems will not be easy. Many professional organizations are lobbying for less government regulation. They also want EHRs to be redesigned to support patients and clinicians rather than supporting healthcare administrators with compliance and billing. A relatively new office in the Centers for Medicare and Medicaid Services (CMS), the Office of Healthcare Experience and Interoperability (OHEI), is attempting to reduce clinicians' administrative obligations.

Some proposed solutions are technological. For example, artificial intelligence can streamline EHR use before, during, and after patient visits. Smart EHRs can summarize a patient's medical history, pull out relevant health information, and suggest potential diagnoses (Waldren and Billings 2024). During the visit, AI assistants can act as scribes using speech recognition and natural language processing technology to record information in real time, make documentation suggestions based on what is required for billing, and offer differential diagnoses based on the patient's medical history, diagnostic tests, and the latest research, which will help doctors to make accurate assessments more quickly (Brown 2023).

Many organizations are also addressing clinician shortages with **team-based care models**. With team-based care, physicians take the lead in developing relationships with patients, interpreting available data to make diagnoses, and deciding which treatments to propose. Advanced practitioners, such as physician assistants and nurse practitioners, take on other tasks previously done by physicians, including getting patients' medical histories, reviewing medications, and documenting patient visits in the EHR (known as team documentation or multiple contributor documentation). By sharing information and delegating tasks, physicians carry less of a burden, and other clinicians work to the top of their licenses. The team works collaboratively with patients and their caregivers to achieve shared goals. For example, a patient's breast cancer treatment will often involve radiologists and imaging technicians, pathologists, a breast surgeon, a reconstructive surgeon, anesthesiologists, a medical oncologist, a genetic counselor, infusion nurses for chemotherapy, radiation therapists, several other nurses, a social worker, a mental health counselor, and a nutritionist. A nurse navigator guides the patient through the process. All the team members communicate and have access to the patient's medical records (hence Siegler's worry about confidentiality), thus providing an integrated approach over the full cycle of care.

A team-based approach may or may not lead to better health outcomes, improve patient satisfaction, and decrease costs—the evidence is mixed. However, delegating tasks to other clinicians does seem to reduce physician burnout (DeChant et al. 2019). Dudzinski (2016) reminds us, however, that one can ameliorate moral distress only by identifying and confronting the underlying ethical conflict, not only by trying to improve patient care or making the clinician less stressed. Since moral distress is a systemic issue, it cannot be effectively addressed through individual coping mechanisms such as mindfulness training.

## Conclusion: Moral Tensions in the Patient Encounter

Thorny ethical issues arise in hospitals and clinics. Conflicts occur between patient autonomy and patient well-being, between the rights of patients and the rights of clinicians, between obligations to the patient and obligations to the public, between the wishes of the patient and the wishes of the family, between the demands of one's religion and the needs of the body. Vulnerable patients confront healthcare professionals who have authoritative knowledge but who are also human, with biases and stressors that affect their judgment. Clinician-patient interactions are highly regulated by the government, and treatment decisions are heavily constrained by public and private insurers. At the center of these competing forces, we make some of our most important decisions around personal well-being and meaningful living, life and death, reproduction and parenting.

### REFERENCES

Achey, Thomas S., and Ashley T. Robertson. 2022. "Conscientious Objection: A Review of State Pharmacy Laws and Regulations." *Hospital Pharmacy* 57, no. 2 (April): 268–72. doi:10.1177/00185787211024217.

American Medical Association. 2001. "AMA Principles of Medical Ethics." June. https://code-medical-ethics.ama-assn.org/principles.

———. 2023. "What Is Physician Burnout?" February 16. https://www.ama-assn.org/practice-management/physician-health/what-physician-burnout.

———. n.d. "Code of Medical Ethics." Accessed January 15, 2025. https://code-medical-ethics.ama-assn.org/.

Ancell, Aaron, and Walter Sinnott-Armstrong. 2017. "How to Allow Conscientious Objection in Medicine While Protecting Patient Rights." *Cambridge Quarterly of Healthcare Ethics* 26, no. 1 (January): 120–31. doi:10.1017/S0963180116000694.

Anesi, George L. 2012. "The 'Decrepit Concept' of Confidentiality, 30 Years Later." *Virtual Mentor* 14, no. 9 (September 1): 708–11. doi:10.1001/virtualmentor.2012.14.9.jdsc1-1209.

Arndt, Brian G., John W. Beasley, Michelle D. Watkinson, Jonathan L. Temte, Wen-Jan Tuan, Christine A. Sinsky, and Valerie J. Gilchrist. 2017. "Tethered to the EHR: Primary Care Physician Workload Assessment Using EHR Event Log Data and Time-Motion Observations." *Annals of Family Medicine* 15, no. 5 (September): 419–26. doi:10.1370/afm.2121.

Association of American Medical Colleges. 2024. *The Complexities of Physician Supply and Demand: Projections from 2019 to 2036*. Washington, DC: Association of American Medical Colleges. https://www.aamc.org/media/75236/download.

Baylis, Françoise. 1997. "Errors in Medicine: Nurturing Truthfulness." *Journal of Clinical Ethics* 8, no. 4 (Winter): 336–40. doi:10.1086/JCE199708403.

Beauchamp, Tom L., and James F. Childress. 2019. *Principles of Biomedical Ethics*. 8th ed. New York: Oxford University Press.

Beltran-Aroca, Cristina M., Eloy Girela-Lopez, Eliseo Collazo-Chao, Manuel Montero-Pérez-Barquero, and Maria C. Muñoz-Villanueva. 2016. "Confidentiality Breaches in Clinical Practice: What Happens in Hospitals?" *BMC Medical Ethics* 17: article no. 52. doi:10.1186/s12910-016-0136-y.

Blackhall, Leslie J., Gelya Frank, Sheila Murphy, and Vicki Michel. 2001. "Bioethics in a Different Tongue: The Case of Truth-Telling." *Journal of Urban Health* 78, no. 1 (March): 59–71. doi:10.1093/jurban/78.1.59.

British Medical Association. 2024. *Ethics Toolkit: The Doctor-Patient Relationship*. January. https://www.bma.org.uk/media/nalcxoal/the-doctor-patient-relationship2024.pdf.

Brown, N. Adam. 2023. "AI Won't Replace Doctors. But It May Help with Burnout." *MedPage Today*. July 19. https://www.medpagetoday.com/opinion/prescriptionsforabrokensystem/105540.

Centeno-Cortés, Carlos, and Juan M. Núñez-Olarte. 1994. "Questioning Diagnosis Disclosure in Terminal Cancer Patients: A Prospective Study Evaluating Patients' Responses." *Palliative Medicine* 8, no. 1 (January): 39–44. doi:10.1177/026921639400800107.

Childress, James F. 2020. *Public Bioethics: Principles and Problems*. Oxford: Oxford University Press. doi:10.1093/med/9780199798483.001.0001.

Dean, Wendy, Simon Talbot, and Austin Dean. 2019. "Reframing Clinician Distress: Moral Injury Not Burnout." *Federal Practitioner* 36, no. 9 (September): 400–402. https://pmc.ncbi.nlm.nih.gov/articles/PMC6752815/.

DeChant, Paul F., Annabel Acs, Kyu B. Rhee, Talia S. Boulanger, Jane L. Snowdon, Michael A. Tutty, Christine A. Sinsky, and Kelly J. Thomas Craig. 2019. "Effect of Organization-Directed Workplace Interventions on Physician Burnout: A Systematic Review." *Mayo Clinic Proceedings: Innovations, Quality & Outcomes* 3, no. 4 (December): 384–408. doi:10.1016/j.mayocpiqo.2019.07.006.

Dinelli, John A. 2022. "Conscientious Objection Based on Patient Identity: A Virtue Ethics Argument against LGBTQ+ Discrimination." *Voices in Bioethics* 8. https://journals.library.columbia.edu/index.php/bioethics/article/view/10098#_edn14.

Doggett, Lisa. 2023. "Doctors Have Their Own Diagnosis: 'Moral Distress' from an Inhumane Health System." *NPR*. August 2. https://www.npr.org/sections/health-shots/2023/08/02/1191446579/doctors-have-their-own-diagnosis-moral-distress-from-an-inhumane-health-system.

Dudzinski, Denise Marie. 2016. "Navigating Moral Distress Using the Moral Distress Map." *Journal of Medical Ethics* 42, no. 5 (May): 321–24. doi:10.1136/medethics-2015-103156.

Eberl, Jason T. 2019. "Protecting Reasonable Conscientious Refusals in Health Care." *Theoretical Medicine and Bioethics* 40, no. 6 (December): 565–81. doi:10.1007/s11017-019-09512-w.

Edwards, Griffin Sims. 2010. "Database of State *Tarasoff* Laws." *Social Science Research Network*. February. https://ssrn.com/abstract=1551505.

Fiala, Christian, and Joyce H. Arthur. 2017. "There Is No Defence for 'Conscientious Objection' in Reproductive Health Care." *European Journal of Obstetrics & Gynecology and Reproductive Biology* 216 (September): 254–58. doi:10.1016/j.ejogrb.2017.07.023.

Foreman, Judy. 2006. "At Risk of Exposure." *L.A. Times*. June 26. http://articles.latimes.com/2006/jun/26/health/he-privacy26.

Gallagher, Thomas H., Jane M. Garbutt, Amy D. Waterman, David R. Flum, Eric B. Larson, Brian M. Waterman, W. Claiborne Dunagan, Victoria J. Fraser, and Wendy Levinson. 2006. "Choosing Your Words Carefully: How Physicians Would Disclose Harmful Medical Errors to Patients." *Archives of Internal Medicine* 166, no. 15 (August): 1585–93. doi:10.1001/archinte.166.15.1585.

Gallagher, Thomas H., Michelle M. Mello, Wendy Levinson, Matthew K. Wynia, Ajit K. Sachdeva, Lois Snyder Sulmasy, Robert D. Truog, et al. 2013. "Talking with Patients about Other Clinicians' Errors." *New England Journal of Medicine* 369, no. 18 (October 31): 1752–57. doi:10.1056/NEJMsb1303119.

Gawande, Atul. 2014. *Being Mortal: Medicine and What Matters in the End*. New York: Picador.

Gazelle, Gail, Jane M. Liebschutz, and Helen Riess. 2015. "Physician Burnout: Coaching a Way Out." *Journal of General Internal Medicine* 30, no. 4 (April): 508–13. doi:10.1007/s11606-014-3144-y.

Han, Shasha, Tait D. Shanafelt, Christine A. Sinsky, Karim M. Awad, Liselotte N. Dyrbye, Lynne C. Fiscus, Mickey Trockel, and Joel Goh. 2019. "Estimating the Attributable Cost of Physician Burnout in the United States." *Annals of Internal Medicine* 170, no. 11 (June 4): 784–90. doi:10.7326/M18-1422.

Health Professions Council of South Africa. 2021. *Guidelines for Good Practice in the Healthcare Professions.* Booklet 5, *Confidentiality: Protecting and Providing Information.* December. https://www.hpcsa.co.za/Uploads/professional_practice/ethics/Booklet_5_Confidentiality_Protecting_and_Providing_Information_vDec_2021.pdf.

"Hippocratic Oath." 2002. Translated by Michael North. National Library of Medicine, National Institutes of Health. https://www.nlm.nih.gov/hmd/greek/greek_oath.html.

Indian Medical Council. 2002. "(Professional Conduct, Etiquette and Ethics) Regulations." https://upload.indiacode.nic.in/showfile?actid=AC_CEN_12_13_00007_1956102_1517807321142&type=regulation&filename=10.Ethics%20Regulations-2002.pdf.

James, Eric, James Lioi, and Francis Yang. 2022. "Conscientious Objection and the Impact on Transgender Patients: A Response to 'Identifying and Addressing Barriers to Transgender Healthcare.'" *Journal of General Internal Medicine* 37, no. 4 (March): 971. doi:10.1007/s11606-021-07317-z.

Jameton, Andrew. 1984. *Nursing Practice: The Ethical Issues.* Englewood Cliffs, NJ: Prentice Hall.

Kaldjian, Lauris C., Elizabeth W. Jones, Barry J. Wu, Valerie L. Forman-Hoffman, Benjamin H. Levi, and Gary E. Rosenthal. 2007. "Disclosing Medical Errors to Patients: Attitudes and Practices of Physicians and Trainees." *Journal of General Internal Medicine* 22, no. 7 (July): 988–96. doi:10.1007/s11606-007-0227-z.

Kazdaglis, G. A., C. Arnaoutoglou, D. Karypidis, G. Memekidou, G. Spanos, and O. Papadopoulos. 2010. "Disclosing the Truth to Terminal Cancer Patients: A Discussion of Ethical and Cultural Issues." *Eastern Mediterranean Health Journal* 16, no. 4: 442–47. https://www.emro.who.int/emhj-volume-16-2010/volume-16-issue-4/article-18.html.

Kelly, William D., and Stanley R. Friesen. 1950. "Do Cancer Patients Want to Be Told?" *Surgery* 27, no. 6 (June): 822–26. https://www.surgjournal.com/article/0039-6060(50)90252-2/abstract.

Kushnir, Talma, Dan Greenberg, Nir Madjar, Israel Hadari, Yuval Yermiahu, and Yaacov G. Bachner. 2014. "Is Burnout Associated with Referral Rates among Primary Care Physicians in Community Clinics?" *Family Practice* 31, no. 1 (February): 44–50. doi:10.1093/fampra/cmt060.

Lamb, Rae M., David M. Studdert, Richard M. J. Bohmer, Donald M. Berwick, and Troyen A. Brennan. 2003. "Hospital Disclosure Practices: Results of a National Survey." *Health Affairs* 22, no. 2 (March–April): 73–83. doi:10.1377/hlthaff.22.2.73.

Litz, Brett T., Nathan Stein, Eileen Delaney, Leslie Lebowitz, William P. Nash, Caroline Silva, and Shira Maguen. 2009. "Moral Injury and Moral Repair in War Veterans: A Preliminary Model and Intervention Strategy." *Clinical Psychology Review* 29, no. 8 (December): 695–706. doi:10.1016/j.cpr.2009.07.003.

Mayer, D. K., S. K. Parsons, N. Terrin, H. Tighiouart, S. Jeruss, K. Nakagawa, Y. Iwata, J. Hara, and S. Saiki-Craighill. 2005. "School Re-entry after a Cancer Diagnosis: Physician Attitudes about Truth Telling and Information Sharing." *Child: Care, Health and Development* 31, no. 3 (May): 355–63. doi:10.1111/j.1365-2214.2005.00522.x.

Merry, Alan F. 2009. "How Does the Law Recognize and Deal with Medical Errors?" *Journal of the Royal Society of Medicine* 102, no. 7 (July 1): 265–71. doi:10.1258/jrsm.2009.09k029.

Mizrahi, Terry. 1984. "Managing Medical Mistakes: Ideology, Insularity and Accountability among Internists-in-Training." *Social Science & Medicine* 19, no. 2: 135–46. doi:10.1016/0277-9536(84)90280-6.

Mystakidou, Kyriaki, Christina Liossi, Lambros Vlachos, and Joannis Papadimitriou. 1996. "Disclosure of Diagnostic Information to Cancer Patients in Greece." *Palliative Medicine* 10, no. 3 (July): 195–200. doi:10.1177/026921639601000303.

National Center for Health Workforce Analysis. 2022. "Nurse Workforce Projections, 2020–2035." November. https://bhw.hrsa.gov/sites/default/files/bureau-health-workforce/Nursing-Workforce-Projections-Factsheet.pdf.

National Conference of State Legislatures. 2022. "Mental Health Professionals' Duty to Warn." March 16. https://www.ncsl.org/health/mental-health-professionals-duty-to-warn.

Novack, Dennis H., Robin Plumer, Raymond L. Smith, Herbert Ochitill, Gary R. Morrow, and John M. Bennett. 1979. "Changes in Physicians' Attitudes toward Telling the Cancer Patient." *JAMA: Journal of the American Medical Association* 241, no. 9 (March 2): 897–900. doi:10.1001/jama.1979.03290350017012.

Oken, Donald. 1961. "What to Tell Cancer Patients: A Study of Medical Attitudes." *JAMA: Journal of the American Medical Association* 175, no. 13 (April 1): 1120–28. doi:10.1001/jama.1961.03040130004002.

Panagioti, Maria, Keith Geraghty, Judith Johnson, Anli Zhou, Efharis Panagopoulou, Carolyn Chew-Graham, David Peters, Alexander Hodkinson, Ruth Riley, and Aneez Esmail. 2018. "Association between Physician Burnout and Patient Safety, Professionalism, and Patient Satisfaction: A Systematic Review and Meta-analysis." *JAMA Internal Medicine* 178, no. 10 (September 4): 1317–31. doi:10.1001/jamainternmed.2018.3713.

Pellegrino, Edmund D. 1994. "Patient and Physician Autonomy: Conflicting Rights and Obligations in the Physician-Patient Relationship." *Journal of Contemporary Health Law and Policy* 10, no. 1: 47–68. https://scholarship.law.edu/jchlp/vol10/iss1/8.

Perlin, Michael L. 2006. "'You Got No Secrets to Conceal': Considering the Application of the *Tarasoff* Doctrine Abroad." *University of Cincinnati Law Review* 75, no. 2 (Winter): 611–30. https://digitalcommons.nyls.edu/fac_articles_chapters/767/.

"Primary Care Health Professional Shortage Areas (HPSAs)." 2024. Kaiser Family Foundation. Last modified April 1, 2024. https://www.kff.org/other/state-indicator/primary-care-health-professional-shortage-areas-hpsas/.

Reis-Dennis, Samuel, and Abram L Brummett. 2022. "Are Conscientious Objectors Morally Obligated to Refer?" *Journal of Medical Ethics* 48, no. 8 (August): 547–50. doi:10.1136/medethics-2020-107025.

Rosenberg, Abby R., Helene Starks, Yoram Unguru, Chris Feudtner, and Douglas Diekema. 2017. "Truth Telling in the Setting of Cultural Differences and Incurable Pediatric Illness." *JAMA Pediatrics* 171, no. 11 (November 1): 1113–19. doi:10.1001/jamapediatrics.2017.2568.

Rothstein, Mark A. 2010. "The Hippocratic Bargain and Health Information Technology." *Journal of Law, Medicine & Ethics* 38, no. 1 (Spring): 7–13. doi:10.1111/j.1748-720X.2010.00460.x.

Savulescu, Julian. 2006. "Conscientious Objection in Medicine." *BMJ* 332, no. 7536 (February 4): 294–97. doi:10.1136/bmj.332.7536.294.

Siegler, Mark. 1982. "Confidentiality in Medicine—a Decrepit Concept." *New England Journal of Medicine* 307, no. 24 (December 9): 1518–21. doi:10.1056/NEJM198212093072411.

Smith, Martin L., and Heidi P. Forster. 2000. "Morally Managing Medical Mistakes." *Cambridge Quarterly of Healthcare Ethics* 9, no. 1 (January): 38–53. doi:10.1017/s0963180100901051.

Sokol, Daniel K. 2006. "How the Doctor's Nose Has Shortened over Time: A Historical Overview of the Truth-Telling Debate in the Doctor-Patient

Relationship." *Journal of the Royal Society of Medicine* 99, no. 12 (December): 632–36. doi:10.1177/014107680609901212.

Sulmasy, Lois Snyder, and Thomas A. Bledsoe. 2019. *American College of Physicians Ethics Manual.* 7th ed. *Annals of Internal Medicine* 170, no. S2 (January 15): S1–32. doi:10.7326/M18-2160.

Surbone, Antonella, Claudio Ritossa, and Antonio G. Spagnolo. 2004. "Evolution of Truth-Telling Attitudes and Practices in Italy." *Critical Reviews in Oncology/Hematology* 52, no. 3 (December): 165–72. doi:10.1016/j.critrevonc.2004.09.002.

Sweet, Matthew P., and James L. Bernat. 1997. "A Study of the Ethical Duty of Physicians to Disclose Errors." *Journal of Clinical Ethics* 8, no. 4 (Winter): 341–48. doi:10.1086/JCE199708404.

Thomasma, David C. 1994. "Telling the Truth to Patients: A Clinical Ethics Exploration." *Cambridge Quarterly of Healthcare Ethics* 3, no. 3 (Summer): 375–82. doi:10.1017/s096318010000520x.

Waldren, Steven E., and Edmund Billings. 2024. *AI Assistant for Clinical Review and Value-Based Care.* American Academy of Family Physicians. January. https://www.aafp.org/dam/AAFP/documents/practice_management/innovation_lab/report-navina-ai-clinical-review-phase2.pdf.

Wang, Hongchun, Fang Zhao, Xiangling Wang, and Xiaoyang Chen. 2018. "To Tell or Not: The Chinese Doctors' Dilemma on Disclosure of a Cancer Diagnosis to the Patient." *Iranian Journal of Public Health* 47, no. 11 (November): 1773–74. https://ijph.tums.ac.ir/index.php/ijph/article/view/15171.

Warner, David Michael II, and Arunab Harish Mehta. 2021. "Identifying and Addressing Barriers to Transgender Healthcare: Where We Are and What We Need to Do about It." *Journal of General Internal Medicine* 36, no. 11 (November): 3559–61. doi:10.1007/s11606-021-07001-2.

Weisleder, Pedro. 2023. "Moral Distress, Moral Injury, and Burnout: Clinicians' Resilience and Adaptability Are Not the Solution." *Annals of the Child Neurology Society* 1, no. 4 (December): 262–66. doi:10.1002/cns3.20048.

Wicclair, Mark R. 2011. *Conscientious Objection in Health Care: An Ethical Analysis.* Cambridge: Cambridge University Press. doi:10.1017/CBO9780511973727.

Willard-Grace, Rachel, Margae Knox, Beatrice Huang, Hali Hammer, Coleen Kivlahan, and Kevin Grumbach. 2019. "Burnout and Health Care Workforce Turnover." *Annals of Family Medicine* 17, no. 1 (January): 36–41. doi:10.1370/afm.2338.

World Medical Association. 2022. "WMA International Code of Medical Ethics." https://www.wma.net/policies-post/wma-international-code-of-medical-ethics/.

Wu, Albert W., Thomas A. Cavanaugh, Stephen J. McPhee, Bernard Lo, and Guy P. Micco. 1997. "To Tell the Truth: Ethical and Practical Issues in Disclosing Medical Mistakes to Patients." *Journal of General Internal Medicine* 12, no. 12 (December): 770–75. doi:10.1046/j.1525-1497.1997.07163.x.

Zahedi, Farzaneh. 2011. "The Challenge of Truth Telling across Cultures: A Case Study." *Journal of Medical Ethics and History of Medicine* 4. https://jmehm.tums.ac.ir/index.php/jmehm/article/view/68.

## Further Reading

DeVita, Michael A., and Mark P. Aulisio, eds. 2001. Special issue, *Kennedy Institute of Ethics Journal* 11, no. 2 (June). https://muse.jhu.edu/issue/1100.
  This special issue gathers five presentations from a conference on medical mistakes held at the University of Pittsburgh Medical Center in 2000. The papers consider how errors have been defined and responses to them, both at the institutional and legal levels. Several of the authors argue that medical errors should be more fully disclosed, and they offer recommendations for how to encourage transparency.

Fainzang, Sylvie. 2016. *An Anthropology of Lying: Information in the Doctor-Patient Relationship*. London: Routledge.
  Analyzes the exchange of information between clinicians and patients at several hospitals in France. Fainzang documents how significantly the disclosure of diagnosis, prognosis, and treatment options diverge from the ideal conditions of supporting autonomous decision-making described by much of medical ethics discourse, to the extent that patients often can only offer "resigned consent." She argues that the power differentials between patients and clinicians in hospital settings impede effective communication, typically in unacknowledged and therefore unaddressed ways.

Frezza, Eldo E. 2020. *The Moral Distress Syndrome Affecting Physicians: How Current Healthcare Is Putting Doctors and Patients at Risk*. New York: Routledge. doi:10.4324/9781003034766.
  Discusses the growing problem of moral distress among physicians by documenting what causes moral distress and its effects on clinicians, patients, and institutions. Through a fictional dialogue between two physicians, the author uses current research to illuminate how healthcare organizations may exacerbate moral distress and its consequences for them, in the form

of burnout, medical error, and turnover. Frezza suggests ways to lessen moral distress, both at individual and organizational levels.

Giubilini, Alberto, and Julian Savulescu, eds. 2017. "Conscientious Objection in Healthcare: Problems and Perspectives." Special section, *Cambridge Quarterly of Healthcare Ethics* 26, no. 1 (January): 3–158. doi:10.1017/S096318011600075X.

A collection of thirteen previously unpublished articles on conscientious objection/refusal. The authors discuss whether there is a right to conscientious objection, the conflict between individual conscience and professional duties, whether conscientious objections must be reasonable, the obligation to refer to other clinicians, and how clinicians should handle specific cases, such as treating sex offenders for sexual dysfunction.

Halper, Thomas. 1996. "Privacy and Autonomy: From Warren and Brandeis to *Roe* and *Cruzan*." *Journal of Medicine and Philosophy* 21, no. 2 (April): 121–35. doi:10.1093/jmp/21.2.121.

Considers the constitutional right to privacy as it has developed in cases related to healthcare—particularly abortion and the right to refuse treatment. Halper traces the evolution of the legal concept of privacy and argues that protecting autonomy needs to be the most important goal of medical law.

Hébert, Philip C. 2021. *Doing Right: A Practical Guide to Ethics for Medical Trainees and Physicians*. 4th ed. New York: Oxford University Press.

Examines the foundational theories of medical ethics that are then applied to a range of issues through a discussion of specific cases. With an intended audience of medical students, the authors offer an eight-step method for resolving ethical problems based on professional and legal expectations. This book provides an illuminating contrast to medical ethics texts written primarily for philosophers and bioethicists.

Jackson, Jennifer. 2001. *Truth, Trust and Medicine*. London: Routledge.

A thorough investigation of the moral basis of the "core virtue" of truthfulness and its implications for medical professionals. Jackson provides a history of truth and lies in medicine, what it means to lie, and when deception is excused or justified in clinical practice and medical research. The book incorporates the work of many philosophers (Augustine, Kant, Alasdair MacIntyre, Sissela Bok, and others) and discusses many concrete cases.

Rhodes, Rosamond. 2020. *The Trusted Doctor: Medical Ethics and Professionalism*. Oxford: Oxford University Press. doi:10.1093/med/9780190859909.001.0001.

Critiques the dominance of the principlist approach in medical ethics and instead claims that the clinician's overriding obligation is earning the patient's trust. Rhodes elaborates on the duties that follow from this obligation, including prioritizing altruism, honesty, and evidence-based approaches. The book argues that this image of the "good doctor" more accurately mirrors the moral experience of clinicians and more effectively resolves common ethical issues in medical practice.

Rubin, Susan B., and Laurie Zoloth, eds. 2000. *Margin of Error: The Ethics of Mistakes in the Practice of Medicine.* Hagerstown, MD: University Publishing Group.

Examines various aspects of medical error by considering specific cases, both their causes and consequences. The authors discuss how medical error should be defined and how clinicians and institutions should be held accountable for their mistakes. Finally, the book offers an extended examination of the role of ethics consultations in responding to errors and what happens when ethics consultations themselves are implicated.

Werth, James L. Jr., Elizabeth Reynolds Welfel, and G. Andrew H. Benjamin, eds. 2009. *The Duty to Protect: Ethical, Legal, and Professional Considerations for Mental Health Professionals.* Washington, DC: American Psychological Association. doi:10.1037/11866-000.

Examines the obligations that therapists have to patients and wider communities. Intended for practitioners, the contributed chapters focus on the moral and legal standards for the duty to protect and then apply those standards to situations in which patients may be at risk of harming themselves or others, or in which clinicians may be harmed. It suggests how mental health professionals may practice effective self-care when confronting these problems and maps out emerging issues in this field.

# CHAPTER 5
# The Ethics and Legality of Abortion

**Key topics in this chapter:**
- Whether the fetus is a person and whether that resolves the moral question of abortion
- Two competing frameworks for interpreting the U.S. Constitution and their implications for the legality of abortion
- The impact of the *Dobbs* decision overturning *Roe*, especially for clinicians
- Global trends in abortion laws

## Introduction

One would think that abortion is not a pressing moral issue for most medical professionals, since most abortion providers are obstetrician-gynecologists (OB/GYNs), a small percentage of clinicians are OB/GYNs, and only about 18 percent of OB/GYNs perform abortions (Frederiksen et al. 2023). The legal status of abortion, however, raises ethical problems beyond this relatively small group of abortion providers. This is especially true in the U.S. after the 2022 *Dobbs v. Jackson Women's Health Organization* decision, since states are now passing abortion laws that impact clinicians more generally. For example, in Washington state, abortion is permitted to the point of viability, and the Reproductive Privacy Act requires all public hospitals that provide maternity services also to provide "substantially equivalent" abortion services (RCW 9.02.100, 9.02.160 [1991]). By contrast, Arkansas's Human Life Protection Act prohibits abortion in all cases, even in cases of rape or incest, except "to save the life of a pregnant woman in a medical emergency" (Act 180 [2019]). Under the circumstances, many clinicians find themselves forced to take a stand: in Washington, to decide whether to opt out of providing abortion services on moral grounds, and in Arkansas, to determine when a pregnant woman who wants or needs an abortion has destabilized to a life-threatening medical emergency. Clinicians may have to make difficult decisions about where to work based on this legal complexity. Ethics committees in states with abortion bans may have to advise clinicians about when the woman's life is truly at risk, and boards of trustees in Washington and elsewhere have to credential some clinicians who will not conscientiously object to performing abortions.

The post-*Roe* legal landscape implicates all medical professionals in this debate, not only abortion providers. But philosophers have focused on the morality of abortion for decades. A section on abortion is routinely included in textbooks and anthologies on applied ethics. Apart from its moral importance, abortion raises several perennial philosophical issues that may account for this sustained level of interest. Philosophers consider the meaning and extent of individual rights, the proper role of government, the meaning of motherhood, and the moral status of the fetus. One reason why abortion is such a complicated issue is because the biological process of sexual reproduction, including gestation inside of a woman, means that there is a gray area around the issue of personal identity. There are not two unambiguously separate individuals. Rather, there is a process of growth by which a couple of cells turn into a rational, basically self-sufficient person, from the moment of conception up to somewhere in childhood.

Before we begin, we have two notes about language. First, we recognize that trans men and gender-nonconforming people may become pregnant and seek abortions. But because the majority of people in these situations are women, for simplicity of reference, we use the term "women" and feminine pronouns. This usage also calls attention to the significance of gendered norms in legal and moral debates around abortion: the gender of the pregnant person impacts how their personhood is understood, culturally and politically. Additionally, in writing on abortion, philosophers tend to refer only to "the fetus," so we often adopt that simpler language here. However, the appropriate language to describe it changes during its development. Within the first two weeks post-conception (the germinal stage), the fertilized egg transitions from a zygote to a blastocyst, it becomes an embryo at approximately three weeks of development, and it is a fetus from the ninth week until birth. We emphasize this point because it is precisely the gradual development from zygote to newborn infant that makes moral judgments about abortion so difficult.

## Common Arguments on the Morality of Abortion

The most well-known positions on the ethics of abortion focus on personhood and rights, or how the woman is obligated to treat the fetus—whether it is a special obligation that she has taken on or whether it is on par with her obligations to other, full-fledged persons. The standard argument against abortion claims that because the embryo or fetus is a person, it has a right to life, and because it has a right to life, it would be wrong to abort it. If we give the argument a valid form, it looks like this:

P1  The fetus is a person from the moment of conception.

P2  Every person has a right to life.

P3  The pregnant woman is a person.

P4  Every person has a right to control what happens in and to their own body.

C1  Therefore, the fetus has a right to life, and the pregnant woman has a right to control what happens in and to her own body.

P5  These rights come into conflict if the woman seeks an abortion.

P6  The right to life is stronger than the right to decide what happens in and to one's own body.

C2  Therefore, the fetus's right to life is stronger than the pregnant woman's right to bodily self-control.

P7  If an action involving a rights claim violates a stronger rights claim, then the action is immoral.

C3  Therefore, abortion is immoral.

Proponents of this argument do not deny that women can control their bodies, only that there is a limit to that control based on the harm principle: as John Stuart Mill puts it, "the only purpose for which power can be rightfully exercised over any member of a civilized community, against his will, is to prevent harm to others" (1978, 9). The exercise of the woman's right over her body extends to the point where it would harm another person—in this case, the fetus. Although bringing the fetus to term may get in the way of the woman's other pursuits, aborting the fetus would end its life, which is a more significant harm.

Opponents and supporters of abortion often focus on the first premise of this argument: they disagree about whether the fetus is a person. For example, in their argument against abortion, Patrick Lee and Robert George (2005) claim that an embryo or fetus has the same three characteristics that define each of us as human beings: it has its own distinct genetic profile, it is a member of the human species, and it is a complete organism that develops according to its own genetic code. Thus, the embryo or fetus is a human being just like we are, albeit in a very early stage of development, so it has the human rights that all of us have, including the right to life (see also George and Tollefsen 2011). Other philosophers use different but similar strategies to establish the fetus's personhood, grounded in the probability of it developing humanity (Noonan 1970) or the beginning of brain function (Brody 1975).

This appeal to the fetus's humanity is the dominant strategy for opposing abortion in nonphilosophical contexts as well. Anti-abortion activists often display pictures of aborted fetuses during protests to show how similar they are to grown human beings: they have bodies that are like ours, and they have been murdered. Billboards claim that an embryo has a detectable heartbeat six weeks after conception—even though it lacks cardiac valves that, in infants, children, and adults, produce a heartbeat; the sound that is supposedly a heartbeat is manufactured by the ultrasound machine (Simmons-Duffin and Feibel 2022; American College of Obstetricians and Gynecologists, n.d.). Nonetheless, laws in several states, such as the Texas Heartbeat Act (SB 8 [2021]) and Florida's Heartbeat Protection Act (SB 300 [2023]), ban abortion after six weeks of pregnancy—the idea being that this physical characteristic makes someone a distinct, individual human being with a right to life rather than just a clump of cells. For years, anti-abortion groups have provided funds for ultrasound machines at "pregnancy resource centers," and some states legally require abortion providers to perform ultrasounds on pregnant women and to show or describe the images to them (Coe and Altman 2012). They assume a woman will be less likely to have an abortion after she has seen the ultrasound image since, even in the early stages of development, an embryo takes on some of the characteristics of a newborn baby: arms and legs appear by week eight, at week nine the embryo starts to move, and at eleven weeks it can hiccup. Some states have passed abortion bans that include "fetal personhood" provisions, including ones that criminalize women's behavior that might endanger fetuses. For example, Georgia's Living Infants Fairness and Equality Act (HB 481), which was passed in 2019 and went into effect after *Dobbs*, defines an "unborn child" as "a member of the species Homo sapiens at any stage of development who is carried in the womb." Women who use alcohol or drugs while pregnant may be accused of "prenatal abuse," which healthcare practitioners are required to report to state authorities (Ga. Code § 15-11-2 [56], § 19-7-5).

Other philosophers focus on the same premise—the claim that the fetus is a person—but draw the opposite conclusion. Mary Anne Warren (1973), for example, says that the traditional argument against abortion asserts as obvious that the fetus is a person from the moment of conception because it has the same genetic material as other *Homo sapiens*. But personhood, in the sense that would confer rights on someone, is a moral rather than a biological claim. Warren argues that fetuses are not full members of the moral community because they lack the five characteristics that typically distinguish persons from nonpersons: consciousness, especially the capacity to feel pleasure and pain (sentience); reasoning; self-motivated activity; the capacity to communicate; and the presence of self-concepts, individual and/or racial. Other philosophers use different but similar strategies to deny that the fetus is a person, saying that it lacks a concept of self (Tooley 1972) or that it has no conscious interests until late in gestation (at around twenty-eight weeks) (Steinbock 2011). Because a fetus is not a person (in this morally weighty sense of the term) through most or all of its development, we have few or no direct moral obligations to it—any more than we have to something with the same level of awareness, such as (Warren says) a newborn guppy.

Many supporters of abortion rights seem to adopt this position when they affirm, "My body, my choice." They realize that the right over our bodies is limited by the harm principle; however, they claim that it does not apply in this case: "My body, my choice—because whether I choose to continue a pregnancy does not harm another person or violate their rights." The assumption among abortion rights activists, then, is that the fetus is not a person and has no rights, so it does not impose any restrictions on the woman's right to bodily self-control.

Of course, one could have indirect obligations to the fetus insofar as the woman values it as a potential human life. One wrongs the woman if one ends the life of a wanted fetus, even if it is not a person. According to

Elizabeth Harman (2019), the woman's attitude toward the fetus is crucial for determining how we should feel, say, about miscarriages as opposed to abortions. And a fetus's moral status changes over the course of the pregnancy. Aborting a fetus early in its development is morally and emotionally different from being forced to carry a child to term and give it up for adoption. In the latter case, the woman is made to take on a relationship with what becomes a child.

Other theorists claim that we can address the abortion issue without settling the metaphysical question of whether the fetus is a person. In her canonical defense of abortion, Judith Jarvis Thomson (1971) says that even if we grant (for the sake of argument) that the fetus is a person with a right to life, that does not imply that it should not be killed at all, only that it should not be killed unjustly (see also Boonin 2019). And there are many cases where ending the fetus's life would not violate that restriction. Thomson first considers "involuntary pregnancy" (as a result of rape), and she gives the following analogy: A famous violinist has a kidney ailment that will kill him unless he has someone else's kidneys filter his blood for him. Since only you have the right blood type, his friends kidnap you and surgically attach you to him so your kidneys perform this function. After nine months, his kidneys will have healed, and they will be able to detach him. In such a case, Thomson says that the violinist has no right to your kidneys, even if it would be nice of you—"a great kindness"—to let him use your body for nine months (1971, 48–49). The right to life is not a right to all the conditions that would allow someone to live. It is a right only to the things that someone is owed. In cases of involuntary pregnancy as well as cases where the woman's life is at risk or the pregnancy is semivoluntary (that is, it occurs despite precautions taken not to get pregnant, such as failures of birth control), the fetus, even if it is a person, has no right to the woman's body. It is morally permissible to abort it. Thomson thus challenges the truth of the sixth premise in the traditional anti-abortion argument, the claim that the right to life is stronger than the right to decide what happens in and to one's own body.

Don Marquis (1989) devises an anti-abortion argument that also does not depend on whether the fetus is a person. He claims that abortion is wrong for the same reason that murder is wrong: both of them deprive someone of a future like ours. Killing someone is wrong because it cuts short a life in which they would have experiences that they value, and so does aborting a fetus. Note that Marquis is not saying that the fetus should be treated as a person because it is a potential person. Rather, he is saying that a future of possible goods is denied to both an aborted fetus and a murdered adult. Potentiality is operative in both cases, only with regard to a possible future rather than personhood (see also Hendricks 2019).

Much of the philosophical debate revolves around the question of whether a fetus can make moral demands of the woman on par with the demands that other people can make of her, and what those demands entail if the fetus is a full-fledged person. Opponents of abortion say that if we determine that the fetus has the requisite characteristics—the right genes, brain activity, consciousness, self-awareness, a future like ours, etc.—then it is a being to whom the woman has obligations. Just as "my right to swing my fist stops where another man's nose begins"—a legal adage attributed to Oliver Wendell Holmes Jr.—the woman's right over her body stops where the fetus's life begins. The situations are identical, a simple application of the harm principle. A fetus is essentially like us, like any other potential murder victim, at least in a moral sense.

Defenders of abortion have contested this reasoning either by denying that fetuses have rights or by arguing that any rights they have do not amount to an absolute right to life. They claim that fetuses are not persons but potential persons, and to treat them as full-fledged persons is a kind of logical mistake. After all, we should not treat an acorn like an oak tree (Thomson 1971, 47–48), and a prince does not have the same rights as a king (Singer 2011, 138). Mere potentiality relegates someone or something to a lesser status, either with no rights at all or with rights that are less pressing than the rights of an actual person, such that the woman's existing rights will always override a fetus's potential rights (Warren 1973, 47–48). In addition, the mere fact that someone needs what you have—your kidneys (Thomson 1971) or your bone marrow (Boonin 2019)—does not mean that denying it to them would treat them unjustly unless you have voluntarily taken on that obligation. In either case, the woman's right over her body is paramount.

## Constitutional Interpretation and the Legality of Abortion in the U.S.

Whether abortion should be legal is a separate question from whether abortion is ethically permissible. Plenty of things are morally wrong that are legal, such as lying to a friend or shouting Nazi slogans on a Seattle street corner. Whether abortion should be legal depends on how the government conceives of its function and the legal standing of the fetus. In a liberal political system such as the United States, where the purpose of government is to protect the rights of its citizens, the standard philosophical questions about abortion linger in the background: Does the woman have a right to an abortion, does the fetus have a right to life, and what does each entail about how they ought to be treated? More specifically, does the U.S. Constitution include a right to privacy that entails that women have a right to abortion, or do fetuses have all the rights, including the right to equal protection under the law, that other persons have?

### 1. Dworkin's interpretivism

Two opposing theories of constitutional interpretation—interpretivism and textualism—have dominated the conversation and have validated the landmark Supreme Court cases on abortion. **Interpretivism**, also called law as integrity or the moral reading of the Constitution, is associated most with Ronald Dworkin, who claims that when the law or some provision in the Constitution is vague, judges have discretion to interpret it, and in doing so they must consult principles that are separate from the rules that are codified in the law, since the rules themselves give no guidance. To inform their interpretation, judges should draw on principles of justice, fairness, respect for rights, or some other dimension of morality—the values that justify the law for us. Dworkin lists two classes of principles. As a threshold requirement, an interpretation of the law must be consistent with judgments that have come before it, what he calls "fit" with the common law (the body of law created by prior court decisions/precedents). It must also advance "political morality," including "equal concern" and "basic liberty" (Dworkin 1986, 225–38; 1993, 119–21, 128; 1996, 72–75, 80–81, 83).

Based on this approach, Dworkin (1996) argues in favor of a constitutionally protected right to get an abortion, in effect defending *Roe v. Wade*. The fact that a right to privacy or a right to abortion is not explicitly stated in the Constitution is irrelevant, since it is contained in the existing language of the Constitution once we give it our best reading—that is, according to principles. Dworkin's argument for abortion rights has several steps to it.

P1     A woman has a right over her own body.

Earlier Supreme Court decisions have recognized that a person has a right to control their own role in procreation. For example, married people can buy and use contraceptives without government restriction (*Griswold v. Connecticut*, 381 U.S. 479 [1965]), as can unmarried people (*Eisenstadt v. Baird*, 405 U.S. 438 [1972]); and the government cannot forcibly sterilize prisoners (*Skinner v. State of Oklahoma*, 316 U.S. 535 [1942]). The idea is that decisions about sex, procreation, family, and marriage are such personal, intimate issues—they are so bound up with a person's deep religious and moral convictions—that they should be left to a person's own conscience.

P2     A right can only be overridden by a competing right or a compelling state interest.

If someone has a right, it can only be limited for two reasons: either two rights conflict, so only one right can be protected, or there is a **compelling state interest**. The former condition is encapsulated in Holmes's adage and Mill's harm principle, since violating a person's rights is a kind of harm. With regard to the latter condition, the state may restrict a right (as little as possible) only if it achieves some crucial (not merely legitimate or important) governmental interest. So, the question becomes: Is there a competing right that would restrict a woman's right over her own body, or is there a compelling state interest that justifies limiting that right?

Dworkin sets aside the question of whether the fetus is a metaphysical person (with moral status) (85–86, 90–92) or a theological person (with a soul) (46) and focuses on whether it is a **constitutional person**.

P3     A fetus is not a constitutional person. (Dworkin 1996, 87–89)

If the fetus were a constitutional person, it would have rights on par with any fully functioning adult, including the right to equal protection under the law, so it could not be killed except in very rare circumstances (perhaps only to save the pregnant woman's life). However, Dworkin says that since fetal personhood would entail that abortion would have to be outlawed everywhere and would be legally equivalent to infanticide, something few critics of a general right to abortion are claiming, then even they do not believe a fetus is a constitutional person. In addition, as the Supreme Court says in *Roe*, the Court has never asserted that a fetus is a person; the existence of permissive abortion laws in several states in the nineteenth and twentieth centuries, which were not struck down by the Court, implies that fetuses are not covered by the Equal Protection Clause of the Fourteenth Amendment. Furthermore, states like Georgia that try to grant personhood to fetuses by statute cannot restrict a woman's constitutional rights by majority vote (Dworkin 1996, 88).

> C1  Therefore, a fetus does not have competing rights that restrict a woman's control over her body (derivative view). (84–85)

On what Dworkin calls the derivative view, a person's rights are derived from their status as a constitutional person. Since a fetus is not a constitutional person, a fetus does not have rights that conflict with the rights of the pregnant woman.

But there is also what Dworkin calls the detached view. This is the idea that there are objective and intrinsic goods that we ought to promote, the state has a compelling interest in promoting such goods, and we can only promote them by outlawing abortion.

> P4  The government has an obligation to promote respect for the intrinsic value of human life (detached view). (Dworkin 1996, 84–85, 93–95)

Dworkin himself says that, just because the fetus is not a person, it does not mean that it has no moral status or that choosing to abort a fetus carries no moral weight (1993, 12; 1996, 114). There is something significant about a developing human life that deserves our respect, even if the fetus itself has no legal rights or interests. Fetuses resemble persons in the sense that they are living things. Following this line of thinking, some opponents of abortion say that the government should restrict abortion to cultivate respect for human life.

> P5  The state can promote respect for the intrinsic value of human life without prohibiting abortion. (Dworkin 1996, 112–14)

A **strict scrutiny test** is applied when a proposed law would violate a person's right—in this case, the right a woman has over her own body. As mentioned earlier, the interest furthered by the law must be compelling in the sense that it is necessary to further a crucial government interest, *and* the law must be narrowly tailored, meaning it restricts the right as little as possible to accomplish the end. Dworkin addresses the latter point, claiming that the state can promote respect for life without completely banning abortion. For example, a state could prohibit abortion after the fetus is viable (able to survive outside of the womb). This respects a woman's right to choose before that—it gives her time to make this important decision—but it also recognizes the value of fetal life when it resembles a living baby more than just a clump of cells (113–14).

> P6   Prohibiting abortion out of respect for the intrinsic value of human life would violate our First Amendment rights. (98–109)

Among other things, the First Amendment forbids the establishment of religion by the government and allows individuals the free exercise of religion. There is strong disagreement about why human life has intrinsic value and when it becomes morally significant. Such fundamental questions are tied inextricably to our moral, spiritual, and religious beliefs. If the state were to prohibit abortion, it would force on its citizens a particular position on the value of (unborn) human life. Just as the Court has protected access to contraception, thus taking no position on whether procreation is the only purpose of sex (103), it should not determine when and under what conditions life has intrinsic value.

> C2   There is no compelling state interest that would justify prohibiting abortion.

Dworkin concludes that the state does not have to prohibit abortion to promote the intrinsic value of human life.

> C3   Therefore, the state would violate a woman's right over her own body if it outlawed abortion.

Because the fetus has no constitutional rights and because outlawing abortion is unnecessary to promote the value of human life, abortion should be permitted, at least at earlier stages of the pregnancy. The woman's right to procreative autonomy is constitutionally protected.

## 2. Roe v. Wade *(1973)*

Dworkin's view aligns with the Supreme Court's reasoning in *Roe v. Wade* (410 U.S. 113 [1973]), which set limits to state laws on abortion for fifty years. There, the Court concluded that states could impose "virtually no restriction" on abortions in the first trimester, states could regulate abortions in the second trimester (to protect the life of the woman), and states could (if they chose) prohibit abortions after the point of viability (when the fetus can survive outside of the womb, around twenty-three to twenty-four weeks) because of their legitimate interest in protecting potential life. To recognize the right of women to get abortions, the Court majority appealed to the right to privacy. Every person has a private sphere within which they can decide how to live. In this case, the Court said that an abortion is a personal decision that a woman has as to how to manage her own body. Although the right to privacy is not explicitly recognized in the Constitution, the Court ruled that it is implied by the Due Process Clause of the Fourteenth Amendment, which restricts the reach of government when it comes to people's personal liberties, and the Ninth Amendment, which says that just because a right is not listed, it does not mean there is no such right retained by the people. It is also a background assumption behind the rights that are enumerated. Dworkin would say that recognizing the right to privacy protects the fundamental principle of basic liberty.

Although *Planned Parenthood v. Casey* (505 U.S. 833 [1992]) later replaced the strict scrutiny test with an undue burden standard—states cannot "place a substantial obstacle in the path of a woman seeking an abortion" (877)—it reaffirmed the "essential holding" of *Roe*: "The right of the woman to choose to have an abortion before viability and to obtain it without undue interference from the State" (846). Once again, this is entailed by the right to privacy: "'If the right of privacy means anything, it is the right of the *individual*, married or single, to be free from unwarranted governmental intrusion into matters so fundamentally affecting a person as the decision whether to bear or beget a child'" (896; quoting *Eisenstadt v. Baird*, 405 U.S. 438 [1972], at 453).

*Roe* was prompted by a challenge to a Texas law that criminalized abortion, and in their arguments for the ban, Texas had claimed that life begins at conception. In the Court's decision, the majority noted that there are many different opinions on this issue: some people believe that life begins at conception, some believe it begins at the point of quickening (a medieval notion that the fetus is "ensouled" when it first moves voluntarily), some think it begins at viability, others think it begins with live birth, and still others think that there is no clear point when the fetus becomes a person. People disagree, and people's opinions have changed over time. For example, although the Catholic Church now strictly opposes abortion because they claim that life begins at conception, that view only became official Church doctrine in 1869, with Pope Pius IX's *Apostolicae Sedis*. Before then, the Church followed Aristotle and Aquinas, claiming that abortions were permissible prior to the point of quickening, which occurs at about eighteen to twenty-one weeks of fetal development. In light of the longstanding uncertainty regarding the personhood question, the Supreme Court took no position on this controversial issue. It also found no common law precedent in which the Fourteenth Amendment had been applied to the unborn. Given the fact that abortions were legally permitted in some states before and after the Fourteenth Amendment was ratified, the Court concluded that the fetus had no constitutional rights that conflicted with the woman's right to privacy.

## *3. Scalia's textualism and originalism*

While Dworkin's approach to constitutional interpretation provided retroactive support for the Court's reasoning in *Roe v. Wade*, Justice Antonin Scalia's textualism and originalism heavily influenced the Justices who would later sign on to the majority opinion in *Dobbs*, which overturned *Roe*. To defend his view, Scalia begins with the uncontroversial claim that we need a rule to interpret the Constitution. A rule ensures uniformity in the Court's rulings: that like cases are treated alike and different cases differently, that clear precedents are set, and that there is predictable meaning to the law (Scalia 2020, 6–7). Some common bases of legal interpretation are unsuited to provide such a rule. Judicial discretion leaves the decision up to the subjective moral commitments of the individual judge, which varies from judge to judge and from moment to moment, thus providing no uniformity. A judge who decides what is best acts like a legislator and thus violates the separation of powers (9–10, 28). Appeals to legislative intent look at lawmakers' notes, floor debates, and committee reports to determine what Congress meant by the law; appeals to legislative history look at the process by which the law came to exist, and that process is supposed to tell us something about what it means. However, Scalia says that this is not only anti-democratic—the people would be bound to something that few of them are aware of—but also misunderstands the process by which something becomes law. Only the text of the law matters because that text, not notes or histories, passed both houses of Congress and was signed into law by the President (26–29). The only clear rule is provided by textualism and originalism. According to **textualism**, the law means what the text of the statute says: "When the text of a statute is clear, that is the end of the matter" (25). When it is unclear, judges must adopt an interpretation compatible with previously enacted laws (26). According to **originalism**, the text of a statute means what it meant when it was originally enacted because that is how legislators understood what they were approving at the time (12). When the original meaning of the Constitution is unclear, we can look at how it was interpreted by state legislatures in the years after the Constitution was written (21–22).

Applying textualism to abortion law, Scalia claims that there is no right to privacy and no right to abortion because "the Constitution says absolutely nothing about it" (2020, 155). Applying originalism, he says that such rights are not somehow contained in the Due Process Clause of the Fourteenth Amendment (as the majority in *Roe* claim) because, when the Fourteenth Amendment was ratified in 1868, three-quarters of the states prohibited abortion at any point in the pregnancy. Since the people and the courts, including the Supreme Court, allowed those laws to stand—"the longstanding traditions of American society have permitted [abortion] to be legally proscribed"—they clearly did not think that the Due Process Clause covered a woman's unqualified right over her body, such that abortion was constitutionally protected (155). Indeed, no right to privacy or right to abortion was ever mentioned prior to the twentieth century. The majority in *Roe* read their own personal moral convictions into the Constitution and made new law rather than interpreting existing law, which is the risk of any appeal to judicial discretion. Since the Constitution and the common law are silent about abortion, the decision about whether to prohibit abortion to protect unborn human life should be left to the states: "Value judgments, after all, should be voted on, not dictated" (157).

### 4. Dobbs v. Jackson Women's Health Organization *(2022)*

In 2022, the U.S. Supreme Court overturned both *Roe* and *Casey*. *Dobbs v. Jackson Women's Health Organization* (597 U.S. \_\_\_ [2022]) reflects the deep impact that Scalia's textualism and originalism had on the Court's relatively new conservative majority. In that decision, the Court found that there is no right to abortion explicitly referenced in the Constitution: "*Roe* . . . held that the abortion right, which is not mentioned in the Constitution, is part of the right to privacy, which is also not mentioned" (slip op. at 2). If these rights are not in the text of the Constitution, then they are not constitutional rights—unless such unenumerated rights were thought to be implicit in the Due Process Clause of the Fourteenth Amendment, as the *Roe* Court thought it was. For this to be the case, the notion would have to be "deeply rooted in this Nation's history and traditions" or "implicit in the concept of ordered liberty" (slip op. at 5, 75 [majority opinion]; quoting *Washington v. Glucksberg*, 521 U.S. 702 [1997], at 721). Since, as noted earlier, many states outlawed abortion before and after the passage of the Fourteenth Amendment, that is not how it was originally understood, and since anti-abortion laws were allowed to stand for many years after that (until 1973), it is not how the courts had understood it (*Dobbs v. Jackson Women's Health Organization*, slip op. at 3, 5, 16, 23, 29 [majority opinion]). Finally, how we define the boundary between competing interests in a scheme of ordered liberty depends on how we balance the interests of pregnant women against the public's interest in protecting prenatal life. Since states may balance those interests differently, it should be left to them, not the Supreme Court, to decide whether the fetus deserves legal protection or whether the woman should be able to control her body even to the point of extinguishing a developing human life.

The majority opinion in *Dobbs* begins with the traditional question of whether there is a conflict of rights:

> Some believe fervently that a human person comes into being at conception and that abortion ends an innocent life. Others feel just as strongly that any regulation of abortion invades a woman's right to control her own body and prevents women from achieving full equality. Still others in a third group think that abortion should be allowed under some but not all circumstances. . . . (slip op. at 1 [majority opinion])

Because this is a contentious claim, the Court ruled that the abortion issue should be left to the states, as it was pre-*Roe*. Still, the personhood question lurks in the background of *Dobbs*. The ruling upheld a Mississippi law that repeatedly refers to the "unborn human being" (MS Code § 41-41-191), and the majority opinion cites several nineteenth-century state laws referring to "unborn children" (slip op. at 90, 92, 100 [majority opinion]). Chief Justice John Roberts refers twice to the "unborn child" in his concurring opinion, using his own words—that is, not quoting the Mississippi law (slip op. at 3 [Roberts, C.J., concurring]). And Justice Clarence Thomas, in his concurring opinion, compares the sixty-three million abortions performed since *Roe* to the "immeasurable human suffering" of the Civil War (slip op. at 6-7 [Thomas, J., concurring]).

Nonetheless, the Court claims to remain agnostic on the personhood question, writing: "Our opinion is not based on any view about if and when prenatal life is entitled to any of the rights enjoyed after birth" (slip op. at 38 [majority opinion]). And in November 2022, the Supreme Court also denied certiorari (review of a lower court decision) for a group of anti-abortion activists who had petitioned on behalf of fetuses to claim constitutional protections (*Doe as Next Friend Doe v. McKee*, 143 S. Ct. 309 [2022]). Although, like the *Roe* Court, the *Dobbs* majority takes no official stand on fetal personhood, it comes to a very different conclusion: *Roe* let individual women decide for themselves, whereas *Dobbs* says that states can, if they want, recognize the personhood of the fetus and prohibit abortions entirely, since there is no right to privacy or abortion that conflicts with such laws. As the dissenters in the *Dobbs* case put it, "the Court . . . says that from the very moment of fertilization, a woman has no rights to speak of" (slip op. at 2 [dissenting opinion]).

## 5. Outstanding legal issues post-*Roe*

The *Dobbs* decision has raised many thorny legal questions. Do state laws prohibiting abortion, some of which automatically went into effect after *Roe* was overturned (so-called trigger laws), violate their state constitutions? Challenges to such laws have appealed to liberty, due process, and privacy; the free exercise of religion; or the individual's right to make healthcare decisions, which, ironically, was initially put in place as a constitutional amendment in some conservative states to block the Affordable Care Act's individual mandate (Felix, Sobell, and Salganicoff 2023). Some challenges have already succeeded. For example, South Carolina's state supreme court struck down an anti-abortion statute based on the right to privacy enshrined in the state constitution (Zernike 2023b). This is just the beginning. Does the FDA's approval of mifepristone preempt state law banning its use for medication abortions? Can a state government prohibit companies outside of the state from mailing mifepristone or other abortion medications to people in the state? Can states enforce a federal statute from 1948 (the Comstock Act, 18 USC § 1461) that considers "every article or thing designed, adapted, or intended for producing abortion, or for any indecent or immoral use . . . nonmailable matter"? The

U.S. Attorney General's Office, as of this writing, says that mifepristone cannot be prohibited since the sender lacks the intent that the drug will be used unlawfully (Schroeder 2022). Can Texas punish a Texas resident for getting a legal abortion in Colorado and then returning to Texas, where it is illegal? Can Texas punish family members and friends who help women, financially or otherwise, to obtain an abortion elsewhere? Can Colorado clinicians who perform abortions in Colorado on women from Texas be extradited to Texas? Some states have enacted shield laws to protect abortion providers and women who obtain legal abortion services from extradition and prosecution in other states (e.g., Colorado SB 23-188). Will the courts allow women to continue obtaining prescriptions for abortion pills through telemedicine (virtual consultations with clinicians)? Do prohibitions on the use of state resources to "promote" abortion (for example, in Idaho) have a chilling effect on the discussion of abortion at state universities and thus infringe on academic freedom? Although the same law makes it illegal for healthcare professionals to "assist" in an abortion or attempted abortion, a federal judge ruled in July 2023 that prohibiting healthcare professionals from referring patients to out-of-state abortion services violates their free speech rights (Johnson and Komenda 2023).

## Clinicians' Professional and Legal Obligations

In addition to the moral issues, clinicians face various interpretations of what their professional obligations are, and they have to navigate the complex and unstable patchwork of legislation now regulating abortion in the U.S.

### 1. Hippocratic Oath

Opponents of abortion have long noted that, unlike the Constitution's silence on the right to privacy, the Hippocratic Oath explicitly prohibits providing women with a pessary to induce abortion ("Hippocratic Oath" 2002). A pessary is a device, often made of cloth like a tampon, inserted into the vagina, which may be filled with medicines of various kinds. The Hippocratic Oath is not a legally binding obligation for physicians, but it is often taken to be the founding document of medical ethics in Western cultures, and some medical students still take the Oath upon graduation. So, are doctors implicitly or explicitly committed to the position that abortion violates their professional duties?

Because there is some debate about how to interpret this apparent ban on abortion in ancient Greek medicine, the answer is not clear. Pessaries were only one method used to induce abortion, so the specificity of this element of the Oath does not entail a prohibition against abortion in general. Ludwig Edelstein notes that, even if the Oath does include a general prohibition on performing abortions, it is the view of only one school of ancient thought, namely the Pythagoreans (1943, 15–18). The majority opinion in *Roe* calls attention to this and notes that both Plato and Aristotle approved of abortion (410 U.S. 113 [1973], at 130–32; see Plato 1961, 854 [149c–d]; Aristotle 2013, 219 [7.16, 1335b24–27]). Finally, the Hippocratic Oath also prohibits the use of surgery and any required payment for medical education, elements that have been conveniently de-emphasized as the science and industry of medicine have changed. Indeed, the modern version of the Hippocratic Oath, written by Louis Lasagna (1964), includes no reference to abortion, either for or against. The appeal to the Hippocratic Oath thus resolves nothing. We should also recognize that the Hippocratic Oath was not central to modern discussions of medical ethics until it was introduced as a standard part of medical education in the 1920s. Therefore, appeals to the Hippocratic Oath do not necessarily carry any argumentative weight, and we should attend to the selectiveness of those appeals.

## 2. American Medical Association

In the nineteenth century, many physicians believed that abortion was contrary to the Hippocratic Oath, so they directed women to nonprofessional abortion providers and midwives. The American Medical Association (AMA) formally adopted an anti-abortion position in 1859. Its condemnation of abortion not only represented the position of most of its members but also consolidated its power as gatekeeper of the profession. Anti-abortion activist Dr. Horatio Robinson Storer, who had led the movement within the AMA, then used the position to mount a public campaign that resulted in its widespread criminalization.

The AMA officially changed its stance in 1970, and its Code of Medical Ethics includes the following position on abortion:

> Abortion is a safe and common medical procedure, about which thoughtful individuals hold diverging, yet equally deeply held and

well-considered perspectives. Like all health care decisions, a decision to terminate a pregnancy should be made privately within the relationship of trust between patient and physician in keeping with the patient's unique values and needs and the physician's best professional judgment. (American Medical Association, n.d., 4.2.7)

Post-*Dobbs*, the AMA reaffirmed this position in November 2022, voicing its opposition to "governmental interference in the practice of medicine, especially for well-established, medically necessary treatments." Since "reproductive care is health care," criminalization of abortion attempts to prevent clinicians from fulfilling their professional duties. The AMA's amended ethical guidance permits physicians to perform abortions when, in their opinion, it is necessary to protect the safety and health of pregnant women, even when it is against the law. It also acknowledges the autonomy of clinicians by recognizing the range of moral positions on abortion and affirming the legitimacy of conscientious refusal (American Medical Association 2022; see also Wynia 2022).

### 3. *What counts as a threat to the pregnant woman's life?*

Perhaps the most difficult problem facing healthcare practitioners post-*Roe* is what to do when a pregnancy threatens a woman's life, health, or well-being. The majority in *Dobbs* says that there must be a "rational basis" for thinking that an abortion prohibition serves "legitimate state interests" (slip op. at 77 [majority opinion]). The dissent in *Dobbs*, however, notes that a "rational basis" is the "lowest level of scrutiny known to the law," so that a concern for fetal life could justify just about any restriction (*Dobbs v. Jackson Women's Health Organization*, slip op. at 2 [dissenting opinion]). Justice William Rehnquist's dissent in *Roe* says that the Fourteenth Amendment "does place a limit" on abortion laws: for example, "If the Texas statute were to prohibit an abortion even where the mother's life is in jeopardy, I have little doubt that such a statute would lack a rational relation to a valid state objective" (*Roe v. Wade*, at 173 [Rehnquist, W., dissenting]). However, the dissenting Justices in *Dobbs* question the concreteness of this criterion: "How much risk to a woman's life can a State force her to incur, before the Fourteenth Amendment's protection of life kicks in?" (*Dobbs v. Jackson Women's Health Organization*, slip op. at 35-36 [dissenting opinion]).

The post-*Roe* rush to pass anti-abortion legislation and trigger laws that had been in place for years without being carefully evaluated have generated medically vague language regulating when doctors can legally perform abortions to protect pregnant women, since these laws were written by politicians and lawyers rather than doctors. This lack of clarity puts women at risk of severe injury and death, and it puts doctors at risk of violating the law or failing to fulfill their moral obligation to safeguard patients. For example, although virtually all abortion bans throughout the world have what is called "an exception to criminalization" to preserve the woman's life, the conditions under which abortion is allowed are described differently in different jurisdictions. Sometimes the specific exceptions are codified in the legislation itself, such as allowing abortions when there is an ectopic pregnancy or the woman has cervical cancer; sometimes courts have carved out exceptions in their rulings on abortion laws. The European Court of Human Rights has said that whether the woman's life is at risk should be decided by the woman's physician or an emergency room doctor.

Vague standards remain in many places, however, especially in the United States. For example, the Texas law makes exceptions for "medical emergency," which "places the woman in danger of death or a serious risk of substantial impairment of a major bodily function" (HS 171); an abortion may be performed in Mississippi "in the case where necessary for the preservation of the mother's life" (MS Code § 41-41-45); and Louisiana makes an exception to prevent "death or substantial risk of death" or "permanent impairment of a life-sustaining organ" (Act 467). Physicians are left wondering which conditions meet these standards or, more practically, whether their patients have reached a state of crisis that would, in the eyes of prosecutors and state medical boards, meet these standards. Making a mistake on this point could cost them civil penalties, the removal of their medical licenses, or criminal prosecution—in Texas, a prison sentence of up to ninety-nine years and a minimum $100,000 fine.

Because of this, most physicians in states where abortion is severely restricted simply refuse to discuss abortion as a medical option. Those who are willing to discuss it often suggest that pregnant women travel to states where abortion is legal. Anyone who is pregnant may be impacted by these consequences, not only women who want to end their pregnancies. Here is an illustrative case: A Texas woman's water broke when she was nineteen weeks pregnant. The fetus would not survive, and if the pregnancy continued, the woman risked an infection, which could lead to sepsis and kill her. Because there was still a fetal heartbeat, however, the doctors worried about the legality of aborting the fetus. And the woman did not have sepsis yet. So, did the likelihood of eventually getting sepsis put the woman "in danger of death or a serious risk of substantial impairment of a major bodily function"? The doctors were not sure, so they recommended that she fly to Colorado to get an abortion, which she did. She sat next to the bathroom on the flight in case she went into labor ("Moral Danger for Mothers" 2022). Delays in being able to travel, to afford the procedure, to take time off work or away from children, or to schedule appointments put women at further risk. If women are victims of intimate partner violence or if they are teenagers whose parents would be unsupportive of an abortion, their access is further impeded.

Even when exceptions to protect the life of the woman are in place, the vague language in the statutes has the opposite effect: women are denied treatment until death is imminent. In other words, the law forces doctors to choose a riskier option than they otherwise would. For example, another Texas woman had a premature rupture of membranes, which resulted in the loss of amniotic fluid. The fetus had virtually no chance of surviving, but a fetal heartbeat remained. The woman had cramps and yellow discharge, and she passed clots of blood, but she was told that it had to be worse to indicate an infection called chorioamnionitis, which can lead to blood clots (in the pelvis and lungs) and sepsis. Even though she had wanted the pregnancy, she was in the position of wishing that her fetus would die just so she could get the care she needed. Only when the infection got worse was labor induced. The baby was stillborn, and the woman was finally treated. A similar case, which caused the death of a pregnant woman in Ireland in 2012, rallied public opinion in favor of abortion rights and led in part to the overturning of Ireland's abortion ban in 2018. In 2024, two women died in Georgia after experiencing complications from the abortion pill, complications that, with routine reproductive care, would not have been life-threatening. In one case, the patient's fear seems to have stopped her from seeking follow-up care; in the other, the patient was too ill to travel to another state, and doctors at the Georgia hospital felt compelled to wait until an infection endangered her life (Surana 2024). As one obstetrician claims, these laws functionally "isolate" reproductive care from the rest of healthcare and thereby risk pregnant women's lives, in some of the same ways that back-alley abortions did prior to the *Roe* decision (Karkowsky 2024). Even when the pregnant woman lives, having to carry a fetus that everyone knows will not survive and having to subject herself to worsening symptoms compounds the pregnant woman's sense of loss and causes psychological trauma in addition to the physical trauma: "It's just really unimaginable to be in a position of having to think: How close to death am I before somebody is going to take action and help me?" (Feibel 2022).

In March 2023, five women who had experienced miscarriages or other health complications during pregnancy sued the state of Texas (*Zurawski v. State of Texas*, No. D-1-GN-23-000968), claiming that they had been denied abortions despite the risks to their lives from hemorrhage or life-threatening infections. They demanded that the state clarify when physicians can make exceptions to the state's abortion ban (Zernike 2023a). In May 2024, the Texas Supreme Court rejected the challenge, ruling that the language by which clinicians determine whether exceptions are justified—"reasonable medical judgment"—is sufficiently clear.

These are acute medical conditions, but there are other, more common health risks that all pregnant women face. A woman carrying a child to term is fourteen times more likely to die from complications around pregnancy and childbirth than a woman who has an induced abortion (8.8 deaths per 100,000 live births versus 0.6 deaths per 100,000 abortions) (Raymond and Grimes 2012). In *Roe*, the Court acknowledged that mortality rates are lower for abortions during the first trimester than they are for carrying the child to term, which is one reason why they said that the state had no power to restrict it: doing so would force women to take on that risk (149, 163). Similarly, every common maternal morbidity (short- or long-term health problems resulting from pregnancy and childbirth) is higher for live birth compared to abortion: relative risks were 1.3 times greater for mental health conditions, 1.8 times greater for urinary tract infections, 4.4 times greater for postpartum hemorrhages, 5.2 times greater for obstetric infections, 24 times greater for hypertensive disorders of pregnancy, 25 times greater for antepartum hemorrhages, and 26 times greater for anemia (Bruce et al. 2008). This is especially worrisome in the United States because abortion bans exacerbate an existing problem: the U.S. ranks last among developed countries in maternal health (GBD 2015 Maternal Mortality Collaborators 2016; Tikkanen et al. 2020). In fact, those U.S.

states that have banned or are trying to ban abortion have the worst maternal and child health outcomes compared to other states and are least likely to invest in at-risk populations (Badger, Sanger-Katz, and Miller 2022).

Being forced to carry a child to term especially impacts women of color. In the U.S., Black women are over three times more likely than white women to die from pregnancy-related complications (Hill et al. 2024), and Black-serving hospitals have higher rates of maternal complications than other hospitals (Creanga et al. 2014; see also Creanga et al. 2017). These outcomes arise from longstanding forms of medical discrimination based on race: people of color are less likely to be trusted by medical professionals, and they are less likely to trust and form lasting relationships with medical professionals. Some of that lack of trust is historical. Medical experiments such as the Tuskegee syphilis study and J. Marion Sims's gynecological experiments treated Black people as specimens for the purpose of improving medical outcomes for whites (Washington 2008). Some of that lack of trust has more contemporary origins. During pregnancy and after childbirth, Black women are less likely to be believed when they share concerns with their clinicians. They are less likely to have access to health insurance, comprehensive sex education, and birth control (Ross and Solinger 2017). When their clinicians share their racial identity, patients of color are more likely to agree to preventive care, more likely to take medications as prescribed, and more likely to self-report higher care quality. But doctors are disproportionately white (González, Vega, and Tarraf 2010; Traylor et al. 2010; Alsan, Garrick, and Graziani 2019; Gonzalez et al. 2022). For these reasons, women of color face a spectrum of problems in obtaining adequate gynecological and obstetrical care. The intersection of race and socioeconomic status is important here: the ability to access high-quality prenatal care requires not only health insurance to cover medical care but also time off of work for regular appointments, childcare or eldercare, transportation, and accommodations for unpredictable and varying effects of pregnancy, such as morning sickness—all of which Black women, who are disproportionately poor, are less likely to have (Ross and Solinger 2017). Abortion bans in the U.S. result in an unfair distribution of burdens, imposed disproportionately on society's least well-off.

To fully assess whether the government ought to prohibit abortion (or, in the U.S., ought to allow it to be legally prohibited at the state level), we should consider the real-world effects that an abortion ban would have or that existing abortion bans do have. This will help us decide whether abortion bans violate the harm principle and whether a liberal government ought to force women to risk their health for the sake of embryos and fetuses whose legal status is in question.

## The Legality of Abortion outside the U.S.

Globally, there has been a trend toward more liberal abortion laws, especially in the developed world. Abortion on demand is available in most of Europe, Canada, Australia, Argentina, South Africa, Russia, China, and several other countries. However, this trend obscures their many differences. **Gestational limits** vary, often depending on the circumstances of the pregnancy. And the laws that exist arose out of very different legal histories. For example:

- In Canada, a woman can get an abortion for any reason up to twelve weeks and six days after conception in Prince Edward Island and Yukon and up to twenty-three weeks and six days in British Columbia, Ontario, and Quebec. In the landmark case *R. v. Morgentaler* ([1988] 1 S.C.R. 30), the Supreme Court of Canada struck down abortion prohibitions in the criminal code.

- In Russia, a woman can get an abortion for any reason up to twelve weeks after conception, up to twenty-two weeks in cases of rape, and at any point if the pregnancy is life-threatening. Russia was the first country to make abortion legal for any reason when the Soviet government issued the Decree on Women's Healthcare in 1920. To encourage population growth, abortion was banned in 1936, but the ban was lifted in 1955, after Stalin's death. It has remained legal since then.

- In France, a woman can get an abortion for any reason up to fourteen weeks after conception and at any point to prevent mental or physical harm to the woman, to protect the woman's life, or if the child will have a severe, incurable illness. The French parliament initially legalized abortion with a ten-week limit in 1975 (Law 75-17), later expanding it to twelve weeks (in 2001) and fourteen weeks (in 2022).

There is no typical abortion law, and there is no typical evolution of abortion laws.

Many countries prohibit abortion but allow exceptions for different reasons, including the woman's poor economic and social circumstances (e.g., Ethiopia, Finland, India), cases of fetal abnormalities (e.g., Great Britain, Mexico, Turkey), to preserve the woman's physical or mental health (e.g., Algeria, Colombia, Thailand), to preserve the woman's physical health (e.g., Peru, Poland, Saudi Arabia), or to save the woman's life (e.g., Brazil, Egypt, Myanmar)—with many of these countries adopting several such exceptions. And although it is rare, some countries have complete prohibitions on abortion, with no exceptions codified in the law. They include El Salvador and Honduras in Central America; the Dominican Republic and Haiti in the Caribbean; Iraq; several countries in Africa, including Angola, Congo-Brazzaville, Congo-Kinshasa, Gabon, Madagascar, Mauritania, and Senegal; and Laos and the Philippines in Southeast Asia. In countries with restrictive regulations, women often get unsafe, illegal abortions that result in medical complications, including hemorrhage, infection, and damage to internal organs. In Africa, where an estimated 93 percent of women of reproductive age live in countries with restrictive abortion laws, 48 percent of abortions are done in the least safe conditions, and 1.6 million women are treated annually for complications resulting from unsafe abortions, accounting for at least 9 percent of maternal deaths and the highest number of abortion-related deaths of any world region (Ganatra et al. 2017; Guttmacher Institute 2018). Even where abortion is legally allowed, women may not have access because they are unable to pay for abortions, or there are few local clinicians, for instance. This is why a 2018 Irish law both increased the gestational age during which abortion is legal and established that abortions would be free for all women (Health [Regulation of Termination of Pregnancy] Act 2018).

The United Nations has consistently claimed that access to safe abortion services is a human right. In 1994, the International Conference on Population and Development's (ICPD) Programme of Action asserted that reproductive rights are human rights. It called on countries to address unsafe abortion practices, to ensure access when abortion is legal (by removing legal barriers and confronting cultural stigma), and to deliver post-abortion care after both legal and illegal abortions. The U.N. Committee on the Rights of the Child has insisted that abortion be decriminalized out of respect for women's autonomy. And in *Mellet v. Ireland* (2016), the U.N. Human Rights Committee, which monitors international treaties, concluded that international human rights law precludes the criminalization of abortion. Regional human rights courts, including the European Court of Human Rights, the Inter-American Court of Human Rights, and the African Commission on Human and Peoples' Rights, have come to the same conclusion: access to safe abortions is a human right (Fine, Mayall, and Sepúlveda 2017; Council on Foreign Relations 2022).

## Conclusion: The Challenge of Polarization

Perhaps because the dominant positions are so divergent, there has been little progress in resolving ethical and legal disagreements on abortion. Those who claim that abortion is permissible insist that fetuses have little or no moral standing. Protecting safe, legal, and easy access to abortion respects a woman's autonomy and is part of a right to basic healthcare. Abortion is equivalent to contraception: nothing of greater moral significance is lost in respecting a woman's right to terminate a pregnancy, especially in its early stages. By contrast, anti-abortion advocates believe that, from the moment of conception, fetuses are human beings, just like newborn infants or adults, only at earlier stages of development. Since the law is supposed to protect the vulnerable, it ought to protect not only newborns, the cognitively disabled, and adults with dementia—all of whom lack some qualities of fully formed persons—but also unborn children, who are least able to defend themselves. On this view, the practice of abortion is equivalent to the Holocaust, the deliberate mass killing of one kind of person. There is no compromise between these two positions that would both respect a woman's right to privacy and respect a fetus's right to life. Legal abortion with gestational limits—six weeks, twelve weeks, twenty-three weeks, or whatever—tries to take a middle position but does not resolve the core philosophical dilemmas posed by abortion. Are embryos/fetuses before the gestational limit so morally insignificant as to be expendable? Are women after that time mere instruments for reproduction (unwilling human incubators à la *The Handmaid's Tale*)?

Healthcare professionals and legislators stand in the middle of this battleground. Clinicians who assist women in obtaining abortions are either providing an essential component of women's healthcare or participating in genocide. U.S. states are seemingly making clinicians' decisions for them—except that clinicians in states prohibiting abortion have to decide when a pregnant woman's life is at risk, and clinicians in states allowing abortion have to decide whether to conscientiously refuse. Healthcare systems that are religiously affiliated raise additional challenges, including whether clinicians should even inform their patients when abortion is an option—supporting patient autonomy but perhaps encouraging what the system considers a wrongful killing. Under the circumstances, what does it mean to do no harm?

## References

Alsan, Marcella, Owen Garrick, and Grant Graziani. 2019. "Does Diversity Matter for Health? Experimental Evidence from Oakland." *American Economic Review* 109, no. 12 (December): 4071–111. doi:10.1257/aer.20181446.

American College of Obstetricians and Gynecologists. n.d. "ACOG Guide to Language and Abortion." Accessed January 15, 2025. https://www.acog.org/contact/media-center/abortion-language-guide.

American Medical Association. 2022. "AMA Announces New Adopted Policies Related to Reproductive Health Care." November 16. https://www.ama-assn.org/press-center/press-releases/ama-announces-new-adopted-policies-related-reproductive-health-care.

———. n.d. "Code of Medical Ethics." Accessed January 15, 2025. https://code-medical-ethics.ama-assn.org/.

Aristotle. 2013. *Aristotle's "Politics."* Translated by Carnes Lord. 2nd ed. Chicago: University of Chicago Press.

Badger, Emily, Margot Sanger-Katz, and Claire Cain Miller. 2022. "States with Abortion Bans Are among Least Supportive for Mothers and Children." *New York Times (The Upshot).* July 28. https://www.nytimes.com/2022/07/28/upshot/abortion-bans-states-social-services.html.

Boonin, David. 2019. *Beyond Roe: Why Abortion Should Be Legal—Even If the Fetus Is a Person.* Oxford: Oxford University Press.

Brody, Baruch. 1975. *Abortion and the Sanctity of Human Life: A Philosophical View.* Cambridge, MA: MIT Press.

Bruce, F. Carol, Cynthia J. Berg, Mark C. Hornbrook, Evelyn P. Whitlock, William M. Callaghan, Donald J. Bachman, Rachel Gold, and Patricia M. Dietz. 2008. "Maternal Morbidity Rates in a Managed Care Population." *Obstetrics & Gynecology* 111, no. 5 (May): 1089–95. doi:10.1097/AOG.0b013e31816c441a.

Coe, Cynthia D., and Matthew C. Altman. 2012. "Mandatory Ultrasound Laws and the Coercive Use of Informed Consent." *Techné: Research in Philosophy and Technology* 16, no. 1 (Winter): 16–30. doi:10.5840/techne20121613.

Council on Foreign Relations. 2022. "How the U.S. Compares with the Rest of the World on Abortion Rights." *PBS News Hour*. July 1. https://www.pbs.org/newshour/politics/how-the-u-s-compares-with-the-rest-of-the-world-on-abortion-rights.

Creanga, Andreea A., Brian T. Bateman, Jill M. Mhyre, Elena Kuklina, Alexander Shilkrut, and William M. Callaghan. 2014. "Performance of Racial and Ethnic Minority-Serving Hospitals on Delivery-Related Indicators." *American Journal of Obstetrics & Gynecology* 211, no. 6 (December): 647.e1–16. doi:10.1016/j.ajog.2014.06.006.

Creanga, Andreea A., Carla Syverson, Kristi Seed, and William M. Callaghan. 2017. "Pregnancy-Related Mortality in the United States, 2011–2013." *Obstetrics & Gynecology* 130, no. 2 (August): 366–73. doi:10.1097/AOG.0000000000002114.

Dworkin, Ronald. 1986. *Law's Empire*. Cambridge, MA: Belknap.

———. 1993. *Life's Dominion: An Argument about Abortion, Euthanasia, and Individual Freedom*. New York: Knopf.

———. 1996. *Freedom's Law: The Moral Reading of the Constitution*. Cambridge, MA: Harvard University Press.

Edelstein, Ludwig. 1943. *The Hippocratic Oath: Text, Translation, and Interpretation*. Baltimore: Johns Hopkins Press.

Feibel, Carrie. 2022. "Because of Texas Abortion Law, Her Wanted Pregnancy Became a Medical Nightmare." *NPR*. July 26. https://www.npr.org/sections/health-shots/2022/07/26/1111280165/because-of-texas-abortion-law-her-wanted-pregnancy-became-a-medical-nightmare.

Felix, Mabel, Laurie Sobel, and Alina Salganicoff. 2023. "Legal Challenges to State Abortion Bans since the Dobbs Decision." Kaiser Family Foundation. January 20. https://www.kff.org/womens-health-policy/issue-brief/legal-challenges-to-state-abortion-bans-since-the-dobbs-decision/.

Fine, Johanna B., Katherine Mayall, and Lilian Sepúlveda. 2017. *Health and Human Rights Journal* 19, no. 1 (June 2). https://www.hhrjournal.org/2017/06/the-role-of-international-human-rights-norms-in-the-liberalization-of-abortion-laws-globally/.

Frederiksen, Brittni, Usha Ranji, Ivette Gomez, and Alina Salganicoff. 2023. "A National Survey of OBGYNs' Experiences after *Dobbs*." Kaiser Family Foundation. June 21. https://www.kff.org/womens-health-policy/report/a-national-survey-of-obgyns-experiences-after-dobbs/.

Ganatra, Bela, Caitlin Gerdts, Clémentine Rossier, Brooke Ronald Johnson Jr., Özge Tunçalp, Anisa Assifi, Gilda Sedgh, et al. 2017. "Global, Regional, and

Subregional Classification of Abortions by Safety, 2010–14: Estimates from a Bayesian Hierarchical Model." *Lancet* 390, no. 10110 (November 25): P2372–81. doi:10.1016/S0140-6736(17)31794-4.

GBD 2015 Maternal Mortality Collaborators. 2016. "Global, Regional, and National Levels of Maternal Mortality, 1990–2015: A Systematic Analysis for the Global Burden of Disease Study 2015." *Lancet* 388 (October 8): 1775–812. doi:10.1016/S0140-6736(16)31470-2.

George, Robert P., and Christopher Tollefsen. 2011. *Embryo: A Defense of Human Life*. 2nd ed. Princeton, NJ: Witherspoon Institute.

Gonzalez, Dulce, Genevieve M. Kenney, Marla McDaniel, and Claire O'Brien. 2022. "Racial, Ethnic, and Language Concordance between Patients and Their Usual Healthcare Providers." Urban Institute, Robert Wood Johnson Foundation. March 23. https://www.rwjf.org/en/library/research/2022/03/racial-ethnic-and-language-concordance-between-patients-and-their-usual-healthcare-providers.html.

González, Hector M., William A. Vega, and Wassim Tarraf. 2010. "Health Care Quality Perceptions among Foreign-Born Latinos and the Importance of Speaking the Same Language." *Journal of the American Board of Family Medicine* 23, no. 6 (November–December): 745–52. doi:10.3122/jabfm.2010.06.090264.

Guttmacher Institute. 2018. "Fact Sheet: Abortion in Africa." https://www.guttmacher.org/sites/default/files/factsheet/ib_aww-africa.pdf.

Harman, Elizabeth. 2019. "The Ever Conscious View and the Contingency of Moral Status." In *Rethinking Moral Status*, edited by Steve Clarke, Hazem Zohny, and Julian Savulescu, 90–107. Oxford: Oxford University Press. doi:10.1093/oso/9780192894076.001.0001.

Hendricks, Perry. 2019. "Even If the Fetus Is Not a Person, Abortion Is Immoral: The Impairment Argument." *Bioethics* 33, no. 2 (February): 245–53. doi:10.1111/bioe.12533.

Hill, Latoya, Alisha Rao, Samantha Artiga, and Usha Ranji. 2024. "Racial Disparities in Maternal and Infant Health: Current Status and Efforts to Address Them." Kaiser Family Foundation. October 25. https://www.kff.org/racial-equity-and-health-policy/issue-brief/racial-disparities-in-maternal-and-infant-health-current-status-and-efforts-to-address-them/.

"Hippocratic Oath." 2002. Translated by Michael North. National Library of Medicine, National Institutes of Health. https://www.nlm.nih.gov/hmd/greek/greek_oath.html.

Johnson, Gene, and Ed Komenda. 2023. "Idaho Health Care Providers Can Refer Patients for Abortions out of State, Federal Judge Rules." *Associated Press*. August 1. https://apnews.com/article/abortion-referral-idaho-ruling-b989a9561a988667d4b360dabb58ecc8.

Karkowsky, Chavi Eve. 2024. "Abortion Pills Are Safe. Post-Roe America Isn't." *New York Times*. October 24. https://www.nytimes.com/2024/10/24/opinion/abortion-pills-us-roe.html.

Lasagna, Louis. 1964. "The Hippocratic Oath: Modern Version." https://www.pbs.org/wgbh/nova/doctors/oath_modern.html.

Lee, Patrick, and Robert P. George. 2005. "The Wrong of Abortion." In *Contemporary Debates in Applied Ethics*, edited by Andrew I. Cohen and Christopher Heath Wellman, 13–26. Malden, MA: Blackwell.

Marquis, Don. 1989. "Why Abortion Is Immoral." *Journal of Philosophy* 86, no. 4 (April): 183–202. doi:10.2307/2026961.

Mill, John Stuart. 1978. *On Liberty*. Edited by Elizabeth Rapaport. Indianapolis: Hackett.

"Moral Danger for Mothers." 2022. *Economist*. July 23, p. 23.

Noonan, John T. Jr. 1970. "An Almost Absolute Value in History." In *The Morality of Abortion: Legal and Historical Perspectives*, edited by John T. Noonan Jr., 51–59. Cambridge, MA: Harvard University Press.

Plato. 1961. *Theatetus*. In *The Collected Dialogues of Plato*, edited by Edith Hamilton and Huntington Cairns, 845–919. Princeton, NJ: Princeton University Press.

Raymond, Elizabeth G., and David A. Grimes. 2012. "The Comparative Safety of Legal Induced Abortion and Childbirth in the United States." *Obstetrics & Gynecology* 199, no. 2 (February): 215–19. doi:10.1097/AOG.0b013e31823fe923.

Ross, Loretta J., and Rickie Solinger. 2017. *Reproductive Justice: An Introduction*. Oakland: University of California Press.

Scalia, Antonin. 2020. *The Essential Scalia: On the Constitution, the Courts, and the Rule of Law*. Edited by Jeffrey S. Sutton and Edward Whelan. New York: Crown Forum.

Schroeder, Christopher H. 2022. "Application of the Comstock Act to the Mailing of Prescription Drugs That Can Be Used for Abortions," 46 Op. O.L.C. __ (Dec. 23, 2022). https://www.justice.gov/olc/opinion/file/1560596/download.

Simmons-Duffin, Selena, and Carrie Feibel. 2022. "The Texas Abortion Ban Hinges on 'Fetal Heartbeat.' Doctors Call That Misleading." *NPR*. May 3. https://www.npr.org/sections/health-shots/2021/09/02/1033727679/fetal-heartbeat-isnt-a-medical-term-but-its-still-used-in-laws-on-abortion.

Singer, Peter. 2011. "Taking Life: The Embryo and Fetus." In *Practical Ethics*, 3rd ed., 123–54. Cambridge: Cambridge University Press. doi:10.1017/CBO9780511975950.007.

Steinbock, Bonnie. 2011. "Abortion." In *Life before Birth: The Moral and Legal Status of Embryos and Fetuses*, 2nd ed., 36–107. Oxford: Oxford University Press. doi:10.1093/acprof:oso/9780195341621.003.0010.

Surana, Kavitha. 2024. "Abortion Bans Have Delayed Emergency Medical Care. In Georgia, Experts Say This Mother's Death Was Preventable." *ProPublica*. September 16. https://www.propublica.org/article/georgia-abortion-ban-amber-thurman-death.

Thomson, Judith Jarvis. 1971. "A Defense of Abortion." *Philosophy & Public Affairs* 1, no. 1 (Autumn): 47–66. https://www.jstor.org/stable/2265091.

Tikkanen, Roosa, Munira Z. Gunja, Molly FitzGerald, and Laurie Zephyrin. 2020. "Maternal Mortality and Maternity Care in the United States Compared to 10 Other Developed Countries." Commonwealth Fund. November 18. https://www.commonwealthfund.org/publications/issue-briefs/2020/nov/maternal-mortality-maternity-care-us-compared-10-countries.

Tooley, Michael. 1972. "Abortion and Infanticide." *Philosophy & Public Affairs* 2, no. 1 (Autumn): 37–65. https://www.jstor.org/stable/2264919.

Traylor, Ana H., Julie A. Schmittdiel, Connie S. Uratsu, Carol M. Mangione, and Usha Subramanian. 2010. "Adherence to Cardiovascular Disease Medications: Does Patient-Provider Race/Ethnicity and Language Concordance Matter?" *Journal of General Internal Medicine* 25, no. 11 (November): 1172–77. doi:10.1007/s11606-010-1424-8.

Warren, Mary Anne. 1973. "On the Moral and Legal Status of Abortion." *Monist* 57, no. 1 (January): 43–61. doi:10.5840/monist197357133.

Washington, Harriet A. 2008. *Medical Apartheid: The Dark History of Medical Experimentation on Black Americans from Colonial Times to the Present*. New York: Harlem Moon.

Wynia, Matthew K. 2022. "Professional Civil Disobedience—Medical-Society Responsibilities after *Dobbs*." *New England Journal of Medicine* 387, no. 11 (September 15): 959–61. doi:10.1056/NEJMp2210192.

Zernike, Kate. 2023a. "Five Women Sue Texas over the State's Abortion Ban." *New York Times*. March 6. https://www.nytimes.com/2023/03/06/us/texas-abortion-ban-suit.html.

———. 2023b. "South Carolina Constitution Includes Abortion Right, State Supreme Court Rules." *New York Times*. January 5. https://www.nytimes.com/2023/01/05/us/south-carolina-abortion-supreme-court.html.

## FURTHER READING

Boonin, David. 2002. *A Defense of Abortion*. Cambridge: Cambridge University Press. doi:10.1017/CBO9780511610172.

> Critiques all the major anti-abortion arguments, focusing especially on the claim that a fetus is a person with a right to life. Boonin also argues that even if the fetus does have a right to life, it would still be permissible to

abort it. In a separate chapter, he addresses non-rights-based approaches such as Marquis's future-like-ours argument.

Feinberg, Joel, ed. 1984. *The Problem of Abortion*. 2nd ed. Belmont, CA: Wadsworth.
>Collects sixteen of the most important philosophical essays on abortion (at the time of publication), as well as brief excerpts from *Roe v. Wade*. In addition to the essays by Noonan, Thomson, Warren, and Tooley mentioned in this chapter's References, the book includes essays by applied ethicists such as L. W. Sumner, S. I. Benn, Joel Feinberg, Jane English, and Sissela Bok.

Finnis, John, and Robert P. George. 2022. "Equal Protection and the Unborn Child: A *Dobbs* Brief." *Harvard Journal of Law & Public Policy* 45, no. 3 (Summer): 927–1031. https://journals.law.harvard.edu/jlpp/wp-content/uploads/sites/90/2022/10/7-JLPP-45_3-Finnis-George.pdf.
>An amicus curiae brief filed in the *Dobbs* case by two philosophers who oppose abortion rights. Finnis and George argue that fetuses are constitutional persons covered by the Equal Protection Clause of the Fourteenth Amendment. They argue against the reasoning in *Roe* and *Casey* for denying fetuses constitutional personhood, and they respond to claims in amicus briefs submitted on behalf of the other side in *Dobbs*.

Foster, Diana Greene. 2021. *The Turnaway Study: Ten Years, a Thousand Women, and the Consequences of Having—or Being Denied—an Abortion*. New York: Scribner.
>A landmark sociological study that follows a thousand women who sought abortions in the U.S., either successfully or unsuccessfully, and how their lives changed as a result. The book includes both hard data and narratives that illustrate why, for example, some women do not realize they are pregnant until the second trimester and what motivates women to get abortions. It gives a picture of what it is like to seek an abortion and the obstacles women face, especially financial pressures, even when abortion is technically available.

Greasley, Kate. 2017. *Arguments about Abortion: Personhood, Morality, and Law*. Oxford: Oxford University Press. doi:10.1093/acprof:oso/9780198766780.001.0001.
>Argues that the morality of abortion cannot be settled without establishing whether the fetus is a person. Greasley claims that one becomes a person through the gradual development of psychological and emotional capacities, and that once a minimum threshold of personhood is achieved,

all persons have equal moral status—that is, personhood is a "range property." She concludes that when a fetus achieves personhood, it is morally impermissible to kill it, except under very rare circumstances.

Hursthouse, Rosalind. 1991. "Virtue Theory and Abortion." *Philosophy & Public Affairs* 20, no. 3 (Summer): 223–46. https://www.jstor.org/stable/2265432.
Argues that we do not have to settle the issue of whether the fetus is a person to determine whether abortion is wrong or right. From the perspective of virtue ethics, we must evaluate each abortion by looking at how it affects (or would affect) human flourishing. Some women who get abortions are virtuous, and some are vicious, depending on whether they are trying to live a worthwhile life, whether they recognize that the fetus is a life (and not just a thing), and which attitudes or character traits are manifested in the decision.

Kaczor, Christopher. 2011. *The Ethics of Abortion: Women's Rights, Human Life, and the Question of Justice.* New York: Routledge. doi:10.4324/9781003305217.
Argues that all human beings, including embryos and fetuses, should be respected as persons and concludes that all intentional abortions, even in cases of rape or incest, are morally wrong. Kaczor engages the arguments of many other philosophers writing on the abortion issue, including Warren, Boonin, McMahan, and Thomson.

Little, Margaret Olivia. 2003. "Abortion." In *A Companion to Applied Ethics*, edited by R. G. Frey and Christopher Heath Wellman, 313–25. Malden, MA: Blackwell. doi:10.1002/9780470996621.ch23.
Contends that ending assistance to a fetus whose life depends on the woman, even if it is a person, is not "wrongful interference." Nonetheless, since the fetus is a "burgeoning human life," the abortion issue is morally weighty. Whether aborting a fetus is morally decent depends on the relationship between the woman and her fetus—whether she wants to take on motherhood as a "practical identity," which will affect her future commitments and obligations, or whether she has already taken on the "norms of parenthood."

McMahan, Jeff. 2002. *The Ethics of Killing: Problems at the Margins of Life.* Oxford: Oxford University Press. doi:10.1093/0195079981.001.0001.
Approaches the ethics of killing by considering personal identity and what makes us the kind of entities we are. McMahan asserts that we are embodied minds and that the badness of death is proportional to the strength of our time-relative interest in continuing to live. Since fetuses have little psychological unity, it is worse to kill an adult human than it is to kill a

fetus. And prior to the fetus's developing consciousness (around twenty weeks), abortion is morally indistinguishable from contraception.

Watson, Katie. 2018. *Scarlet A: The Ethics, Law, and Politics of Ordinary Abortion*. Oxford: Oxford University Press.

Attempts to change the conversation around abortion by focusing on "ordinary abortion" rather than abortions sought due to rape or incest, fetal abnormalities, or life-threatening conditions. Watson suggests that we put abortion in its social context (e.g., abortion is a family issue, since most women who get abortions are already mothers), recognize when we smuggle moral assumptions into our vocabulary (e.g., whether the fetus is a "life" or a "potential life"), and acknowledge how abortion is stigmatized (e.g., legally requiring doctors to read counseling scripts to women considering abortions, under the guise of informed consent).

# CHAPTER 6
# Pregnancy and Reproductive Technologies

**Key topics in this chapter:**

- The moral status of embryos and fetuses in disability-selective abortion, in vitro fertilization, and stem cell research
- How the liberal model of procreative autonomy is qualified by parental obligations and considerations of justice in genetic enhancement and surrogate motherhood
- Political, legal, and regulatory issues around pregnancy and reproduction, including the criminalization of behavior by pregnant women
- Commodification of women, embryos, and babies

## Introduction

In the United States and elsewhere, abortion is the dominant focus of reproductive ethics. But the process of reproduction raises other important moral issues: what obligations women have to embryos during pregnancies that they intend to continue; whether reproductive technologies violate the principles of respect for autonomy, nonmaleficence, beneficence, and justice; and what kinds of embryonic research can be justified, if any. Many of these questions have become prominent in ethical and legal debates only in the last several decades, as new medical technologies have made possible greater surveillance of pregnant women and fetuses, offered people wider options for becoming parents, and created new genetic pathways to prevent and treat disease. The ethical ramifications of these technologies raise the same questions that we find elsewhere in medical ethics: Who or what is morally considerable? How do we weigh respect for autonomy against nonmaleficence, beneficence, and justice? And how do we balance competing claims to autonomy or beneficence?

## The Criminalization of Pregnancy

In pregnancy, there is no self-evident point at which we are dealing with two morally considerable beings rather than one. The continuous development of the fetus inside of a woman's body generates fraught questions about the extent to which her bodily autonomy takes moral precedence over the future autonomy and current well-being of the fetus, even when a woman intends to carry the pregnancy to term. Since the 1980s, pregnant women have, in many U.S. states, been legally charged with fetal endangerment as an extension of child endangerment laws. This legal shift came about as a result of three concurrent but distinct political forces: (1) the pro-life movement, which (typically) argues that life begins at conception and therefore that fetuses should be understood as "unborn children" with the same rights as other people; (2) laws initially designed to protect pregnant women from domestic violence, which sharpened penalties for abusers who also harm fetuses; and (3) the war on drugs, which especially targeted the poor and people of color as threats to the health of the larger society. The 1980s and early 1990s were characterized by social panic around infants born with prenatal exposure to crack, the crystallized form of cocaine. This panic did not extend to infants prenatally exposed to powder cocaine, which is chemically identical and was typically used by whites and people of higher socioeconomic status. There were fears that a generation of "crack babies" would grow up with profound cognitive and physical impairments: "The inner-city crack epidemic is now giving birth to the newest horror: a bio-underclass" (Besharov 1989, B1). The rhetoric of "unfit mothers" legitimized medical surveillance of pregnant women and the legal criminalization of behaviors taken to cause prenatal harm (Ross and Solinger 2017, 171–72).

In response, thirty-eight states passed feticide laws and have prosecuted thousands of pregnant women for child neglect or abuse, or (in some states) murder, primarily on the assumption that drug use endangers fetuses—even though the vast majority of fetuses involved in such cases are born healthy. Low-income and Black women are much more likely to be screened for illicit drug use by primary care physicians and hospitals during pregnancy—often without their knowledge or consent—and then arrested for such crimes (Paltrow and Flavin 2013; Dirks 2022). In some hospitals, police officers train nurses on how to collect medical evidence to prosecute these cases. Sometimes women are screened for drug use during labor and arrested within hours after giving birth (Goodwin 2020, 111). The crime is not drug use—only drug possession, not use of the drug, is criminalized in the United States—but endangerment of the fetus. In 1999, Regina McKnight was convicted of homicide following a stillbirth after using illegal drugs: "Without her knowledge or consent, McKnight's doctors turned her medical records and tests over to the police, who, without scientific support, claimed that the stillbirth she endured must have resulted from the illicit substance" (16). McKnight's conviction was overturned on appeal, but only after she had served seven years in prison (Goodwin 2017, S21).

In these cases, typically no medical or scientific evidence is offered that using a drug has directly harmed the fetus. The crime is framed in terms of endangerment, not actual harm. But here too the medical evidence is inconsistent with the criminalization of pregnancy: although there is some evidence that binge drinking during early pregnancy harms the fetus (Henderson, Kesmodel, and Gray 2007), there is no systematic evidence that use of crack cocaine (for instance) during pregnancy endangers future children's health (Gómez 1997, 24; see also Paltrow and Flavin 2013, 796–97). Nonetheless, it has been much more common for women to be arrested for drug use during pregnancy than for alcohol use. The "crack baby epidemic" is now acknowledged to be a myth (Okie 2009). Social determinants of health, such as quality of housing and access to healthcare, have a much greater impact on long-term outcomes for children, whether they have been exposed prenatally to drugs or not (Hurt et al. 1995).

This logic of limiting pregnant women's rights to protect fetuses has also been extended to nondrug incidents. Women have been prosecuted after suffering pregnancy loss as a result of accidents such as falling down a flight of stairs, suicide attempts, or intimate partner violence. A woman was referred to law enforcement after confidentially disclosing to clinicians a "prior reliance on pain medication," considering "abortion as an option early on in [the] pregnancy," and preferring "a vaginal birth over cesarean section," which were used to undermine her decision-making authority (Goodwin 2017, S22). In 2004, Melissa Rowland was charged with child endangerment and murder after refusing a cesarean section, resulting in the stillbirth of one of her twins. Furthermore, in some instances when pregnant women disagree with their clinicians about treatment, such as bed rest (as in the case of Samantha Burton in 2010) or cesarean birth (as in the case of Laura Pemberton in 1999), they have been taken into custody so that their clinicians' treatment plans can be enforced, on the justification that their fetuses must be protected. A court may assign a **guardian ad litem** to make medical decisions on behalf of the fetus if a judge believes that a pregnant woman is not acting in the fetus's best interests (Cohen 2018, 1299). Referral to law enforcement also typically means that child protective services will investigate whether the woman should retain custody of the newborn infant and any other children she has.

These laws mean that some actions only count as crimes for pregnant women, and there are forms of autonomy, such as the right to confidentiality or the right to refuse treatment recommended by a physician, that are suspended during pregnancy. In no other context does discussing one's medical history, considering options, or expressing a preference for treatment—even before coming to a decision—trigger criminal charges. In ethical terms, the criminalization of pregnancy is typically justified on the basis that the present and future well-being of the child outweighs the autonomy of the pregnant woman (Haack 2008, 146–47). Although parents have obligations to promote the well-being of their children, those obligations do not directly limit what they can do to their own bodies. Pregnancy criminalization laws frame pregnant women as means to a reproductive end rather than autonomous agents in their own right. They also draw on the cultural image of the "good mother" who is willing to sacrifice any of her interests for her children and to defer to medical authority. As Howard Minkoff and Lynn Paltrow argue, "When physicians' concerns about fetal well-being are allowed to supersede both a woman's judgment about what is best for her family and her right to safeguard her bodily integrity, then there is no principled limitation on state power to police pregnancy and punish pregnant women" (2004, 1235).

Two arguments challenge the practices of surveilling and punishing pregnant women for the sake of fetal welfare. First, respecting the autonomy of the pregnant woman is almost always in the long-term best interests of both mother and child. Most medical organizations oppose the criminalization of pregnancy out of concern that women who already receive little prenatal care will avoid it if they see clinicians as arms of the criminal justice system rather than patient advocates (Gómez 1997, 49). A second argument is that these legal prosecutions usually have not demonstrated direct harm to the child as a result of the pregnant woman's behavior. In short, such practices neither prevent harm (nonmaleficence) nor promote well-being (beneficence).

This legal trend can also be criticized by an appeal to justice, not only in the sense that people who are pregnant can be held legally liable in ways that nonpregnant people cannot, but also because certain groups of pregnant people, especially poor and unhoused people, have been disproportionately charged with fetal endangerment and related crimes when they have sought treatment at state-subsidized clinics or hospitals. A second, more variable factor has been race. Until the height of the opioid epidemic, fetal endangerment laws tended to target women of color (Bridges 2020, 775). At one South Carolina hospital in the late 1980s and early 1990s, for example, forty-nine out of fifty women referred to law enforcement were Black, and the fiftieth was a white woman on whose medical chart a nurse noted: "Lives with her boyfriend who is a Negro" (Goodwin 2020, 201). In recent decades, white women have been more likely to face charges of fetal endangerment for substance abuse, in keeping with the higher frequency of opioid use among whites (Bridges 2020, 820–25). The inconsistent and inequitable enforcement of these laws is itself a problem of justice. Many of the charges against pregnant women end up being overturned on appeal, but some women have pled guilty and have endured the consequences of criminal records, including loss of custody of their children.

Alongside the legal criminalization of pregnancy are moral questions of reproductive responsibility: What are a pregnant woman's obligations to the fetus? How should those obligations be weighed against the woman's autonomy and well-being? As with other moral issues related to reproduction, these questions would be easier to answer if we could clearly establish when the fetus becomes a person—at conception, at viability, at birth? The moral and legal status of the fetus, at any point during its development, would determine the duties of the pregnant woman and concomitant restrictions on her behavior. Prior to the fetus becoming a person (assuming that point is not conception), the principles of respect for autonomy, nonmaleficence, beneficence, and justice apply to the woman alone, with the usual emphasis on patient self-determination. Information about fetal alcohol syndrome and addiction treatment options may be offered to her, but ultimately she decides what happens to and in her body. Her privacy must be protected by the same rules around confidentiality that apply to every other patient: confidentiality may only be breached if they are an imminent danger to themselves or others. After the fetus achieves the status of personhood, however, clinicians must advocate for two patients. It makes more sense, after that point, to acknowledge and address the possibility that the pregnant woman's choices may be a threat to the fetus's future autonomy and present well-being.

Given the continuing debate about the personhood of the fetus and the grounds of personhood itself, we are left with moral ambiguity about the woman's obligations. This problem is intensified by the fact that, even if we could establish a clear line at which the fetus gains this moral status, what happens before that point may medically affect what happens after that point. For instance, binge drinking in early pregnancy may impact physical and cognitive development prenatally and postnatally. So, concern for the future child's well-being seems to justify restrictions on the woman's current behavior, even before the fetus becomes a person. Julian Savulescu (2007a) argues that a pregnant woman has obligations to refrain from behaviors that will harm the fetus and to allow medical treatments that will benefit it as long as these actions do not significantly harm her—what he calls the duty of easy rescue. All the moral conflicts that are raised with abortion also emerge in this issue.

One thing that seems clear is that laws and moral obligations should be established on objective medical evidence. The panic about "crack babies" and fetal alcohol syndrome seems to have been based on limited studies, and a more complex picture of the health effects of prenatal alcohol and drug use has emerged in more recent research. A second guiding principle is that incarcerating pregnant women and new mothers is unlikely to maximize the well-being of those women, their children, or other women dealing with addiction who are thinking of seeking prenatal care. Advocating for fetuses need not conflict with advocating for mothers. Generally, seeing those needs as shared supports the long-term well-being and autonomy of both. Minkoff and Paltrow conclude that "the best protection for a fetus lies in the protection of the rights of the individual best positioned and most highly motivated to defend its interests: an informed and empowered mother" (2004, 1236). This may mean putting women in touch with addiction services, including harm reduction services, and helping them gain access to quality healthcare, housing, nutrition, and education rather than sending them to jail. With those principles in mind, the closer a fetus is to being able to live outside of the woman's body, the higher

her procreative responsibility—obligations derived from the principles of respect for autonomy, nonmaleficence, beneficence, and justice. Within healthcare institutions, advocating for fetuses should still take the form of attempting to forge common ground between clinicians and pregnant women. Those alliances, both early and late in pregnancy, are most likely to build trust with the woman and effectively improve health outcomes for both her and the future child.

## In Vitro Fertilization

Whereas the criminalization of pregnancy deals with the moral and legal obligations of pregnant women, the development of reproductive technologies has raised moral issues about the processes of becoming pregnant in the first place. Many technological innovations can help couples reproduce who are unable to conceive through unassisted sexual intercourse. Intrauterine (artificial) insemination and ovarian stimulation are two examples. Setting aside the question-begging claim that such interventions are unnatural and therefore wrong, such methods raise broad questions about justice. For example, is it unfair that richer couples can afford these treatments and poorer couples cannot? Should we devote our limited economic resources to creating new babies, or would it be better to care for the many children in our underfunded foster care system? Is it arrogant and selfish for couples to go to such lengths just so they can raise children with their own genes? Although these are interesting philosophical questions, deeper ethical and legal issues arise with what the U.S. Centers for Disease Control and Prevention (CDC) (2019) calls **assisted reproductive technology (ART)**. The CDC defines ART as "all fertility treatments in which either eggs or embryos are handled," most notably **in vitro fertilization (IVF)**.

Research on external fertilization began with marine animals in the 1890s and continued with mice and rabbits in the 1930s. M. C. Chang (1959) fertilized and developed a rabbit egg in vitro in 1947. The first human baby produced through IVF, Louise Brown, was born in 1978 in England (Steptoe and Edwards 1978). By 2021, 2.3 percent of all infants born in the U.S. (86,146 infants) were conceived through IVF (U.S. Department of Health and Human Services 2024).

IVF is a treatment for infertility. The process usually begins with the controlled stimulation of a woman's ovaries: follicle-stimulating hormone

(FSH) increases production of oocytes (superovulation), luteinizing hormone (LH) matures the eggs, and exogenous human chorionic gonadotropin (hCG) triggers final maturation. A needle is then inserted trans-vaginally to extract the follicles containing the eggs. A number of eggs (up to fifteen) are retrieved. Clinicians also subject sperm to the process of capacitation, which raises the chance of fertilization by increasing motility and making the membrane more permeable. The eggs are then fertilized with sperm in a culture medium (a solution that supports cell growth); sometimes the sperm is injected directly into the egg (intracytoplasmic sperm injection). The fertilized egg is typically incubated for five days, when it reaches the blastocyst stage. The processes of external fertilization and incubation happen "in glass" (hence the term "in vitro" or the more colloquial "test tube baby") rather than within the woman's body. The early-stage embryos then may undergo preimplantation genetic testing (PGT) to screen for genetic disorders. When the woman is ready to be pregnant, an embryo is loaded into a transfer catheter, which is passed through the cervix and into the endometrial cavity of the uterus, where the embryo is implanted. Typically, only one embryo is implanted (Jain and Singh 2024). The remaining embryos are usually frozen (cryopreserved) and can remain frozen indefinitely. Retrieving and freezing multiple embryos increases the chances of live birth (because backup embryos are available in case of miscarriage), allows for more than one pregnancy, makes younger eggs available in the future, reduces financial costs, and avoids the health risks of another oocyte retrieval. A single cycle of IVF treatment typically costs between $15,000 and $30,000, and some people need to go through multiple cycles to give birth successfully (Conrad and Grifo 2023).

In vitro fertilization has several benefits: it overcomes infertility and sterility; it allows women who are undergoing chemotherapy to save eggs for later use, since cancer treatment may cause ovaries to stop releasing eggs; it increases the chances of carrying a child to term, since embryos may be screened for chromosomal abnormalities that cause miscarriage; and it is available to anyone, including same-sex couples, single people (with egg or sperm donors), and transgender people. With developing technology, the risks of IVF treatment have diminished. Multiple-embryo transfer has been used to increase the chances of at least one successful implantation, but it poses more of a risk to maternal health than single-embryo transfer, since multifetal pregnancies are more likely to produce complications such as preterm labor and antenatal conditions such as hypertension. To reduce multifetal gestations, the Practice Committee of the American Society for Reproductive Medicine (2017) recommends that multiple-embryo transfer (with two or three at most) only be used in older women, for whom it is less likely to result in a multiple-gestation birth. When multifetal gestations do occur, patients may opt for selective reduction, where some of the fetuses are aborted to reduce the pregnancy to a twin or singleton pregnancy. In 2017, the rate of twin pregnancies dropped to less than 7 percent of in vitro fertilizations (Katler et al. 2022). The other most common maternal health risk, ovarian hyperstimulation syndrome, happens in only 1–5 percent of cases (Steward et al. 2014). Although severe cases can be fatal, treatment in a hospital, including IV fluids and anticoagulant medications, greatly reduces the risk of death. Studies of the risk to maternal health from singleton IVF pregnancies are inconclusive, as are studies of the risk of birth defects (Jackson et al. 2004; Hansen et al. 2013). In sum, improvements to IVF technology over the last few decades have reduced risks to women's well-being.

There are two main moral objections to in vitro fertilization. First, those who believe in fetal personhood object to the destruction of unused embryos. When an IVF pregnancy is successfully carried to term, many of the blastocysts that were produced and frozen as backups are not needed. In this situation, usually the unused embryos are eventually thawed and discarded or donated for scientific research. Some of the same arguments against abortion also apply here. For example, Robert George and Christopher Tollefsen (2011) claim that an embryo is a human being that is developing according to its unique genetic code, so it has a right to life just like we do. Not only does this entail that abortion is morally wrong, but it also means that we should not produce spare embryos for IVF. According to George and Tollefson, all successfully created embryos should be implanted in the woman or "adopted" by others, not destroyed (50–51, 214).

In a February 2024 decision that gained national attention, the Alabama Supreme Court ruled that "the Wrongful Death of a Minor Act applies on its face to all unborn children, without limitation" and that the act contains no exception for "extrauterine children—that is, unborn children who are located outside of a biological uterus at the time they are killed" (*LePage v. The Center for Reproductive Medicine, P.C.*, SC-2022-0579 [2024], at 7, 3). The Alabama legislature then quickly passed a bill (SB 159) to protect IVF clinics from liability. When the governer signed the bill into law, she said that the state "works to foster a culture of life" because it helps parents "grow their families through IVF" (Nazzaro 2024). All this happened against the backdrop of Alabama's total ban on abortion, which defines "unborn child, child, or person" as "a human being, specifically including an unborn child in utero at any stage of development, regardless of viability" (Ala. Code § 26-23H-3 [2023]). The Alabama Supreme Court doubted whether prenatal protections could apply to some embryos and not others based merely on their "physical location" (*LePage v. The Center for Reproductive Medicine, P.C.*, at 11). Other states with fetal personhood laws may well run into the same legal conundrum about how to handle embryos produced through IVF.

If early-stage frozen embryos are not already human beings or persons, the potential to become persons may or may not be enough to generate moral obligations. Potentiality was emphasized in the U.K. Department of Health and Social Security's *Report of the Committee of Inquiry into Human Fertilisation and Embryology* (commonly called the **Warnock Report**, after committee chair Mary Warnock) (1984), which was convened to recommend how to regulate IVF and embryological research following the birth of Louise Brown. Although it concluded that all human embryos have a "special status" and "should be afforded some protection in law" (11.17), the Warnock Report did not prohibit all embryonic research, opting instead for a fourteen-day rule, which allows such research only until the fourteenth day after fertilization. The committee's reasoning was that, at that point, the embryo can no longer split into twins, thus serving as a mark of individuality, and the "primitive streak" appears, a precursor of the brain and spinal cord (11.5). After that point, the embryo is "a potential human being" (11.2).

In the intervening years, philosophers have debated whether and when embryos' potential personhood makes them morally considerable. For example, Michael Lockwood claims that "a potential for X generates an interest only where there is some individual for whom the development of the potential for X constitutes a *benefit*" (1988, 199). Therefore, embryos only deserve protection when they achieve sentience (after eight weeks). R. M. Hare counters that an embryo's "potential lies in the fact that if it prospers there will, in consequence, in the future, grow up an ordinary grown human person who can enjoy all the blessings [of life]"; "the interest of the possible future grown person into whom they might turn that imposes on us, in normal cases, a duty to preserve them" (1988, 225, 217).

He concludes that embryonic research at any point is wrong, which also has implications for IVF. As we saw in the previous chapter, other philosophers are dismissive of the appeal to potential. After all, we should not treat an acorn like an oak tree (Thomson 1971, 47–48). Another common objection to the potentiality argument is that it would require us to respect human gametes (sperm and unfertilized ova), which are also potential persons—a reductio ad absurdum (e.g., Kuhse and Singer 1982, 61).

Philosophers have also addressed the question raised in Alabama recently: whether there is a moral distinction between embryos that are developing in utero and embryos that are cryopreserved for IVF. According to Mary Mahowald (2004), an in utero embryo has the potential to become a full-fledged human person because it contains the genetic blueprint that will make it develop into one, given its presence in the womb, unless its course is disrupted from without (for example, by being aborted). By contrast, cryopreserved embryos "depend crucially on external interventions to reach that end," so they lack "active potency" (210). In Aristotelian terms, they have passive potentiality, not active potentiality. Alfonso Gómez-Lobo (2005) responds that frozen embryos have active potency because they internally contain the power to become human persons and only lack the natural conditions (of being in the uterus) that would allow them to grow and develop. The potential does not have to be given to them from without; they only have to be allowed to actualize their natural potential. If such embryos did not have this potential, Gómez-Lobo says, they would not be suitable for IVF: "The potentiality has to have been already present in the embryo for the embryo to implant" (107). Even in the appeal to potentiality, philosophers attempt to draw a sharp line of moral considerability in a biological process of development that is gradual and continuous.

A second class of objections to in vitro fertilization comes from defenders of disability rights: namely, that screening out some embryos because of genetic disorders assumes that disabled people's lives are not worth living. This conceives of variations from normalcy as problematic, and it reinforces stereotypes by identifying potential people wholly in terms of their disabilities. For many potential parents, the social stigma against even manageable disabilities is likely to motivate them to destroy embryos with disabling conditions. To resist this stigma, individuals in some disability communities select *for* disabilities such as deafness. According to the Ethics Committee of the American Society for Reproductive Medicine, clinicians do not have to do the requested implantation, which respects their autonomy, and they should not implant embryos with "a life-threatening condition that causes severe and early debility with no possibility of reasonable function," thus fulfilling the obligation to do no harm (2017, 1130). However, clinicians may assist parents in implanting embryos with "treatable or effectively manageable" conditions to respect "reproductive liberty and patient autonomy" (2017, 1130, 1132). On their view, clinicians should honor a patient's decision-making process and values. If the patient is willing to raise a disabled child or wants the child to be part of the parent's disability community, the clinician should not act paternalistically by imposing their own view of disability on them. Furthermore, infertile couples should not be treated unequally by being deprived of a choice that is available to fertile couples (who may decide to bring traditionally conceived disabled fetuses to term); they have dispositional authority over the embryos since they belong to them; and by helping patients to conceive, clinicians avoid the harm of depriving future persons, including disabled people, of the goods of life. Since what makes a good life is contested—Elizabeth Barnes (2016) and others defend a value-neutral model of disability as mere difference—it is not clear that one must select against manageable disabilities to promote procreative beneficence (see also Wallis 2020). We discuss the decision to select against disability more thoroughly later in this chapter.

Other objections to IVF have been raised but are less widely accepted. For example, the Catholic Church opposes IVF not only because of the destruction of embryos but because of the artificiality of the procedure. Unlike fertility treatments that help couples to conceive "through an act of love between husband and wife," IVF creates babies "by a laboratory procedure performed by doctors or technicians." It thus does not occur "from the marriage act which by its nature is ordered toward loving openness to life." On this view, it is wrong to take procreation outside of marriage and put it in a petri dish (Haas 1998).

## Surrogate Motherhood

The unnaturalness objection becomes more pronounced when an embryo is implanted in a surrogate. **Surrogate motherhood** allows infertile couples, gay couples, or women who cannot carry fetuses to term (because of severe pelvic disease or repeated miscarriages, for example) to have children with some of their own genetic material. A surrogate mother goes through the pregnancy and delivery for another couple, but unlike adoption, the child is (usually) genetically related to one or both of the people who will raise them. In fact, reproductive technology makes it possible for up to five people to be parents, in one way or another, of one child: an egg donor (genetic mother), a sperm donor (genetic father), a surrogate mother who gestates the fetus (carrying mother), and a couple who raises the child (nurturing, commissioning, or intended parents) (Snowden, Mitchell, and Snowden 1983, 32–35). In *Buzzanca v. Buzzanca* (61 Cal.App.4th 1410, 72 Cal. Rptr.2d 280 [1998]), a California appeals court ruled that when material from anonymous egg and sperm donors is implanted in a surrogate, the intended parents are the lawful parents. Some roles can be combined, of course. For example, sperm from a man who will raise the child may be used to artificially inseminate a woman who is not the intended mother, who then carries the fetus to term (a complete father and a genetic-carrying mother) (Snowden, Mitchell, and Snowden 1983, 32–35). When eggs and sperm from the commissioning mother and father or from donors are used, such that the surrogate has no genetic connection to the baby, it is called full, host, or gestational surrogacy. If the surrogate's egg is fertilized, it is called partial, straight, natural, or traditional surrogacy (Imrie and Jadva 2014).

Because it is often understood as a rights issue, moral and legal questions regarding surrogate motherhood tend to overlap. The *Dobbs* decision notwithstanding, the right to privacy, recognized in *Griswold v. Connecticut* (381 U.S. 479 [1965]) and other Supreme Court cases, seems to make the permissibility of surrogate motherhood in the U.S. relatively straightforward under the law, since the right to privacy entails a right to reproductive freedom. If competent adults freely consent to such an arrangement, then only a compelling state interest—something that is important enough to override the presumption in favor of bodily autonomy—would allow it to be legally restricted or regulated (Robertson 1990). Similarly, from the moral perspective, respecting patient autonomy means that people can do with their sperm, eggs, and uteruses whatever they want, as long as they do not limit other people's autonomy or cause significant harm. Traditional coital reproduction is virtually unregulated for just this reason. If there is a right to be a parent, why should infertile couples have their attempts at reproduction more tightly regulated or even prohibited, as long as they have a willing surrogate?

Despite this apparent simplicity, the case of Baby M exposed the complex moral and legal questions that surrogacy contracts pose. The story began with a possible diagnosis of multiple sclerosis for Elizabeth Stern, after which she and her husband, William, decided that pregnancy would be too risky. Because the rest of his family had been killed in the Holocaust, William was the only chance to continue his bloodline. They contracted with a surrogacy agency, and Mary Beth Whitehead, a married mother of two, answered an advertisement and signed a surrogate parenting agreement, motivated both by a desire to help the Sterns and by the $10,000 contractual fee. She was artificially inseminated with Mr. Stern's sperm, and on March 27, 1986, she gave birth to a baby girl, known in the ensuing court cases as Baby M. Although Whitehead initially relinquished the baby to the Sterns, she quickly changed her mind. When she threatened to kill herself, the Sterns agreed to give her the baby temporarily. Whitehead subsequently refused to give up the baby—including fleeing to Florida—and the Sterns sued for custody. The trial court found the surrogacy contract valid, gave Mr. Stern legal custody, and allowed Mrs. Stern to adopt the child. Whitehead appealed to the New Jersey Supreme Court, which reversed the trial court. It invalidated the surrogacy contract, which it said conflicted with state law, and declared Whitehead to be Baby M's legal mother. However, the court granted custody to Mr. Stern, the baby's legal father, not because of the contract but because it was in the child's best interests (*In the Case of Baby M*, 109 N.J. 396, 537 A.2d 1227 [1988]).

The court decided that surrogacy contracts, by which women agree irrevocably to relinquish their newborn children to others, contradicted state law since the children's best interests played no role in the custody decisions. The court also ruled that such agreements violated the law against baby-selling. The state legislature had prohibited fees for adoption (beyond overhead costs of an approved agency and related medical expenses) because they took advantage of women's economic desperation and substituted the profit motive for a concern for children's well-being. **Commercial surrogacy** raises the same concerns. Finally, the court said that such agreements were degrading to women—although they did not specify how. The court did say that a woman could agree to act as a surrogate provided that she was not compensated beyond necessary expenses related to the pregnancy (**altruistic surrogacy**) and she was not legally compelled to give up the child when it was born.

In response to the court's judgment, five states immediately passed laws banning commercial surrogacy. Today, there is a patchwork of different laws. Some states prohibit compensation for surrogates and refuse to enforce commercial surrogacy contracts. Some states allow pre-birth parentage orders, depending on who is genetically related to the embryo and other factors, such as whether the couple is married and whether it is a same-sex or heterosexual couple. Some states allow the surrogate to relinquish the child only days after birth. Some states enforce such contracts unless they are contrary to a child's best interests. And some states allow enforceable gestational carrier agreements, even with compensation. Outside of the U.S., there is also a lot of variation. China, France, and Germany ban both commercial and altruistic surrogacy; Australia, Canada, and India allow only altruistic surrogacy; and Russia, Ukraine, and Georgia allow both commercial and altruistic surrogacy. The European Union prohibits commercial surrogacy based on the European Convention on Bioethics (Article 21) and the Charter of Fundamental Rights of the European Union (Article 3), both of which prohibit the use of the human body and its parts for financial gain.

Some of the moral issues around surrogate motherhood were first raised in the Warnock Report, which considers at least six objections:

1. "To introduce a third party into the process of procreation . . . is an attack on the value of the marital relationship."

2. "It is inconsistent with human dignity that a woman should use her uterus for financial profit and treat it as an incubator for someone else's child."

3. To deliberately become pregnant with "the intention of giving up the child" distorts "the relationship between mother and child."

4. It may harm the child, who has natural bonds with the birth mother.

5. It is degrading to the child because it is being sold for money.

6. "Since there are some risks attached to pregnancy, no woman ought to be asked to undertake pregnancy for another, in order to earn money." (Department of Health and Social Security 1984, 44–45)

As Bonnie Steinbock (1990) notes, none of these arguments against surrogacy is successful without modification. People donate or sell blood, and they lease their bodies out to employers all the time. We do plenty of things for money, including risky occupations such as logging and meatpacking. Since, in many cases, the baby's biological parent wants to take custody, the child "belongs" to them already. Anyway, it is a custody agreement, not an ownership agreement (Steinbock 1990, 129–31). The parents cannot treat the child as property; for one thing, they have legal and moral obligations to promote the child's well-being (Hanna 2010). Furthermore, appealing to the mother-child relationship rests on gender stereotypes, commits a naturalistic fallacy (assuming that what is natural is good), and presupposes that the woman is not acting altruistically—namely, helping a baby to have a good home with people who desperately want to be parents. If surrogate mothers were somehow violating their natural role, then giving one's child up for adoption would also be morally wrong—and indeed worse, since women presumably have more of a connection with their postnatal children—something that no one is claiming. Surrogate mothers are often motivated by a desire to help infertile couples, and most surrogates do not suffer psychologically (Imrie and Jadva 2014). Finally, although Catholic philosophers oppose surrogacy because it "separates the unitive and procreative aspects of [the] marital act" (Aznar and Martínez Peris 2019, 61), this depends on a particular view of marriage that not everyone accepts.

The themes raised by the Warnock Report, however, reappear in more sophisticated ways in several common philosophical arguments against surrogacy. For example, one challenge to the liberal model is that the surrogate mother cannot give what we would consider informed consent. Women who have never had children may not understand the risks and discomfort that come with pregnancy, and women who have had children may not be able to anticipate what it is like to surrender their newborn babies to other couples. Thus, the decision to become a surrogate may not be fully informed. The counter to this objection is that it risks treating women paternalistically, as if we have to protect them against the bad consequences of their own choices. The same objection applies to all pregnancies: women giving birth for the first time may have little idea of what becoming a parent entails, women giving birth to a second child may not know how multiple children will impact their lives, and so on. On some liberal feminist accounts, the right of women over their own bodies entails the right to have a baby (or not), the right to have someone else's baby, and the right to profit financially from it (Andrews 1990). Christine Straehle (2024) defends a liberal model that defines surrogacy as reproductive labor covered under the right to freedom of occupational choice (see also Cooper and Waldby 2014, 37–88).

But even if surrogate mothers take themselves (rightly or wrongly) to be informed, do they freely consent? Although it is not universally the case, surrogate mothers tend to be poorer, less well-educated, and live in less developed countries than most commissioning mothers and fathers. A situation in which poor women are compelled by economic necessity or otherwise manipulated to sell their bodies to rich couples may be coercive. As Kant would put it, they are treated merely as means because the pressure to survive economically means that they must consent to take on others' ends. In this case, the end is obvious: they are being used as gestational vessels—"an incubator for someone else's child"—so that rich couples can continue their bloodlines. In Marxist terms, surrogate motherhood is a form of veiled slavery because the woman is forced to do it out of economic necessity, and it turns both the product of her labor (the baby) and the woman herself into commodities. The connection to Marx, however, raises an obvious challenge to this objection. There is nothing uniquely morally problematic about surrogate motherhood if economic exploitation is a general feature of all work under capitalism. Surrogate motherhood is only impermissible if all other wage labor is impermissible (Parry 2018; Wilkinson 2023).

At least two things make surrogacy different from other jobs, however. First, surrogate mothers are not only paid to be pregnant but to relinquish their babies to other people after the babies are born. The commodification of workers is not unique; the commodification of babies is. As Steinbock notes, "Mr. Stern did not agree to pay Ms. Whitehead merely to *have* his child, but to provide him with a child" (1990, 131). Someone cannot sell their one-year-old child to another family. Why would it be any different for a one-day-old child? If commercial surrogacy is child-selling, then it would seem to be morally wrong and legally prohibited (Rae 1994; Dickenson 2017, 65–87). This is one reason why altruistic surrogacy is more commonly accepted than commercial surrogacy.

A second difference from other employment is that surrogate mothers are typically women, and the objectification of women as baby-makers exemplifies and reinforces gender stereotypes. Historically, the reduction of women to breeders of children has undermined their status as autonomous persons. Enslaved and poor women in particular have been forced to give up their reproductive freedom for the benefit of others. In short, surrogacy takes reproduction, which is an essential attribute of women's personhood, and turns it into a "fungible exchangeable object" (Radin 1996, 84; see also Cavaliere 2022).

A symptom of this instrumentalization is the control that commissioning parents often assert over many aspects of surrogate mothers' lives. Surrogates undergo weeks of hormone injections, tests to determine if fallopian tubes are blocked, and the embryo transfer procedure, some of which is uncomfortable or even painful. Unlike other jobs, a pregnant woman then works twenty-four hours a day for nine months, all of which is regulated. In the case of Baby M, Mary Beth Whitehead agreed not to smoke cigarettes, drink alcohol, or take illegal drugs, and she agreed not to take medications without her doctor's written consent. She had to keep a regular schedule of medical examinations and follow all medical instructions from the inseminating physician and her own obstetrician. She agreed not to have an abortion unless her own life was at risk, and she agreed to have an abortion "upon demand" of the genetic father if the fetus was diagnosed with a genetic or congenital disorder ("Surrogate Parenting Agreement" 1985).

Another objection is that children produced through surrogacy are psychologically harmed as a result of being treated like commodities and separated from their natural mothers. As we have noted, people have rights over their own bodies, but those rights are limited when they infringe on other people's rights—in this case, by causing harm to children. Although there is no evidence of a correlation between psychological problems and being born via surrogacy (Söderström-Anttila et al. 2016; Yau et al. 2021; Kneebone, Beilby, and Hammarberg 2022), this objection has fueled a new movement in support of an international treaty to outlaw surrogacy, which they say violates the U.N. Convention on the Rights of the Child, specifically the prohibition on the sale of children (Winfield 2024). Anca Gheaus (2024) concedes that surrogate children are not always harmed in either an absolute sense (some live perfectly good lives) or in a relative sense (some live as good or better lives than they would with their gestational mothers). However, she says that allocating control rights over them through private agreements harms them in the same way that slaves are harmed even when they are owned by benevolent masters. In these ways, surrogacy, like IVF, provokes debate about the objectification of pregnant women's bodies, the commodification of children, and the moral status of embryos.

## Disability-Selective Abortion

Both IVF and surrogacy use **prenatal screening** to control the kinds of embryos that will be brought to term, but prenatal screening has become an almost ubiquitous practice in pregnancy more generally. And prenatal screening raises the question of which embryos are valued and therefore which children are worth having. Many pregnant women with access to reproductive services undergo prenatal testing to determine whether the developing fetuses have abnormalities associated with disease or disability. This can be done with ultrasound, which allows clinicians to examine a fetus by sonar; chorionic villus sampling (CVS), which uses a needle to take a sample of tissue from the placenta; or amniocentesis, where a needle is inserted into the uterus to extract some of the amniotic fluid, which contains fetal cells. Ultrasound is used to monitor the development of the body, including organs and other body parts. It can detect several congenital conditions, including anencephaly (a fatal condition where parts of the brain and skull do not fully develop) and spina bifida (where the spine and membranes around the spinal cord do not fully close). Because it is more invasive and thus more dangerous, CVS or amniocentesis is only performed on pregnant women who have increased chances of having babies with genetic or chromosomal conditions. It can detect such conditions as Down syndrome (where an extra chromosome causes developmental delays and sometimes physical disabilities), cystic fibrosis (where thick mucus interferes with lung and intestinal function), and Tay-Sachs disease (where a fatty substance in the brain destroys nerve cells, leading to loss of muscle function, loss of vision and hearing, and paralysis). With recent improvements in medical technology, clinicians can now perform noninvasive prenatal testing (NIPT), a screening that isolates cell-free DNA shed from the placenta and circulating in maternal blood. This screening is not definitive; it indicates whether the risk of having certain conditions such as Down syndrome is increased or decreased. A positive result calls for additional testing.

Prenatal screening is commonly considered a form of prenatal care to ensure that one will have a healthy baby. Although some impairments can be corrected with surgery in utero—for example, closing a spinal defect resulting from spina bifida—many cannot. And researchers have not yet tried gene therapy to correct genetic impairments in utero (which raises other ethical questions that we address later in this chapter). When fetal abnormalities can be diagnosed but not corrected, a pregnant woman faces a choice: either to abort the fetus or to deliver a disabled baby.

The ethical questions that arise with **disability-selective abortions** (also called fetal abnormality abortions) are different from abortion in general. If abortion is permissible, then a woman may decide to terminate a pregnancy because she does not want another child, because a child would interfere with her career, because she cannot afford it, or for any number of reasons. In those cases, the woman does not want a baby, so she aborts the fetus. By contrast, with disability-selective abortion, the pregnant woman wants a baby but does not want *this* baby. The question then becomes: Is it permissible for a woman to abort an otherwise-wanted fetus because it is disabled? In England and Wales, which tracks statutory grounds for abortion, 1.6 percent of all abortions in 2021 were performed because of fetal abnormalities (3,370 out of 214,256) (Office for Health Improvement and Disparities 2024). Are those morally different—more justified or less justified—than "normal" abortions?

The two sides on the disability-selective abortion debate often focus on the same facets of the issue but have radically different interpretations and evaluations. To begin, there is the question of how we should perceive **disabilities**. Is a disability a bad thing to be avoided or merely a difference whose negative value is primarily caused by social factors? Adrienne Asch (1999) takes the latter position. Nondisabled people often assume that disabled people live miserable lives because of their limitations, so we should abort them for their own good. But people with disabilities usually adapt to them, experiencing them as the normal conditions under which they approach the world. This disjunction between public perception of disability and the subjective experience of people with disabilities is known as the **disability paradox** (Albrecht and Devlieger 1999; National Council on Disability 2019). Someone with cystic fibrosis cannot climb mountains (without adequate adaptive tools), and someone with Down syndrome may not be able to understand *The Critique of Pure Reason*, but they can have other experiences that are just as fulfilling (some of which may not be accessible to people without such disabilities). On Asch's view, this is no different from other physical and mental variations. Someone who is five feet tall may not be able to dunk a basketball and many otherwise smart people also struggle to understand Kant, but they probably do not wish that they had never been born. We all get along with what we have. In this sense, disabilities are neutral traits rather than negative ones, and it is only within social situations and within socially established norms of health that such characteristics function as impairments (see also Barnes 2016, 78–118).

When people with disabilities do suffer, it has more to do with the built environment in which they find themselves. If people in wheelchairs cannot access buildings or there are no enriching jobs for people with cognitive impairments, then those disabilities become **handicaps**. When an employer perceives an applicant with cerebral palsy as generally incompetent, the biological trait becomes an obstacle to greater self-sufficiency—not because of the trait itself but because of the employer's prejudice. Disability-selective abortion is only a solution if disability itself, rather than social stigma against disability, is framed as the problem. Even if ultimately we support access to abortion, we can make disability-selective abortion less likely by adequately funding social programs for disabled children and adults, and by removing disincentives to meaningful employment (Ziegler 2017). The challenges facing people of color provide an illuminating parallel. On average, Black people in the U.S. have worse health outcomes and shorter life spans, and they are more likely to end up in poverty and go to prison. To address these problems, we should confront the enduring legacy of racism, not encourage Black women to get abortions.

Opponents of disability-selective abortion also claim that normalizing the practice produces more discrimination by sending the message that disabled people cannot live worthwhile lives. Erik Parens and Adrienne Asch call this the expressivist argument (1999, S2). Marsha Saxton puts it this way: "The message at the heart of widespread selective abortion on the basis of prenatal diagnosis is the greatest insult: some of us are 'too flawed' in our very DNA to exist; we are unworthy of being born" (2013, 98; see also Kittay and Kittay 2000). Prenatal genetic screening is framed by medical professionals in ways that portray disability inaccurately and reinforce negative stereotypes (Klein 2011; Gould 2020). It does the same thing as other forms of prejudice: it defines a person wholly in terms of one devalued property (gender, skin color, ethnicity, mental or physical ability, and so on) or reduces the fetus to "a single trait [that] stands in for the whole" (Parens and Asch 1999, S2; see also Asch and Wasserman 2005). Disability rights activists call attention to the fact that devaluing the lives of one kind of person and using that as a reason to kill them (or prevent their existence) is "a similar eugenic ideology" as Nazism: "determining who should and should not inhabit the world" under the guise of doing it for their own good (because they cannot be happy) or for the good of society (because of the cost of caring for them) (Hubbard 2013, 81–82; see also Saxton 2013). Prior to the *Dobbs* ruling, some U.S. states had legally prohibited abortions based on a fetal diagnosis of disability, ostensibly because of its connection to eugenics—although there is reason to believe that it was simply part of a larger anti-abortion strategy (Smith 2019). When Indiana's disability-selective abortion ban was challenged in 2019, Justice Clarence Thomas's concurrence in the denial of certiorari claimed that the law was constitutional because it "promote[s] a State's compelling interest in preventing abortion from becoming a tool of modern-day eugenics" (*Box v. Planned Parenthood of Indiana and Kentucky, Inc.*, 587 U.S. ___, 139 S.Ct. 1780 [2019], at 1783).

Another argument against disability-selective abortion, what Parens and Asch call the parental attitude argument, is that it reflects a morally problematic view of parenthood (1999, S5–S6; see also Asch and Wasserman 2005). In wanting only a nondisabled child, one would not only be defining the future child wholly in terms of their disability but would also be holding on to the "fantasy—and fallacy— . . . that parents can guarantee or create perfection for the child" (Asch 1989, 88). In addition, selecting for nondisabled fetuses instrumentalizes reproduction, conceiving of the future child as someone who should be like the parents—to be able to experience what the parents experience and value what they value. It is a selfish and self-centered position: someone who is not enough like me should not exist. However, studies show that disabled people can live happy lives with their own kinds of fulfillment (Crocker 2000), that there is no difference in stress levels between families with and without disabled children (Harris and McHale 1989), and that many families with disabled children find the experience enriching and meaningful (Stainton and Besser 1998). As a remedy to the visions of "perfect" babies that motivate selective abortions, Asch suggests educating parents prior to or after prenatal screening, including discussing the social stigmatization of disability, meeting with other parents who are raising disabled children, and reading the memoirs of people with disabilities (1999, 1655).

Defenders of disability-selective abortion respond that this conception of parenthood as "unconditional welcome" sets up a false dichotomy: either the parents want any child, or they want the perfect child. William Ruddick (2000) says that the former, "maternalist" conception is not the only legitimate way to understand parenthood. Under a "projectivist" conception of parenthood, parents may want a child who can fulfill their hopes and aims, even if the child eventually chooses to pursue other things. For example, parents who enjoy hiking may want to share their experience of nature with a child, so they may select against a fetus who tests positive for hereditary spastic paraplegia. Ruddick also mentions the "familial" conception of parenthood, where the parents hope the child will have their own kids someday and raise a family. It is permissible for parents to select for a fetus who may experience parenthood rather than, say, a fetus with cystic fibrosis who would be sterile. In both cases, parents are not guaranteeing that the child will live out their plans, but they are avoiding having a child who is incapable of pursuing what they take to be meaningful experiences. To be sure, parents can have fulfilling relationships with disabled children. But the benefits of parenthood can also be had with nondisabled children, so selecting against a disabled fetus and conceiving a nondisabled child gets the benefits without the burdens.

Although, as mentioned above, some studies show that disabled children and families can be as happy as everyone else, evidence also suggests that people with physical disabilities are less happy on average (Marinić and Brkljačić 2008). And families with disabled children experience greater financial challenges, poorer social interactions, disruptions to their careers, and negative impacts on their physical and mental health (Singhi et al. 1990; Dyson 1991; Sen and Yurtsever 2007). Having a child with a disability often takes a particular toll on the mother, who, because the woman is usually designated as the primary caregiver, may have to give up her career and devote the rest of her life to caring for the child. Like other abortions, the woman (and the rest of her family) may not be ready for the burden, given the reality in which we currently live. A person who wants to avoid this is not a monster. If the child is never born, there is no harm done to them. But by letting the child be born, parents may have to make significant sacrifices. Although some of these burdens could be socially addressed with greater support for disabled children and their families, the situation as it stands is one that most parents would want to avoid.

On this side of the debate, ethicists reject the contention that disability is just another form of variation like height or vision. Rather than allowing all variations, we usually try to correct harmful deviations from the norm. Steinbock (2000) gives the example of someone with high blood pressure. We do not just say that high blood pressure is a form of variation and that we should respect people with high blood pressure, who are no worse than, only different from, someone with normal blood pressure. Instead, we try to correct it so the person can conform to what is healthy: changing their diet, losing weight, or taking blood pressure medication. If someone has bad eyesight, we give them glasses. When someone breaks their leg, we do not say that we should respect people with broken legs and leave them hobbling around. We set the leg so that it can heal and the person can regain normal functioning. And we try to prevent disabilities. Pregnant women take folic acid to lessen the chances of their children getting spina bifida, and plenty of prescription medications, such as antiepileptic drugs, are not approved for use by pregnant women because they may cause fetal abnormalities. Jeff McMahan (2005) notes that if disability were a neutral trait, then there would be no moral objection to someone knowingly causing one's fetus to be disabled, even if it were the foreseeable side effect of a selfish act. Yet most of us think this is wrong.

On this view, we try to prevent disabilities in our children because disabilities are not good to have, and we should avoid them if we can. Although lack of social accommodations exacerbates limitations caused by disability, we cannot compensate for all physical and mental limitations: as Steinbock says, "not every disability can be overcome by social adaptation" (2000, 114). A person with a severe cognitive disability will not be able to go to college or hold a whole range of jobs, and they may never be able to live independently—not because of our social prejudices but because of their natural limitations. To show that disabilities are not just neutral variations but things we want to avoid, Allen Buchanan poses a thought experiment: "Suppose God tells a couple: 'I'll make a child for you. You can have a child that has limited opportunities due to a physical or cognitive defect or one who does not. Which do you choose?'" (1996, 33–34).

Choosing the nondisabled child is not the result of prejudice or a fantasy about perfection but a realistic assessment that a disabled child's prospects will be limited, regardless of the social circumstances, and a desire to avoid that limitation. While it is true that disabled people can live happy lives, they start with disadvantages that nondisabled children do not have. It makes sense to select for another child who can confront life without these problems. Such reasoning does not express a discriminatory attitude toward the disabled:

> Surely, if the couple says they wish to have a child without defects, this need not mean that they devalue persons with disabilities, or that they would not love and cherish their child if it were disabled. Choosing to have God make a child who does not have defects does not in itself in any way betray negative judgments or attitudes about the value of individuals with defects. (Buchanan 1996, 33–34)

Rather than being based on discrimination, parents may want the child not to suffer because of these limitations, and they may not want to make the necessary sacrifices themselves. When a fetus is shown to have a disability, the parents are, in effect, given that choice by God in the hypothetical situation: Do you want a disabled baby, or do you want to try again for one that is nondisabled? On this view, it is reasonable to try again.

As noted earlier, some disabilities (such as some forms of spina bifida) can be corrected with prenatal surgery, but in the absence of advances in gene therapy, many genetic disabilities, such as Down syndrome, cystic fibrosis, and Tay-Sachs disease, cannot. In such cases, disabled fetuses cannot be brought back to the norm, so the only way to prevent disability is to selectively abort disabled fetuses: "Prenatal screening, along with abortion and embryo selection, can be seen as a form of prevention. It enables prospective parents to prevent an outcome they reasonably want to avoid: the birth of a child who will be sick or have a serious disability" (Steinbock 2000, 118). The point of any kind of testing or screening is to prevent or correct a problem. Adults have their blood pressure tested so clinicians can prevent heart attacks. Prenatal testing is done to find out if the fetus has a disability so that it can be prevented before the fetus is born. Selectively aborting a disabled fetus is not discriminatory; rather, it is the only way to prevent a child from suffering the effects of disability. It is an act of procreative beneficence (Savulescu 2007c).

On this point, the debate over disability-selective abortion overlaps with the ethics of abortion in general and specifically the question of whether the fetus is a person. Is preventing the existence of someone with a disability morally equivalent to correcting a medical disorder or preventing a disability? Some opponents of disability-selective abortion argue that "abortion does not protect the developing fetus from anything. It prevents disability by simply killing the fetus" (Parens and Asch 1999, S3). The disability cannot be prevented because someone (the fetus) is already disabled. Choosing to abort the fetus rejects "the child being created" and refuses "to continue to nurture the life begun" (Asch 2000, 240). Such language sounds a lot like claims that "life begins at conception" and references to "the unborn child" favored by pro-life advocates. Defenders of disability-selective abortion, however, believe that a child is morally considerable and a fetus is not. If a child is born with disabilities, parents have an obligation to care for the child, but they have weaker moral obligations (if any) to a fetus. It is thus permissible to protect a future child from the effects of disability by aborting a disabled fetus and trying to get pregnant again with a nondisabled fetus.

To be sure, not all opponents of disability-selective abortion believe that the fetus is a person. Many of them both defend the right to choose and claim that disability is a bad reason to have an abortion. For example, Marsha Saxton (2013) argues that the social stigma regarding disability, growing out of the eugenics movement and the assumption that disabled children will oppress mothers, pressures women to abort disabled fetuses. Reproductive justice advocates can find common cause with disability rights activists in defending the choice to give birth to disabled children—the right *not* to have an abortion. Similarly, Tom Shakespeare (1998) contends that the real problem is not the woman's right to choose but that the choice seems to be made for her by commonly accepted prejudices against the disabled and social and cultural pressures to abort disabled fetuses. On this view, defenders of disability rights and women's rights can both oppose commonly accepted prejudices against the disabled to support women's free decision-making (see also Asch 1999, 1652; Hall 2013).

Others have questioned whether the disability rights view that opposes selective abortion can be made consistent with feminist defenses of reproductive liberty. For example, Keith Sharp and Sarah Earle (2002) and Bruce Blackshaw (2020) claim that there are "irreconcilable differences."

One cannot say both that a pregnant woman has reproductive control over her body, with the right to terminate a pregnancy for any reason, and that doing so to avoid giving birth to a disabled child is tantamount to eugenics. In these debates, highly abstract notions about personhood, health, and autonomy converge to raise urgent practical questions about when prenatal testing should be offered, how clinicians should present the results to pregnant women, and whether to limit parents' abortion decisions.

## Genetic Enhancement

Human beings have been attempting to improve their health and wellbeing in a variety of ways for millennia: chewing the bark of the cinchona tree to prevent malaria, athletic training, cataract surgery, cochlear implants, and prenatal folic acid supplements to prevent disability are all forms of deliberate enhancement—changing the conditions under which human beings live so they can live better. But a more radical form of intervention has been made possible by recent advancements in genetic technology, which have opened the possibility of modifying or "editing" a person's genome, either prenatally or after birth. The development of CRISPR (Clustered Regularly Interspaced Short Palindromic Repeat) techniques allows for specific genes to be edited; for example, genes that cause leukemia or hemophilia can be deleted from the genome and replaced (Mani 2021).

Genetic modifications tend to be categorized as either **therapies**—preventing or treating disease—or **enhancements**—improving a person's "normal" condition (Murray 2007, 493). The former category is relatively unproblematic. Genetic therapy in the form of bone marrow or stem cell transplants has been used to treat immunodeficiencies for several decades. In December 2023, the U.S. Food and Drug Administration approved two gene modification therapies that address sickle cell disease—one by editing existing genes and one by adding genes—that allow patients to make more hemoglobin (Gibbons and Panepinto 2023). But even this distinction has been contested. In both cases, a person's naturally occurring genes are modified to improve their lives in some way—to address suffering or some form of disadvantage. Pharmacologically, for instance, beta blockers are drugs that treat hypertension and anxiety, but they can also be used by athletes to enhance performance. Some treatments involve both enhancements and therapy in ways that are difficult to disentangle, such as (hypothetically) modifying a genome to create immunity to influenza (Lagay 2001). Even more foundationally, critical disability theorists have argued that some forms of suffering and disadvantage are defined according to "suspect norms," socially prevalent but arbitrary prejudices about what constitutes health (Little 1998, 170). One proposed test for classifying modifications is to examine the "measures of improvement": Are they essentially medical in nature, related to "bodily dynamics," or do they instead involve "social dynamics," such as shyness or athletic competition (Juengst 1998, 43)? Another attempt to delineate therapeutic and nontherapeutic genetic modifications focuses on whether a patient is trying to recover "lost health" or instead is concerned with "non-pathological" traits (Macpherson, Roqué, and Segarra 2019).

A second distinction separates **somatic genetic editing** (genetic engineering that only affects particular cells in an individual patient) from **germline genetic editing** (genetic engineering that affects reproductive cells such as sperm or eggs, such that the edited genome is inherited by future generations). In 2018, a Chinese scientist, He Jiankui, modified the genes of two embryonic twins, a germline modification, to make them immune to HIV. This violated Chinese law (and thus led to his imprisonment) and sparked debates about whether other governments should issue moratoriums on such research (Greely 2019). Currently, germline genetic editing is banned in most European countries, Canada, Japan, and China. In the United States, federal funds cannot be used for research into germline genetic modification. The concerns have to do mostly with the uncertain outcomes across generations. Edited genes may be susceptible to future mutation or introduce unintended vulnerabilities, for instance. Because the risks of such modifications cannot be accurately predicted, either for the existing patient or others in the future, even therapeutic interventions have the status of experiments that may violate the principles of nonmaleficence (because of unintended bad consequences) and respect for autonomy (because, without knowing what will happen, truly informed consent cannot be obtained). To wrestle with these issues, the U.S. National Academies of Science, in conjunction with the U.K. Royal Society and the U.S. National Academy of Medicine, have formed an International Commission on the Clinical Use of Human Germline Genome Editing to create a regulatory framework for future research, including both genetic therapies and genetic enhancements.

Apart from the issue of germline genetic modification, which is generally opposed by researchers and bioethicists, somatic genetic enhancement raises predictable issues around the use of medical technology. As an advocate of **liberal eugenics**, Savulescu (2007b, 2007c) argues that, just as parents have an obligation to prevent and treat disease in their children, they have an obligation to improve their children's lives through genetic enhancement. He sees genetic enhancement as continuous with other kinds of medical and nonmedical interventions, such as people's casual use of caffeine to improve attention, altitude training for athletes, and high blood pressure medications to counteract the natural effects of aging on the circulatory system (Savulescu 2007b, 518). His proposed principle of procreative beneficence means that parents should select "the best child of the possible children one could have" using available genetic tools (Savulescu 2007c, 284). Unlike state-based eugenicist policies, liberal eugenicists like Savulescu appeal to autonomy: medical consumers can determine whether to take advantage of genetic enhancement for themselves and their children according to their own values. The purpose of government regulation is to ensure the safety of such interventions, distribute resources fairly, and establish parameters so that parents are making choices that support their children's future autonomy (Savulescu 2007b, 527–28). But in general we should allow individuals to choose medical interventions, including genetic modification, that prevent or fix naturally occurring conditions that hinder their well-being, as they define it (or as parents define it for their children).

There are several objections to genetic enhancement and to the principle of procreative beneficence in general. As noted earlier, disability rights activists warn that any form of eugenics relies on contingent definitions of health and normalcy that reinforce social stigma against people with disabilities (Asch 2000). In applying the principles of nonmaleficence and beneficence, what counts as well-being needs to be questioned. Other bioethicists raise concerns about the effects of genetic enhancement on basic features of human existence and their significance for how we live—aging, mortality, and finite liberty. For instance, Michael Sandel argues that genetic engineering is "a Promethean aspiration to remake nature, including human nature, to serve our purposes and satisfy our desires" (2004, 54). This "drive to mastery" threatens our ability to confront obstacles, learn humility and resilience, experience effortful achievement, and cultivate empathy for others' limitations. Genetic enhancement seems to treat the person as a set of traits that are valued, instrumentalizing them to bring more of these traits into the world, thereby disrespecting their autonomy—artificially limiting their open-ended pursuit of life-projects—and violating the Kantian prohibition against using someone merely as a means (Habermas 2003; Krimsky 2019, 16). Lastly, since genetic enhancement will have the most powerful effects if done prenatally, this kind of intervention raises the same issues that arise in pediatric research and treatment: How much power should parents have over their child's genome?

Other challenges focus on how genetic enhancements would violate the principle of justice. Positioning patients (or parents) as liberal consumers of medical technology would create inequalities that would intensify across generations. People whose parents could afford genetic enhancements would be privileged in all sorts of ways—intellectually, physically, psychologically—that are not available to those who struggle to access even basic forms of healthcare (Fukuyama 2003; Subica 2023). Related to this concern about justice is how directing resources toward genetic enhancements diverts them from more urgently needed treatments (Murray 2007, 509–10). Finally, it is difficult to anticipate the broad social consequences of genetic enhancement. For instance, it could exacerbate economic inequality or alter definitions of health and normalcy, leading non-enhanced people to identify themselves as disabled (Fukuyama 2003; Wadden 2019).

As with other medical innovations, genetic enhancement is quickly becoming safer and more cost-effective, but bioethical and political debates are lagging behind. These debates tend to be framed in terms of two simplistic extremes: that genetic enhancement is morally problematic because it is unnatural, or that genetic enhancement is one more tool that patients (or parents) can choose if it aligns with their priorities and they can afford it. The first conclusion ignores that many medical interventions are unnatural. Advancements such as in vitro fertilization initially raised anxieties about "playing God" or about slippery slopes to *Brave New World* dystopias, and then they were quickly accepted legally and morally.

The second extreme ignores how much the field of bioethics has learned from rejecting the assumptions at work in eugenics. Eugenicists advocate for realizing human improvement (however that is defined) through deliberate human action rather than the slower process of evolution, a goal shared by contemporary **transhumanists** who argue that we have a moral obligation to use genetic enhancement (Bostrom 2003; see also Levin 2018, 37). But how improvement, health, and well-being get defined in these visions is crucial. Leaving individuals to determine what those mean, rather than the state (as in older forms of eugenics), simply reinforces personal or cultural prejudices such as ableism (Kevles 2015).

Genetic enhancement raises crucial questions about the role of bioethics in medical innovation. Should certain kinds of research be legally prohibited? If so, how would such prohibitions be effective, given divergent national laws, variable enforcement of those laws, and scientific incentives to compete for economically profitable innovations? If not, how can intellectual freedom be balanced with ethical concerns? What kind of informed consent would be necessary? How could benefits to current patients be balanced against long-term consequences for future generations (Cribbs and Perera 2017)? Although consequentialist reasoning, weighing risks and benefits, dominates genetic enhancement debates, there is also room to consider how these interventions impact autonomy. How might they expand the range of ways that parents can promote children's emerging autonomy or exercise their own reproductive freedom? On the other hand, how might they reduce autonomy to consumerist notions of liberty or reinforce existing social biases and forms of discrimination? The core moral issues—balancing autonomy, well-being, and justice—consistently emerge in the history of bioethics. As researchers rapidly expand the scope of genetic enhancement, philosophers must take a more public role in the political debate about how the technology can be ethically applied.

## Stem Cell Research

The question of fetal personhood has implications not only for women's reproductive rights but also for the ethics of medical research on human embryonic stem cells. **Stem cells** are special cells that can differentiate into other kinds of cells, thus generating skin, muscle, nerve, and bone cells. Implanting stem cells into a particular kind of tissue activates genes that make them differentiate into that kind of cell. Stem cells repair injuries and generate new blood cells in all human bodies, but these multipotent cells are less versatile than the pluripotent stem cells found in very young embryos (three to five days old), where they give rise to all the different cells found in the newborn infant. Pluripotent stem cells can also be found in umbilical cord blood and amniotic fluid.

At the beginning of the twentieth century, a Russian hematologist hypothesized that the different types of blood cells (red blood cells, white blood cells, and platelets) must arise from a single kind of "hematopoietic" (blood-making) cell in the bone marrow (Newton 2007, 8). That conclusion was confirmed by researchers in 1963, and further research was done on stem cells in teratomas (a rare kind of tumor made up of various types of body tissue) throughout the 1960s. Stem cells were first isolated and cultured from human embryos in 1998.

It is the plasticity of stem cells that makes them so valuable. Stem cells have the potential to repair or regenerate damaged or diseased tissue, such as heart muscle, spinal neurons, or β-cells in the pancreas, so they may be able to cure heart failure, paralysis, and diabetes, respectively. Apart from these and other regenerative medical uses, stem cells could be used to test the efficacy of new pharmaceutical treatments without posing risks to human subjects. The toxicity of new chemotherapy drugs could be tested on heart tissue generated from stem cells, for instance.

Research on adult stem cells is relatively uncontroversial because they can be removed without harming the person. But those cells are exceedingly rare in the human body and less plastic than embryonic stem cells, so they have less therapeutic potential. Another source of stem cells is "de-differentiated" or reprogrammed cells from adults, in which already specialized cells can be made to act like stem cells. However, it is unclear whether treatment using these cells would cause adverse effects for the patient. Embryonic stem cells are obtained in two different ways: either from existing human embryos (generally, those discarded after in vitro fertilization treatments) or through a cloning process called somatic cell nuclear transfer (SCNT) (Vestal 2008). In both cases, embryos are destroyed through the harvesting of stem cells. It is this step in the process that has led to moral controversy. If life (or more precisely, personhood) begins at conception, then a blastocyst or embryo has the status of a person. On the other hand, if a blastocyst or embryo is a set of cells that is not yet morally considerable, then stem cells can be used to promote the well-being of existing and future persons (Maienschein 2014, 245).

Beyond this central question, moral debates specific to stem cell research concern the timing and nature of informed consent, compensation for donation, and what kind of oversight is appropriate. With regard to the first issue, there is an argument for contemporaneous consent, or consent at the time that embryonic tissue is obtained by researchers, not just consent at the time that embryos are created. Should everyone involved in the creation of the embryo—such as sperm or egg donors—need to consent? The issue of compensation for donated embryonic tissue is linked to the wider issue in research ethics of whether compensation creates coercive conditions or is justified because of the material demands on the donor. Lastly, should ethical oversight of stem cell research take place at a national level, through institutional review boards, or through specialized Embryonic Stem Cell Research Oversight Committees (ESCROs)? These committees can provide more comprehensive scrutiny of research using tissue derived from in vitro fertilization, and they are now required by many journals and organizations funding stem cell research (Hyun 2013, 85–95).

In the United States, stem cell research is federally regulated by two laws. The 1974 Code of Federal Regulations (CFR) prohibits fetal research (covering "the product of conception from implantation until delivery," which includes embryos) unless the health of that particular fetus is "at risk" or "minimal harm" will come to it and the resulting medical knowledge could not otherwise be obtained (45 CFR 46.202, 208). The 1993 version of the U.S. Code allows therapeutic research on fetal and embryonic tissue "after a spontaneous or induced abortion, or after a stillbirth" with the consent of the donor (42 USC 289g-1). In 1995, however, the Dickey-Wicker Amendment was passed, which prohibited the Department of Health and Human Services (HHS), including the National Institutes of Health (NIH), from funding any research that involves "the creation of a human embryo" or "research in which a human embryo or embryos are destroyed, discarded, or knowingly subjected to risk of injury or death greater than that allowed for on research on fetuses in utero" under the 1974 CFR regulation (Balanced Budget Downpayment Act, I, Pub. L. 104–99). In 1997, President Bill Clinton extended this ban to all federal agencies by executive order. In 2001, President George W. Bush attempted to compromise between the moral objections to stem cell research and their medical potential by banning federal funds for research on new stem cell lines but allowing research on existing ones, of which about twenty-one (relatively homogenous) lines turned out to be viable (Murugan 2009). In 2009, President Barack Obama issued an executive order reversing the previous presidential actions and setting up an NIH commission to write a new stem cell research policy. In 2011, an appeals court ruled that the Dickey-Wicker Amendment was ambiguous, and it allowed federal funds to be used to support stem cell research as long as it does not directly destroy an embryo. The NIH allows research on stem cells from embryos that are created through in vitro fertilization for reproductive purposes but are no longer needed, provided they are voluntarily donated by those who underwent the fertilization treatments—in legal terms, the people who own or have custody of the embryos (Kington, n.d.).

Various U.S. states have passed laws promoting or further restricting embryonic stem cell research. For instance, a 2004 California ballot initiative (Proposition 71) made conducting stem cell research a constitutional right, established a process for reviewing research proposals, and funded the California Institute for Regenerative Medicine (CIRM), which was tasked with overseeing grants and loans for stem cell research and developing appropriate regulations. Proposition 71 explicitly bans human cloning as a way of tamping down anxieties about the misuse of stem cells. Lastly, it prohibits treating embryonic stem cells as commodities and establishes procedures for obtaining informed consent from donors. This legislation gained momentum primarily due to patient advocates, especially organizations and individuals focused on diabetes research, arguing that new therapies based on stem cell research were urgently needed (Acosta and Golub 2016). Similar laws have been passed in New Jersey (2004), Massachusetts (2005), Maryland (2006), Missouri (2006), Illinois (2007), Connecticut (2008), and New York (2008). By contrast, other states have moved to ban all fetal and embryonic research or prohibit the use of public funds for stem cell research, including Louisiana (1986), Pennsylvania (1989), North Dakota (2002), and Arkansas (2020). This patchwork of legislation largely mirrors state-level differences in laws regulating abortion.

Internationally, there is also a range of laws governing stem cell research. The United Kingdom was one of the first countries in the world to enact legislation related to stem cell research, perhaps because it was the site of the first baby born using in vitro fertilization (Louise Brown in 1978) and the first nonhuman animal cloning (Dolly the sheep in 1996). The Warnock Report recommended that embryonic research be allowed up to the fourteenth day after fertilization, that trans-species fertilization or gestation be prohibited, and that embryos be "afforded some protection in law," including oversight by ethics committees (Department of Health and Social Security 1984, 84–85). Current British laws permit research on cells derived from both somatic cell nuclear transfer and unused embryos from in vitro fertilization. Singapore is a center of such research and allows research on embryos younger than fourteen days. China allows research using cells from unused embryos produced by in vitro fertilization treatments, from embryos that have been aborted, and from cloned blastocytes (using SCNT). Like U.S. states that support stem cell research, Australia and South Africa ban cloning but allow the use of embryonic stem cells from in vitro fertilization. Over the objections of the Catholic Church, Brazil allows the use of embryonic stem cells derived from in vitro fertilization as long as the embryos have been frozen for more than three years (Dhar and Ho 2009). Other countries, including Portugal, Finland, Germany, and the Philippines, either prohibit cloning (including SCNT) or severely restrict embryonic stem cell research. This fracturing of the legal landscape reflects fundamental anxieties about the moral status of embryos, how embryonic tissue should be produced, and how this technology should be used to improve the health of persons whose moral status is unambiguous.

## Conclusion: Politics of the Body

When new life develops in a woman's body, it becomes a contested political space, and reproductive technologies make it even more complex. One consistent theme is that women's reproductive capacities tend to be politicized, and thus surveillance and regulation are most likely to constrain the bodily autonomy of women. The effects of racial, ethnic, and economic inequalities become more pronounced. Women's rights come into conflict with disability rights. Procreative autonomy fits uneasily in the free market. Can women's capacity to be mothers be bought and sold, or should it only be given away? Are embryos and fetuses persons, potential persons, or commodities? Should unneeded embryos be discarded, adopted, or used for research that may help others? Are selective abortion and genetic enhancement means to a greater humanity or all-too-familiar attempts at creating a master race? In the *Republic*, Plato's ideal state collapses because of the inability to control reproduction. Whether and how to control reproduction and which aspects should be controlled (if any) are now exacerbating some of our deepest social and political divides.

# References

Acosta, Nefi D., and Sidney H. Golub. 2016. "The New Federalism: State Policies Regarding Embryonic Stem Cell Research." *Journal of Law, Medicine & Ethics* 44, no. 3 (September): 419–36. doi:10.1177/1073110516667939.

Albrecht, Gary L., and Patrick J. Devlieger. 1999. "The Disability Paradox: High Quality of Life against All Odds." *Social Science & Medicine* 48, no. 8 (April): 977–88. doi:10.1016/s0277-9536(98)00411-0.

Andrews, Lori B. 1990. "Surrogate Motherhood: The Challenge for Feminists." In *Surrogate Motherhood: Politics and Privacy*, edited by Larry Gostin, 167–82. Bloomington: Indiana University Press.

Asch, Adrienne. 1989. "Reproductive Technology and Disability." In *Reproductive Laws for the 1990s*, edited by Sherrill Cohen and Nadine Taub, 69–124. Clifton, NJ: Humana. doi:0.1007/978-1-4612-3710-5_4.

———. 1999. "Prenatal Diagnosis and Selective Abortion: A Challenge to Practice and Policy." *American Journal of Public Health* 89, no. 11 (November): 1649–57. doi:10.2105/ajph.89.11.1649.

———. 2000. "Why I Haven't Changed My Mind about Prenatal Diagnosis: Reflections and Refinements." In *Prenatal Testing and Disability Rights*, edited by Erik Parens and Adrienne Asch, 234–58. Washington, DC: Georgetown University Press.

Asch, Adrienne, and David Wasserman. 2005. "Where Is the Sin in Synecdoche? Prenatal Testing and the Parent-Child Relationship." In *Quality of Life and Human Difference: Genetic Testing, Health Care, and Disability*, edited by David Wasserman, Jerome Bickenbach, and Robert Wachbroit, 172–216. Cambridge: Cambridge University Press. doi:10.1017/CBO9780511614590.008.

Aznar, Justo, and Miriam Martínez Peris. 2019. "Gestational Surrogacy: Current View." *Linacre Quarterly* 86, no. 1 (February): 56–67. doi:10.1177/0024363919830840.

Barnes, Elizabeth. 2016. *The Minority Body: A Theory of Disability*. Oxford: Oxford University Press. doi:10.1093/acprof:oso/9780198732587.001.0001.

Besharov, Douglas. 1989. "Crack Babies: The Worst Threat Is Mom Herself." *Washington Post*. August 6: B1. https://www.washingtonpost.com/archive/opinions/1989/08/06/crack-babies-the-worst-threat-is-mom-herself/d984f0b2-7598-4dc1-9846-3418df3a5895/.

Blackshaw, Bruce P. 2020. "Genetic Selective Abortion: Still a Matter of Choice." *Ethical Theory and Moral Practice* 23, no. 2 (April): 445–55. doi:10.1007/s10677-020-10080-5.

Bostrom, Nick. 2003. "Human Genetic Enhancements: A Transhumanist Perspective." *Journal of Value Inquiry* 37, no. 4 (December): 493–506. doi:10.1023/b:inqu.0000019037.67783.d5.

Bridges, Khiara M. 2020. "Race, Pregnancy, and the Opioid Epidemic: White Privilege and the Criminalization of Opioid Use During Pregnancy." *Harvard Law Review* 133, no. 3 (January): 770–851. https://harvardlawreview.org/print/vol-133/race-pregnancy-and-the-opioid-epidemic-white-privilege-and-the-criminalization-of-opioid-use-during-pregnancy/.

Buchanan, Allen. 1996. "Choosing Who Will Be Disabled: Genetic Intervention and the Morality of Inclusion." *Social Philosophy and Policy* 13, no. 2 (Summer): 18–46. doi:10.1017/s0265052500003447.

Cavaliere, Giulia. 2022. "Persons and Women, Not Womb-Givers: Reflections on Gestational Surrogacy and Uterus Transplantation." *Bioethics* 36, no. 9 (November): 989–96. doi:10.1111/bioe.13078.

Centers for Disease Control and Prevention. 2019. "What Is Assisted Reproductive Technology?" October 8. https://www.cdc.gov/art/whatis.html.

Chang, M. C. 1959. "Fertilization of Rabbit Ova *In Vitro*." *Nature* 184, no. 4684 (August 8): 466–67. doi:10.1038/184466a0.

Cohen, Laura Beth. 2018. "Informing Consent: Medical Malpractice and the Criminalization of Pregnancy." *Michigan Law Review* 116, no. 7: 1297–316. https://repository.law.umich.edu/mlr/vol116/iss7/4/.

Conrad, Marissa, and James Grifo. 2023. "How Much Does IVF Cost?" *Forbes*. August 14. https://www.forbes.com/health/womens-health/how-much-does-ivf-cost/.

Cooper, Melinda, and Catherine Waldby. 2014. *Clinical Labor: Tissue Donors and Research Subjects in the Global Bioeconomy*. Durham, NC: Duke University Press. doi:10.1215/9780822377009.

Cribbs, Adam P., and Sumeth M. W. Perera. 2017. "Science and Bioethics of CRISPR-Cas9 Gene Editing: An Analysis towards Separating Facts and Fiction." *Yale Journal of Biology and Medicine* 90, no. 4 (December): 625–34. https://pmc.ncbi.nlm.nih.gov/articles/PMC5733851/.

Crocker, Allen C., ed. 2000. Special section on happiness, *American Journal on Mental Retardation* 105, no. 5 (September): 319–416.

Department of Health and Social Security. 1984. *Report of the Committee of Inquiry into Human Fertilisation and Embryology*. London: Her Majesty's Stationery Office. https://www.hfea.gov.uk/media/2608/warnock-report-of-the-committee-of-inquiry-into-human-fertilisation-and-embryology-1984.pdf.

Dhar, Deepali, and John Hsi-En Ho. 2009. "Stem Cell Research Policies around the World." *Yale Journal of Biology and Medicine* 82, no. 3 (September): 113–15. https://pmc.ncbi.nlm.nih.gov/articles/PMC2744936/.

Dickenson, Donna. 2017. *Property in the Body: Feminist Perspectives.* Cambridge: Cambridge University Press. doi:10.1017/9781316675984.

Dirks, Sandhya. 2022. "Criminalization of Pregnancy Has Already Been Happening to the Poor and Women of Color." *NPR.* August 3. https://www.npr.org/2022/08/03/1114181472/criminalization-of-pregnancy-has-already-been-happening-to-the-poor-and-women-of.

Dyson, Lily L. 1991. "Families of Young Children with Handicaps: Parental Stress and Family Functioning." *American Journal on Mental Retardation* 95, no. 6 (May): 623–29.

Ethics Committee of the American Society for Reproductive Medicine. 2017. "Transferring Embryos with Genetic Anomalies Detected in Preimplantation Testing: An Ethics Committee Opinion." *Fertility and Sterility* 107, no. 5 (May): 1130–35. doi:10.1016/j.fertnstert.2017.02.121.

Fukuyama, Francis. 2003. *Our Posthuman Future: Consequences of the Biotechnology Revolution.* New York: Picador.

George, Robert P., and Christopher Tollefsen. 2011. *Embryo: A Defense of Human Life.* 2nd ed. Princeton, NJ: Witherspoon Institute.

Gheaus, Anca. 2024. "Against Private Surrogacy: A Child-Centred View." In *Debating Surrogacy,* by Anca Gheaus and Christine Straehle, 88–148. Oxford: Oxford University Press. doi:10.1093/oso/9780190072162.003.0003.

Gibbons, Gary, and Julie Panepinto. 2023. "FDA Approval of Gene Therapies for Sickle Cell Disease." *National Heart, Lung, and Blood Institute.* December 8. https://www.nhlbi.nih.gov/news/2023/fda-approval-gene-therapies-sickle-cell-disease-dr-gibbons-dr-panepinto.

Gómez, Laura E. 1997. *Misconceiving Mothers: Legislators, Prosecutors, and the Politics of Prenatal Drug Exposure.* Philadelphia: Temple University Press.

Gómez-Lobo, Alfonso. 2005. "On Potentiality and Respect for Embryos: A Reply to Mary Mahowald." *Theoretical Medicine and Bioethics* 26, no. 2 (March): 105–10. doi:10.1007/s11017-005-1235-9.

Goodwin, Michele. 2017. "How the Criminalization of Pregnancy Robs Women of Reproductive Autonomy." In "Just Reproduction: Reimagining Autonomy in Reproductive Medicine," edited by Louise P. King, Rachel L. Zacharias, and Josephine Johnston. Supplement, *Hastings Center Report* 47, no. S3 (December): S19–27. doi:10.1002/hast.791.

———. 2020. *Policing the Womb: Invisible Women and the Criminalization of Motherhood.* New York: Cambridge University Press. doi:10.1017/9781139343244.

Gould, James B. 2020. "Culpable Ignorance, Professional Counselling, and Selective Abortion of Intellectual Disability." *Journal of Bioethical Inquiry* 17, no. 3 (September): 369–81. doi:10.1007/s11673-020-09984-9.

Greely, Henry T. 2019. "CRISPR'd Babies: Human Germline Genome Editing in the 'He Jiankui Affair.'" *Journal of Law and the Biosciences* 6, no. 1 (October): 111–83. doi:10.1093/jlb/lsz010.

Haack, Susan M. 2008. "The Rights and Responsibilities of Pregnant Women." *Ethics & Medicine* 24, no. 3 (Fall): 145–49. https://www.ethicsandmedicine.com/ethics-medicine-volume-243-fall-2008/.

Haas, John M. 1998. "Begotten Not Made: A Catholic View of Reproductive Technology." United States Conference of Catholic Bishops. https://www.usccb.org/issues-and-action/human-life-and-dignity/reproductive-technology/begotten-not-made-a-catholic-view-of-reproductive-technology.

Habermas, Jürgen. 2003. *The Future of Human Nature*. Cambridge: Polity.

Hall, Melinda C. 2013. "Reconciling the Disability Critique and Reproductive Liberty: The Case of Negative Genetic Selection." *International Journal of Feminist Approaches to Bioethics* 6, no. 1 (Spring): 121–43. doi:10.3138/ijfab.6.1.121.

Hanna, Jason K. M. 2010. "Revisiting Child-Based Objections to Commercial Surrogacy." *Bioethics* 24, no. 7 (September): 341–47. doi:10.1111/j.1467-8519.2010.01829.x.

Hansen, Michèle, Jennifer J. Kurinczuk, Elizabeth Milne, Nicholas de Klerk, and Carol Bower. 2013. "Assisted Reproductive Technology and Birth Defects: A Systematic Review and Meta-analysis." *Human Reproduction Update* 19, no. 4 (July–August): 330–53. doi:10.1093/humupd/dmt006.

Hare, R. M. 1988. "When Does Potentiality Count? A Comment on Lockwood." *Bioethics* 2, no. 3 (July): 214–26. doi:10.1111/j.1467-8519.1988.tb00049.x.

Harris, Vicki S., and Susan M. McHale. 1989. "Family Life Problems, Daily Caretaking Activities, and the Psychological Well-Being of Mothers of Mentally Retarded Children." *American Journal of Mental Retardation* 94, no. 3 (November): 231–39.

Henderson, Jane, Ulrik Kesmodel, and Ron Gray. 2007. "Systematic Review of the Fetal Effects of Prenatal Binge-Drinking." *Journal of Epidemiology and Community Health* 61, no. 12 (December): 1069–73. doi:10.1136/jech.2006.054213.

Hubbard, Ruth. 2013. "Abortion and Disability: Who Should and Should Not Inhabit the World?" In *The Disability Studies Reader*, 4th ed., edited by Lennard J. Davis, 74–86. New York: Routledge.

Hurt, Hallam, Nancy Brodsky, Laura Betancourt, Leonard Braitman, Elsa Malmud, and Joan Giannetta. 1995. "Cocaine-Exposed Children:

Follow-Up through 30 Months." *Journal of Developmental & Behavioral Pediatrics* 16, no. 1 (February): 29–35. doi:10.1097/00004703-199502000-00005.

Hyun, Insoo. 2013. *Bioethics and the Future of Stem Cell Research.* Cambridge: Cambridge University Press. doi:10.1017/CBO9780511816031.

Imrie, Susan, and Vasanti Jadva. 2014. "The Long-Term Experiences of Surrogates: Relationships and Contact with Surrogacy Families in Genetic and Gestational Surrogacy Arrangements." *Reproductive BioMedicine Online* 29, no. 4 (October): 424–35. doi:10.1016/j.rbmo.2014.06.004.

Jackson, Rebecca A., Kimberly A. Gibson, Yvonne W. Wu, and Mary S. Croughan. 2004. "Perinatal Outcomes in Singletons Following In Vitro Fertilization: A Meta-analysis." *Obstetrics & Gynecology* 103, no. 3 (March): 551–63. doi:10.1097/01.AOG.0000114989.84822.51.

Jain, Meaghan, and Manvinder Singh. 2024. *Assisted Reproductive Technology (ART) Techniques.* Treasure Island, FL: StatPearls. https://www.ncbi.nlm.nih.gov/books/NBK576409/.

Juengst, Eric. 1998. "What Does Enhancement Mean?" In *Enhancing Human Traits: Ethical and Social Implications,* edited by Erik Parens, 29–47. Washington, DC: Georgetown University Press.

Katler, Quinton S., Jennifer F. Kawwass, Bradley S. Hurst, Amy E. Sparks, David H. McCulloh, Ethan Wantman, and James P. Toner. 2022. "Vanquishing Multiple Pregnancy in In Vitro Fertilization in the United States—A 25-Year Endeavor." *American Journal of Obstetrics & Gynecology* 227, no. 2 (August): 129–35. doi:10.1016/j.ajog.2022.02.005.

Kevles, Daniel J. 2015. "If You Could Design Your Baby's Genes, Would You?" *Politico.* December 9. https://www.politico.com/magazine/story/2015/12/crispr-gene-editing-213425/.

Kington, Raynard S. n.d. "NIH Guidelines for Human Stem Cell Research." National Institutes of Health. Accessed January 15, 2025. https://stemcells.nih.gov/research-policy/guidelines-for-human-stem-cell-research.

Kittay, Eva Feder, and Leo Kittay. 2000. "On the Expressivity and Ethics of Selective Abortion for Disability: Conversations with My Son." In *Prenatal Testing and Disability Rights,* edited by Erik Parens and Adrienne Asch, 165–95. Washington, DC: Georgetown University Press.

Klein, David Alan. 2011. "Medical Disparagement of the Disability Experience: Empirical Evidence for the 'Expressivist Objection.'" *AJOB Primary Research* 2, no. 2: 8–20. doi:10.1080/21507716.2011.594484.

Kneebone, Ezra, Kiri Beilby, and Karin Hammarberg. 2022. "Experiences of Surrogates and Intended Parents of Surrogacy Arrangements: A Systematic Review." *Reproductive BioMedicine Online* 45, no. 4 (October): 815–30. doi:10.1016/j.rbmo.2022.06.006.

Krimsky, Sheldon. 2019. "The Moral Choices on CRISPR Babies." *American Journal of Bioethics* 19, no. 10 (October): 15–16. doi:10.1080/15265161.2019.1644824.

Kuhse, Helga, and Peter Singer. 1982. "The Moral Status of the Embryo: Two Viewpoints." In *Test-Tube Babies: A Guide to Moral Questions, Present Techniques, and Future Possibilities*, edited by William Walters and Peter Singer, 57–63. Oxford: Oxford University Press.

Lagay, Faith. 2001. "Gene Therapy or Genetic Enhancement: Does It Make a Difference?" *AMA Journal of Ethics* 3, no. 2 (February): 37–39. doi:10.1001/virtualmentor.2001.3.2.gnth1-0102.

Levin, Susan B. 2018. "Creating a Higher Breed: Transhumanism and the Prophecy of Anglo-American Eugenics." In *Reproductive Ethics II: New Ideas and Innovations*, edited by Lisa Campo-Edelstein and Paul Burcher, 37–58. Cham: Springer. doi:10.1007/978-3-319-89429-4_4.

Little, Margaret O. 1998. "Cosmetic Surgery, Suspect Norms, and the Ethics of Complicity." In *Enhancing Human Traits: Ethical and Social Implications*, edited by Erik Parens, 162–75. Washington, DC: Georgetown University Press.

Lockwood, Michael. 1988. "Warnock versus Powell (and Harradine): When Does Potentiality Count?" *Bioethics* 2, no. 3 (July): 187–213. doi:10.1111/j.1467-8519.1988.tb00048.x.

Macpherson, Ignacio, María Victoria Roqué, and Ignacio Segarra. 2019. "Ethical Challenges of Germline Genetic Enhancement." *Frontiers in Genetics* 10 (September 3): article no. 767. doi:10.3389/fgene.2019.00767.

Mahowald, Mary B. 2004. "Respect for Embryos and the Potentiality Argument." *Theoretical Medicine and Bioethics* 25, no. 3 (May): 209–14. doi:10.1023/b:meta.0000040065.84498.4c.

Maienschein, Jane. 2014. "Stem-Cell Research Utilizing Embryonic Tissue Should Be Conducted." In *Contemporary Debates in Bioethics*, edited by Arthur L. Caplan and Robert Arp, 237–47. Chichester, UK: Wiley Blackwell.

Mani, Indra. 2021. "CRISPR-Cas9 for Treating Hereditary Diseases." *Progress in Molecular Biology and Translational Science* 181: 165–83. doi:10.1016/bs.pmbts.2021.01.017.

Marinić, Marko, and Tihana Brkljačić. 2008. "Love Over Gold—The Correlation of Happiness Level with Some Life Satisfaction Factors between Persons with and without Physical Disability." *Journal of Developmental and Physical Disabilities* 20, no. 6 (December): 527–40. doi:10.1007/s10882-008-9115-7.

McMahan, Jeff. 2005. "The Morality of Screening for Disability." In "Ethics, Law and Moral Philosophy of Reproductive Biomedicine," edited by Robert G. Edwards, Giuseppe Benagiano, and Edgar Dahl. Supplement, *Reproductive BioMedicine Online* 10, no. S1 (March): 129–32. doi:10.1016/s1472-6483(10)62221-3.

Minkoff, Howard, and Lynn M. Paltrow. 2004. "Melissa Rowland and the Rights of the Pregnant Person." *Obstetrics & Gynecology* 104, no. 6 (December): 1234–36. doi:10.1097/01.AOG.0000146289.65429.48.

Murray, Thomas H. 2007. "Enhancement." In *The Oxford Handbook of Bioethics*, edited by Bonnie Steinbock, 491–515. Oxford: Oxford University Press. doi:10.1093/oxfordhb/9780199562411.003.0022.

Murugan, Varnee. 2009. "Embryonic Stem Cell Research: A Decade of Debate from Bush to Obama." *Yale Journal of Biology and Medicine* 82, no. 3 (September): 101–3. https://pmc.ncbi.nlm.nih.gov/articles/PMC2744932/.

National Council on Disability. 2019. *Quality-Adjusted Life Years and the Devaluation of Life with Disability*. November 6. Washington, DC: National Council on Disability. https://www.ncd.gov/assets/uploads/docs/ncd-quality-adjusted-life-report-508.pdf.

Nazzaro, Miranda. 2024. "Alabama Governor Signs Legislation Protecting IVF Providers into Law." *The Hill*. March 6. https://thehill.com/policy/healthcare/4514729-alabama-governor-signs-legislation-protecting-ivf-providers/.

Newton, David E. 2007. *Stem Cell Research*. New York: Facts on File.

Office for Health Improvement and Disparities, British Department of Health and Social Care. 2024. "Abortion Statistics, England and Wales: 2021." Last modified July 26, 2024. https://www.gov.uk/government/statistics/abortion-statistics-for-england-and-wales-2021/abortion-statistics-england-and-wales-2021.

Okie, Susan. 2009. "The Epidemic That Wasn't." *New York Times*. January 26. https://www.nytimes.com/2009/01/27/health/27coca.html.

Paltrow, Lynn M., and Jeanne Flavin. 2013. "Arrests of and Forced Interventions on Pregnant Women in the United States (1973–2005): The Implications for Women's Legal Status and Public Health." *Journal of Health Politics, Policy and Law* 38, no. 2 (April): 299–343. doi:10.1215/03616878-1966324.

Parens, Erik, and Adrienne Asch. 1999. "The Disability Rights Critique of Prenatal Genetic Testing: Reflections and Recommendations." *Hastings Center Report* 29, no. 5 (September–October): S1–22. doi:10.2307/3527746.

Parry, Bronwyn. 2018. "Surrogate Labour: Exceptional for Whom?" *Economy and Society* 47, no. 2: 214–33. doi:10.1080/03085147.2018.1487180.

Practice Committee of the American Society for Reproductive Medicine. 2017. "Guidance on the Limits to the Number of Embryos to Transfer: A Committee Opinion." *Fertility and Sterility* 107, no. 4 (April): 901–3. doi:10.1016/j.fertnstert.2021.06.050.

Radin, Margaret Jane. 1996. *Contested Commodities: The Trouble with Trade in Sex, Children, Body Parts, and Other Things.* Cambridge, MA: Harvard University Press.

Rae, Scott B. 1994. *The Ethics of Commercial Surrogate Motherhood: Brave New Families?* Westport, CT: Praeger.

Robertson, John A. 1990. "Procreative Liberty and the State's Burden of Proof in Regulating Noncoital Reproduction." In *Surrogate Motherhood: Politics and Privacy*, edited by Larry Gostin, 24–42. Bloomington: Indiana University Press.

Ross, Loretta J., and Rickie Solinger. 2017. *Reproductive Justice: An Introduction.* Oakland: University of California Press.

Ruddick, William. 2000. "Ways to Limit Prenatal Testing." In *Prenatal Testing and Disability Rights*, edited by Erik Parens and Adrienne Asch, 95–107. Washington, DC: Georgetown University Press.

Sandel, Michael J. 2004. "The Case against Perfection." *Atlantic Monthly* 3, no. 293 (April): 51–60. https://www.theatlantic.com/magazine/archive/2004/04/the-case-against-perfection/302927/.

Savulescu, Julian. 2007a. "Future People, Involuntary Medical Treatment in Pregnancy and the Duty of Easy Rescue." *Utilitas* 19, no. 1 (March): 1–20. doi:10.1017/S0953820806002317.

———. 2007b. "Genetic Interventions and the Ethics of Enhancement of Human Beings." In *The Oxford Handbook of Bioethics*, edited by Bonnie Steinbock, 516–35. Oxford: Oxford University Press. doi:10.1093/oxfordhb/9780199562411.003.0023.

———. 2007c. "In Defence of Procreative Beneficence." *Journal of Medical Ethics* 33, no. 5 (May): 284–88. doi:10.1136/jme.2006.018184.

Saxton, Marsha. 2013. "Disability Rights and Selective Abortion." In *The Disability Studies Reader*, edited by Lennard J. Davis, 87–99. New York: Routledge.

Sen, Esine, and Sabire Yurtsever. 2007. "Difficulties Experienced by Families with Disabled Children." *Journal for Specialists in Pediatric Nursing* 12, no. 4 (October): 238–52. doi:10.1111/j.1744-6155.2007.00119.x.

Shakespeare, Tom. 1998. "Choices and Rights: Eugenics, Genetics and Disability Equality." *Disability & Society* 13, no. 5: 665–81. doi:10.1080/09687599826452.

Sharp, Keith, and Sarah Earle. 2002. "Feminism, Abortion and Disability: Irreconcilable Differences?" *Disability & Society* 17, no. 2: 137–45. doi:10.1080/09687590120122297.

Singhi, Pratibha D., Lokender Goyal, Dwarka Pershad, Sunit Singhi, and B. N. S. Walia. 1990. "Psychosocial Problems in Families of Disabled Children." *British Journal of Medical Psychology* 63, no. 2 (June): 173–82. doi:10.1111/j.2044-8341.1990.tb01610.x.

Smith, S. E. 2019. "Disabled People Are Tired of Being a Talking Point in the Abortion Debate." *Vox*. May 29. https://www.vox.com/first-person/2019/5/29/18644320/abortion-ban-2019-selective-abortion-ban-disability.

Snowden, Robert, Geoffrey Duncan Mitchell, and E. M. Snowden. 1983. *Artificial Reproduction: A Social Investigation*. London: Allen and Unwin.

Söderström-Anttila, Viveca, Ulla-Britt Wennerholm, Anne Loft, Anja Pinborg, Kristiina Aittomäki, Liv Bente Romundstad, and Christina Bergh. 2016. "Surrogacy: Outcomes for Surrogate Mothers, Children and the Resulting Families—A Systematic Review." *Human Reproduction Update* 22, no. 2 (March–April): 260–76. doi:10.1093/humupd/dmv046.

Stainton, Tim, and Hilde Besser. 1998. "The Positive Impact of Children with an Intellectual Disability on the Family." *Journal of Intellectual & Developmental Disability* 23, no. 1: 57–70. doi:10.1080/13668259800033581.

Steinbock, Bonnie. 1990. "Surrogate Motherhood as Prenatal Adoption." In *Surrogate Motherhood: Politics and Privacy*, edited by Larry Gostin, 123–35. Bloomington: Indiana University Press.

———. 2000. "Disability, Prenatal Testing, and Selective Abortion." In *Prenatal Testing and Disability Rights*, edited by Erik Parens and Adrienne Asch, 108–23. Washington, DC: Georgetown University Press.

Steptoe, P. C., and R. G. Edwards. 1978. "Birth after Reimplantation of a Human Embryo." *Lancet* 312, no. 8085 (August 12): 366. doi:10.1016/s0140-6736(78)92957-4.

Steward, Ryan G., Lan Lan, Anish A. Shah, Jason S. Yeh, Thomas M. Price, James M. Goldfarb, and Suheil J. Muasher. 2014. "Oocyte Number as a Predictor for Ovarian Hyperstimulation Syndrome and Live Birth: An Analysis of 256,381 In Vitro Fertilization Cycles." *Fertility and Sterility* 101, no. 4 (April): 967–73. doi:10.1016/j.fertnstert.2013.12.026.

Straehle, Christine. 2024. "Defending Surrogacy as Reproductive Labour." In *Debating Surrogacy*, by Anca Gheaus and Christine Straehle, 17–87. Oxford: Oxford University Press. doi:10.1093/oso/9780190072162.001.0001.

Subica, Andrew M. 2023. "CRISPR in Public Health: The Health Equity Implications and Role of Community in Gene-Editing Research and Applications." *American Journal of Public Health* 113, no. 8 (August): 874–82. doi:10.2105/AJPH.2023.307315.

"Surrogate Parenting Agreement." 1985. http://eric_goldman.tripod.com/contracts/babymcontracts.htm.

Thomson, Judith Jarvis. 1971. "A Defense of Abortion." *Philosophy & Public Affairs* 1, no. 1 (Autumn): 47–66. https://www.jstor.org/stable/2265091.

U.S. Department of Health and Human Services. 2024. "Fact Sheet: In Vitro Fertilization (IVF) Use across the United States." March 13. https://www.hhs.gov/about/news/2024/03/13/fact-sheet-in-vitro-fertilization-ivf-use-across-united-states.html.

Vestal, Christy. 2008. "The Science behind Stem Cell Research." Pew Research Center. July 17. https://www.pewresearch.org/religion/2008/07/17/the-science-behind-stem-cell-research/.

Wadden, Jordan Joseph. 2019. "Yesterday's Child, Tomorrow's Therapy Patient: What Are the Roles of Health and Normalcy in Genetic Enhancement?" *American Journal of Bioethics* 19, no. 7 (July): 43–45. doi:10.1080/15265161.2019.1618954.

Wallis, Jacqueline Mae. 2020. "Is It Ever Morally Permissible to Select for Deafness in One's Child?" *Medicine, Health Care and Philosophy* 23, no. 1 (March): 3–15. doi:10.1007/s11019-019-09922-6.

Wilkinson, Stephen. 2023. "Surrogacy: The Ethics of Paid Surrogacy." In *The Routledge Handbook of Commodification*, edited by Elodie Bertrand and Vida Panitch, 303–20. London: Routledge.

Winfield, Nicole. 2024. "Right to Children or Children's Rights? Surrogacy Debate Comes to a Head in Rome." *Associated Press*. April 5. https://apnews.com/article/vatican-surrogacy-ivf-a9229ef32f3c5b4f3b0bb7bd0e08f503.

Yau, Annie, Rachel L. Friedlander, Allison Petrini, Mary Catherine Holt, Darrell E. White II, Joseph Shin, Sital Kalantry, and Steven Spandorfer. 2021. "Medical and Mental Health Implications of Gestational Surrogacy." *American Journal of Obstetrics & Gynecology* 225, no. 3 (September): 264–69. doi:10.1016/j.ajog.2021.04.213.

Ziegler, Mary. 2017. "The Disability Politics of Abortion." *Utah Law Review* 3: 587–631. https://dc.law.utah.edu/ulr/vol2017/iss3/4.

## FURTHER READING

Anomaly, Jonathan. 2024. *Creating Future People: The Science and Ethics of Genetic Enhancement*. 2nd ed. New York: Taylor & Francis.

> An accessible introduction to the bioethical issues raised by genetic enhancement. Anomaly explains the technological background of genetic enhancement and provides an overview of the moral debates around a range of possible enhancements: cognitive, moral (including enhancing social bonding), aesthetic, and immunological. He also addresses the possibility of synthesizing genetic replicas of existing people. These debates lead to discussions of broader moral issues in reproduction and genetics, such as the desire for immortality and respect for autonomy.

Bridges, Khiara M. 2022. "The Dysgenic State: Environmental Injustice and Disability-Selective Abortion Bans." *California Law Review* 110, no. 2: 297–369. doi:10.15779/Z38P843X00.
> Claims that when states both subject people to defect-causing environmental harms and legally prohibit disability-selective abortion, they force the production of impaired citizens—dysgenics rather than eugenics. Bridges argues that people of color are disproportionately affected since they are more often exposed to environmental toxins and are more likely to experience poverty, thus being unable to avoid abortion restrictions.

Howard, Grace E. 2024. *The Pregnancy Police: Conceiving Crime, Arresting Personhood*. Oakland: University of California Press.
> Surveys the trend in the U.S. of charging more pregnant women with crimes against their fertilized eggs, embryos, and fetuses. Howard shows how these recent trends are part of a long history going back to white supremacist eugenics in the early twentieth century. In addition to analyzing the different legal justifications, she also reveals how many healthcare professionals support this practice by reporting their patients.

Human Embryonic Stem Cell Research Advisory Committee, National Research Council and Institute of Medicine. 2010. *Final Report of the National Academies' Human Embryonic Stem Cell Research Advisory Committee and 2010 Amendments to the National Academies' Guidelines for Human Embryonic Stem Cell Research*. Washington, DC: National Academies Press. doi:10.17226/12923.
> The most recent edition of the National Academies' guidelines regulating human embryonic stem cell research. These regulations largely align with the International Society for Stem Cell Research standards. They provide ethical guidance on communicating with gamete and embryo donors, how stem cells should be used, the creation of oversight (ESCRO) committees, and international collaboration between researchers.

International Society for Stem Cell Research. 2021. *ISSCR Guidelines for Stem Cell Research and Clinical Translation*. May. https://www.isscr.org/guidelines.
> Voluntary regulations for stem cell research, written by and for stem cell researchers, regardless of national legal contexts. The guidelines begin with a review of fundamental ethical principles and then apply them to a range of issues specific to stem cell research: obtaining stem cells (including informed consent), using stem cells in human experimentation, and regulatory oversight.

Killian, Caitlin. 2023. *Failing Moms: The Social Condemnation and Criminalization of Mothers*. Cambridge: Polity.

> An analysis of the ideal of motherhood in contemporary society and how it imposes disproportionate expectations and burdens on women before, during, and after pregnancy. Killian uses a reproductive justice lens to examine how women of color and lower socioeconomic class are particularly harmed by these expectations through legal and more informal repercussions. The author discusses various solutions to address these inequities.

Markens, Susan. 2007. *Surrogate Motherhood and the Politics of Reproduction*. Berkeley: University of California Press.

> Uses the Baby M case and a court case in California (*Johnson v. Calvert* [1993]) as lenses to understand America's complex views on parenthood and the state's duty to protect children. Taking a sociological approach, Markens looks at how legislators, judges, women's groups, religious organizations, and the media responded to these cases, and why the resulting policies in New York and California were so different, depending on whether they emphasized the plight of infertile couples or defined surrogacy as baby-selling. She also analyzes the gendered and racial dynamics that shape the politics of reproduction in the U.S.

Parens, Erik, and Adrienne Asch, eds. 2000. *Prenatal Testing and Disability Rights*. Washington, DC: Georgetown University Press.

> A collection of eighteen essays compiled at the end of a two-year project, organized by the Hastings Center, on the disability rights critique of prenatal testing for genetic disability. Chapters describe the history and then-current state of genetic testing in the U.S.; the impact of prenatal testing, selective abortion, and disability on the experience of parenting; whether prenatal testing sends discriminatory messages to disabled people; and policy implications for lawmakers, the courts, and medical professionals.

Schondorf-Gleicher, Anja von, Lyka Mochizuki, Raoul Orvieto, Pasquale Patrizio, Arthur S. Caplan, and Norbert Gleicher. 2022. "Revisiting Selected Ethical Aspects of Current Clinical In Vitro Fertilization (IVF) Practice." *Journal of Assisted Reproduction and Genetics* 39, no. 3 (March): 591–604. doi:10.1007/s10815-022-02439-7.

> A review of the medical literature on IVF from 2010 to 2021, along with an analysis of the ethical issues discussed and neglected. The authors conclude that the following topics need to be reassessed in light of recent changes in clinical practice: whether human embryos are deserving of special consideration; ethical responsibilities of professional organizations; ethical responsibilities of physicians and IVF centers; commercialization

of IVF; data analysis and the peer-review process; and cryopreservation of gametes, embryos, and reproductive tissues.

Tsai, Shelun, Kathryn Shaia, Julia T. Woodward, Michael Y. Sun, and Suheil J. Muasher. 2020. "Surrogacy Laws in the United States: What Obstetrician-Gynecologists Need to Know." *Obstetrics & Gynecology* 135, no. 3 (March): 717–22. doi:10.1097/AOG.0000000000003698.

Surveys the legal history of surrogacy in the U.S. and legislation in different states. Focusing on issues especially relevant to obstetricians and gynecologists, the authors set out the elements of informed consent and propose clinical recommendations for working with surrogates and intended parents at every stage of the surrogacy, including prior to conception, during the pregnancy, and after delivery.

# CHAPTER 7
# Advance Directives and Decision-Making for Incapacitated Patients

**Key topics in this chapter:**

- The distinction between legal competence and medical capacity for decision-making
- How medical decisions are made for incompetent or incapacitated patients using the substituted judgment and best interests standards
- The two kinds of advance directives: substantive directives and proxy directives
- Why advance directives are necessary, and their limitations

## Introduction

As we have discussed, patient autonomy has been the dominant value in medical ethics for the last half-century. But the phrase "patient autonomy" is almost a contradiction. The root of the term "patient," along with "pathology," is passivity, the undergoing of a process, as opposed to being the agent directing a process. Patients are likely to be somewhere on a spectrum of diminished autonomy—to the extreme of being unconscious or cognitively incapacitated when medical decisions need to be made. What should be done when patients are unable to express their wishes? As a way of temporally extending patient autonomy, legal systems and healthcare ethicists have, over the last several decades, recognized the authority of advance care directives, which record patient preferences about who should make decisions or what decisions should be made when a patient is unable to do it themselves.

## Legal Competence versus Medical Capacity

Some of the most difficult medical questions and legal conflicts have been caused by the problem of how to treat incompetent patients. Two terms that tend to be used interchangeably in informal settings are important to distinguish here: **competence** refers to the legal determination that one can make decisions for oneself, whereas **capacity** describes the ability to participate in medical decision-making, which clinicians assess situationally. Competence is a "global assessment" of the legal status of the person, whereas capacity is a "functional assessment" of what they can do (Hegde and Ellajosyula 2016). Competence is a binary category: one is either competent or incompetent. Adults (over eighteen) are presumed to be competent unless they are legally determined not to be. By contrast, capacity is a spectrum, defined by the same cognitive abilities that allow for informed consent: the abilities to (1) communicate one's choices clearly, either verbally or nonverbally; (2) understand the alternatives relevant to their current situation; (3) appreciate the overall significance of those alternatives, not only the facts; and (4) engage in reasoning about those alternatives—for instance, considering their risks and benefits (Grisso and Applebaum 1998). Understanding the facts of a condition in an abstract sense is different from appreciating the meaning of those facts in one's own case. For example, a patient may understand that stage 4 lung cancer is life-threatening and may acknowledge that they are having trouble breathing while simultaneously denying that their respiratory impairment stems from advanced cancer.

Determining capacity is not a legal finding but a judgment of clinicians and hospital ethics boards—which may spill into legal proceedings to determine competence if patients themselves or family members disagree with clinicians' judgments. The easy cases are infants, people with severe disabilities, people completely unable to communicate their wishes, and people in comas or **persistent vegetative states (PVS)** (also called prolonged vegetative state or unresponsive wakefulness syndrome [UWS], a chronic condition in which the patient has no physical or emotional response and lacks awareness). Easy cases also involve forms of clearly temporary incapacity, such as people who are currently intoxicated or who have suffered a stroke. But how should we treat older children or adolescents, who in a legal sense are presumed to be incompetent until the age of eighteen? What are the rights of minimally conscious patients, who have some awareness of their surroundings and are capable of basic reactions, but are not capable of complex cognition? And what do we do with marginally functional people who are experiencing a gradual but erratic decline in cognitive ability, such as patients suffering from dementia who are sometimes relatively lucid and forceful in expressing their wishes and then confused and incommunicative at other times?

One prevalent method to assess capacity involves healthcare practitioners interviewing patients to measure the four decision-making skills crucial to informed consent, using an instrument such as the MacArthur Competence Assessment Tool for Treatment (MacCAT-T) or the Aid to Capacity Evaluation (ACE). Interviews typically take fifteen to twenty minutes, and after an explanation of their current medical state and their alternatives, clinicians ask patients to paraphrase that information and explain how they weigh the risks and benefits of their options. The questions on the MacCAT-T are specific to the patient's current situation rather than abstract, so the assessment of capacity can be part of the patient's decision-making process (Grisso and Applebaum 1998). Accurately assessing capacity matters so that clinicians can support a patient's autonomy, if they are in fact capable of participating in decision-making to some degree, and can protect their welfare if they are not.

## Substituted Judgment and Best Interests Standards

If a patient is incapacitated and, like a majority of U.S. adults, has not left formal instructions about a **proxy** or **surrogate** who should make medical decisions for them, hospitals or other healthcare professionals try to identify one using a **surrogate hierarchy**. The process is governed by state law, but there is a typical order of people who are considered or asked to serve as proxies:

1. Court-appointed guardian, also called a guardian ad litem, if any. This proxy would be designated as part of a legal decision in which the patient's incompetence has been established, and (usually) some conflict has arisen about whether someone currently serving as a medical proxy is making legitimate decisions on behalf of the patient.
2. Patient-designated healthcare proxy
3. Spouse or domestic partner (even if separated)
4. Adult children

5. Parents
6. Adult siblings
7. Other relatives
8. Close friends
9. Any adult who is familiar with the patient's medical situation, has exhibited care and concern for the patient, and is available to make decisions, as long as the person is not the patient's clinician

If a patient has multiple adult children or multiple adult siblings, the decision of a majority of those willing to serve as medical proxies is binding. The surrogate hierarchy suggests a few ways in which not leaving instructions in advance can complicate medical decision-making: whoever acts as the proxy may have little guidance (either in writing or through previous conversations) about the patient's wishes, people designated as proxies may disagree with each other about what should be done, and people who think that they should be proxies may disagree with the actual proxy's decisions.

In the United States, the more formal process for deciding for incapacitated patients was legally established in a case decided by the Supreme Court of New Jersey in 1985, *In the Matter of Claire C. Conroy* (98 N.J. 321, 486 A.2d 1209). Claire Conroy was an elderly woman suffering from "severe organic brain syndrome" who was deemed incompetent. Due to her physical ailments, she was placed on a feeding tube. Her nephew wanted to have the tube removed, which would result in her death. The court ruled that, when a patient is incompetent, medical decisions should be made by their proxy using two disparate approaches: either (1) interpreting and communicating the priorities of the patient (**substituted judgment**), (2) promoting the current welfare of the patient regardless of their own previously stated wishes (**best interests**), or a combination of the two. The substituted judgment standard emphasizes patient autonomy. Proxies must consider any (even informal) evidence of what the now-incompetent patient would have wanted for themselves. Has the person made claims about whether they would want to live if they were in a persistent vegetative state, were cognitively impaired, or were dependent on a ventilator or feeding tube to prolong their life? In the absence of such evidence, the best interests standard emphasizes nonmaleficence and beneficence. Proxies must make objective judgments about what patients are currently experiencing: if they are in pain and whether that pain can be managed, if they seem to be aware of their environment and how they interact with it, if they can communicate, and if there are things they enjoy. There is a utilitarian underpinning to the latter approach: What benefits and burdens is a person currently experiencing, given their state of consciousness, and do the benefits outweigh the burdens? The majority opinion in *Conroy* makes clear that the person's own interests have to be evaluated, not their "personal worth or social utility" (367). Another way to understand the two approaches is that the first takes another competent person to be responsible for speaking on behalf of the patient subjectively, trying to interpret what their decisions would be from the first-person standpoint, while the second requires that they take the third-person perspective, determining what is objectively best for the patient in their particular medical circumstances.

In trying to take into account both subjective and objective evidence, the *Conroy* case establishes three standards:

1. **Subjective standard**: If a person, while competent, clearly articulated their medical wishes—in an advance directive, or even verbally to a clinician or their medical proxy—those wishes should be followed. Such evidence should be considered in terms of its remoteness, consistency, and thoughtfulness. Were the statements made recently or several decades ago? Has the person steadily maintained those wishes, or are there countervailing statements? Were they made casually or seriously?

2. **Limited-objective standard**: In the absence of clear articulations of the patient's wishes, less formal evidence of what they want can be combined with what is objectively in their best interests to reach a decision: "Life-sustaining treatment may be withheld or withdrawn . . . when there is some trustworthy evidence that the patient would have refused the treatment, and the decision-maker is satisfied that it is clear that the burdens of the patient's continued life with the treatment outweigh the benefits of that life for him" (365).

3. **Pure-objective standard**: If there is no trustworthy evidence about the patient's wishes or the patient has never been competent, then the proxy must use the best interests standard to determine which treatments, if any, will benefit them. In those cases where the person's wishes are completely unknown, then a lot of suffering on one

side of the scale would outweigh the presumption that we should keep them alive.

In other words, the law stipulates that the substituted judgment approach takes priority if the person's wishes can be discerned, and the best interests approach must be used if they cannot.

These two approaches may not be entirely distinguishable, however. Determining what is in the best interests of this particular patient (as opposed to some generic "reasonable" person) can be interpreted to mean taking into account their basic values. Even young children and people with cognitive disabilities are likely to demonstrate preferences about what they find valuable and what they think is worth preserving in their lives. Therefore, establishing a person's best interests, in the broad sense of what supports their well-being, cannot be an entirely objective process (Cantor 2005). Limited capacity does not disqualify a patient from having and communicating their priorities, so we should attempt a "best interpretation" of their will and preferences when possible.

## Case Study: Terri Schiavo

The difficulties of making decisions for incompetent patients using the substituted judgment and best interests standards are dramatically illustrated by the hyper-publicized case of Terri Schiavo. In 1990, at the age of twenty-six, Terri suffered cardiac arrest as the result of an eating disorder. Irreversible brain damage begins after about four minutes of anoxia, and her brain was deprived of oxygen for at least eleven minutes. Resuscitated by emergency medical personnel, she first was comatose and then lapsed into a persistent vegetative state. She left no formal instructions as to whether she wished life-sustaining treatment to continue in these circumstances.

Terri's husband, Michael Schiavo, was designated as her medical proxy, and for the first few years he worked closely with her parents to try to help her recover brain function. In 1993, he accepted the prognosis of Terri's doctors that she would not recuperate from her "wakeful unresponsiveness" (Jennett and Plum 1972, 734): her brain stem was supporting the automatic physiological functions of respiration, heartbeat, sleep-wake cycles, and digestion, but no higher brain function would be recovered. Michael remembered his wife saying that she did not "want to be kept alive on a machine," and he requested a Do Not Resuscitate (DNR) order (Weijer 2005, 1197). In 1998, he petitioned to remove her feeding tube.

Terri's parents opposed his decision based on their Catholic faith. The Catholic Church claims that **ordinary care**, such as nutrition and hydration, is what all human beings need to survive, and it can usually be provided without long-term aggressive or costly interventions. By contrast, **extraordinary care**, such as the use of a respirator that merely prolongs a terminal illness, may involve excessive burdens or offer no hope of benefits. Patients are morally entitled to the former but not the latter (Committee for Pro-Life Activities 1992). Terri's parents also maintained that she was not in a persistent vegetative state but instead had suffered a severe brain injury, from which she could recover and despite which she was at least minimally conscious.

So began a seven-year legal battle about who should function as her medical proxy and whether any legally legitimate preferences could be drawn from Terri's previous casual statements to friends and family members. Accusations of financial incentives and intimate partner violence were made as part of the legal contestation of Michael's role as proxy. Through multiple trials and appeals, both Florida state and federal courts affirmed that Terri was in a persistent vegetative state, that Michael was acting appropriately as her medical proxy, and that she had informally indicated, prior to her incapacity, her desire not to live dependent on artificial support. On this basis, the courts found he had the authority to remove the feeding tube. Terri's parents found physicians who disputed the prognosis, and they claimed that Michael wrongly reported her previously expressed wishes.

As an outgrowth of the legal dispute, Terri's parents increasingly publicized the case and appealed to state and federal politicians, including Florida Governor Jeb Bush and U.S. President George W. Bush. Disability rights advocates and pro-life groups, including the Catholic Church, supported their position, while the right-to-die movement advocated for Michael's choice to end Terri's life. This legal and political turmoil culminated in March 2005, after Terri's feeding tube had been removed by a court order, with a rushed vote by the U.S. Congress to transfer jurisdiction of the case to federal court (Pub. L. 109-3). However, the U.S. Court of Appeals for the Eleventh Circuit denied her parents' petitions to become Terri's medical proxies and continue her hydration and nutrition. The U.S. Supreme Court declined to review the decision of the lower court. So, on March 31, 2005, thirteen days after the removal of her feeding tube and fifteen years after her cardiac arrest, Terri Schiavo was pronounced dead.

An autopsy revealed that much of Terri's brain had atrophied (weighing about half of what a typical adult brain in a person of her size would weigh), presumably as a result of oxygen deprivation, and that she would not have been able to recover higher brain function. In other words, the diagnosis of irreversible, persistent vegetative state was confirmed (Charatan 2005). For incompetent and incapacitated patients, uncertain or conflicting prognoses become especially difficult to navigate. Just as the patient's wishes can be interpreted in contradictory ways by different family members (substituted judgment), so too empirical information about a patient's current condition and medical prospects can be sources of conflict, especially when clinicians offer different judgments based on limited evidence (best interests).

The medical condition of being in a persistent vegetative state raises important questions about our obligations to patients who are not conscious and cannot regain consciousness. Has the person died even though the brain stem continues to direct automatic biological functions? When can organs be harvested for transplant? Is there some value to continued existence if higher brain function cannot be recovered? Should the person be kept alive, such that their body continues to function biologically, or is that demeaning to the person? There are empirical questions alongside the moral ones, including the extent of a patient's brain damage and their prognosis.

Legally, in the U.S. and most of Europe, **whole-brain death**—the irreversible cessation of all brain functions, including the brain stem—is the standard for determining whether someone has died. On this view, Terri Schiavo was alive because she had only lost her higher brain functions—hence the need to make medical decisions on her behalf. But philosophers continue to debate the definition of death, since the basic question of whether a person is alive or dead is a metaphysical, nonempirical issue that rests on highly debated conceptions of what is essential to personhood. Philosophers such as Jeff McMahan (1995), for example, have argued that we should distinguish the death of the person (irreversible loss of the capacity for consciousness) from the biological death of the physical organism (irreversible loss of the organism's functional integrity). Cerebral death is sufficient for the death of the person, even if the brain stem is still functioning. As a way to capture this intuition, the family of Nancy Cruzan (who was severely injured in a car accident and kept alive on artificial support for seven years) recorded two different dates on her tombstone: "departed Jan. 11, 1983" and "at peace Dec. 26, 1990."

Deciding whether to withhold or withdraw life-sustaining treatment for incompetent and incapacitated patients in the absence of advance directives raises the moral question of how to evaluate what kind of life is worth living. Justifications for ending a person's life that invoke compassion and dignity, or that calculate the proper use of scarce healthcare resources, may also be used to support euthanizing people with severe disabilities. In fact, the Catholic Church sided with "moral theologians" who claimed that Terri Schiavo was disabled, not terminally ill, and thus should not have been euthanized: "PVS is best seen as an extreme form of mental and physical disability . . . and not as a terminal illness or fatal pathology from which patients should generally be allowed to die" (Committee for Pro-Life Activities 1992, 43). Our cultural conceptions about what makes a life worthwhile come into play in these discussions, which ideally would function as opportunities to reflect critically on those judgments.

## The History of Advance Directives

The Terri Schiavo case poses such complex questions because she survived the initial medical crisis but remained unresponsive for years afterward, which was made possible by medical advancements that keep people alive in situations that would have quickly led to their deaths for most of human history. Until the twentieth century, decision-making about the circumstances under which someone would live or die was relatively limited. And given the prevailing attitude of paternalism, those decisions were likely to be made by physicians, acting on their interpretation of the principle of beneficence. Those same medical advancements mean that many more people now live long enough to experience diminished cognitive capacity, such that establishing their medical priorities in advance has become more urgent. A major factor here is dementia: Alzheimer's disease alone affects 17 percent of people age seventy-five to eighty-four and 32 percent of people over eighty-five. Emergency medical techniques and artificial support mean that patients can be resuscitated or otherwise survive life-threatening events and then can be almost indefinitely kept alive. If those people are relatively young, they can survive for decades in a persistent vegetative state. Increasingly sophisticated analgesics and sedatives can manage pain, but they also diminish patients' awareness and ability to interact meaningfully with others. This series of changes in medical care began to raise the question in the wider culture about whether prolonging a patient's existence was always morally justified, either because it violated their wishes or did not ultimately benefit them. Finally, more people have experienced firsthand or witnessed diseases associated with old age, such as cancer, dementia, and heart disease, thereby raising questions about which medical interventions would be worthwhile to support their quality of life.

This combination of the emphasis on patient autonomy and increased longevity produces the legal and medical landscape for advance directives. Like other advance directives, such as instructions for organ donation after death or mental health treatment if a patient is incapacitated, advance care directives attempt to establish people's wishes in a legally binding form, while they are still capable of medical decision-making, for what they want or who should make choices regarding their treatment if they lose that capacity at the end of life. In keeping with common practice among bioethicists, we will refer to them simply as **advance directives**. They were first proposed in the late 1960s by Luis Kutner, a human rights lawyer who witnessed the protracted and painful death of a close friend. In association with the Euthanasia Society of America—an organization that advocated not for active euthanasia but for patients' right to choose when and how they die—Kutner proposed what he called a **living will**. He began from the idea that "the law provides that a patient may not be subjected to treatment without his consent" (1969, 550). As Kutner understood it, the living will allows patients to agree or not agree to treatment in advance, and it protects clinicians against liability (typically an issue when withdrawing or withholding life-sustaining treatment) as long as they follow the patient's instructions. Kutner imagined a living will functioning like a property will: a way to claim autonomy over something a person currently controls (their body or their estate) after the person is no longer capable of exercising that autonomy, with the presumption that others will respect those wishes. California adopted the first living will law in 1976, with almost every state following suit over the next decade.

Around this same period of the mid-1970s, a few well-publicized cases of people in persistent vegetative states, including Karen Ann Quinlan and Nancy Cruzan, raised legal and moral questions about whether or when patients who are no longer competent could be removed from life-sustaining treatment. Cruzan was a woman who was severely injured in a car accident and resuscitated by emergency medical technicians but never regained consciousness. She was diagnosed to be in a persistent vegetative state soon after the accident. After five years of treatment, her parents requested that her feeding tube be removed. Her chronic care facility and the state public health department refused. After a series of conflicting legal judgments, the U.S. Supreme Court ruled in June 1990 that competent patients have the right to refuse treatment but that incompetent patients must have provided "clear and convincing" evidence of their wishes (*Cruzan v. Director, Missouri Department of Health*, 497 U.S. 261). In Cruzan's case, a casual remark to a friend before the accident was seen as not meeting that standard, so the hospital's position was affirmed. However, following the decision, the family gathered additional evidence about Cruzan's wishes, and the Missouri Department of Health chose not to oppose the family's request to remove her feeding tube, leading to Cruzan's death in December 1990.

In *Cruzan*, Justice Sandra Day O'Connor specifically recommended using advance directives to avoid such legal disputes. This led Congress to pass the Patient Self-Determination Act (PSDA) (HR 4449 [1990]), which requires states to offer people some form of advance directive: a substantive or proxy directive, or both (McCloskey 1991). Several prominent medical organizations promote advance directives, including the National Council for Death and Dying, the Veterans Administration, and the American Medical Association's Council on Ethical and Judicial Affairs. Healthcare professionals, hospitals, chronic care facilities, and lawyers also encourage the use of advance directives, especially for older adults. Despite several decades of these efforts, as of 2017, only 36.7 percent of American adults had completed advance directives, including 45 percent of people sixty-five and older (Yadav et al. 2017).

## Substantive Directives and Proxy Directives

When a patient is only temporarily incapacitated, clinicians typically wait until the patient can decide for themselves. But when delays would worsen the patient's condition or when the patient permanently lacks decision-making capacity, clinicians consult an advance directive to do what the patient said they would want in these circumstances. There are two kinds of advance directives: substantive directives and proxy directives. **Substantive directives** are living wills. They provide written instructions to healthcare practitioners, typically around what medical interventions are and are not wanted when patients have terminal conditions and are unable to think clearly or communicate their wishes in real time. Since patients complete advance directives before they are incapacitated, substantive directives are often structured by hypotheticals. For example, if a patient has no reasonable expectation of recovery, they may affirm their desire for any necessary artificial hydration and nutrition, as well as palliative care, but no extraordinary measures to prolong their lives, such as ventilators or more aggressive life-prolonging treatments. Ideally, patients should discuss their substantive directives with family members and clinicians, so that those wishes are actually consulted when making decisions. However, directives are not signed by medical professionals because they are legal documents, not medical orders. Templates for advance directives usually suggest that the person's signature be validated by witnesses and notarized to establish the legal standing of the directive. However, advance directives need not be written or recorded in any particular form to be legally binding.

Substantive directives need to be clear and specific to be effective: a refusal of "heroic" measures leaves open a wide array of interpretations, as opposed to the refusal of a ventilator if there is no reasonable chance of recovery. Templates often include prompts to encourage people to articulate what minimum quality of life means to them and then specify treatments they would refuse if their condition falls below that threshold. A typical question provides checklists written in accessible language that also emphasizes medical clarity:

> I desire that my doctor make a concerted effort to return me to an acceptable quality of life using then available treatments and therapies. However, if my quality of life becomes unacceptable as I have defined below, and my doctors have determined that my condition will not improve (is irreversible), I direct that all treatments that extend my life be withdrawn. An unacceptable quality of life means (initial and check all that apply):
>
> _____ ☐ Chronic coma or persistent vegetative state
>
> _____ ☐ No longer able to communicate my needs
>
> _____ ☐ No longer able to recognize family or friends
>
> _____ ☐ Total dependence on others for daily care

_____ ☐ Other: _____.

Initial and check one (1) only:

_____ ☐ Even if I have the quality of life described above, I still wish to be treated with food and water by tube or intravenously (IV).

_____ ☐ If I have the quality of life described above, I do NOT wish to be treated with food and water by tube or intravenously (IV). ("Advance Directive," n.d.)

Such forms also typically allow for open-ended descriptions of the patient's priorities at the end of life.

The language of these forms speaks to the attempt to preserve patient autonomy while curtailing ambiguity so that the patient's wishes can be interpreted accurately. When they are themselves patients, physicians and other clinicians may have an advantage in communicating their wishes in sufficient detail because they are more aware of possible outcomes, the medical options for treatment, and technical language shared with those who will attempt to follow their instructions. A disadvantage shared by all substantive directives, however, is that they ask people to imagine the circumstances under which they would be needed. That anticipation will likely be more accurate after a patient receives a specific diagnosis and prognosis.

Interestingly, about half of U.S. states include an exception invalidating an advance directive if the patient is pregnant, for the duration of the pregnancy. For instance, the Washington state advance directive notes (not offered as a choice): "If I have been diagnosed as pregnant and that diagnosis is known to my physician, this directive shall have no force or effect during the course of my pregnancy" (RCW 70.122.030 [1979]). The legal and political history of reproductive rights in the United States reflects ambivalence about the extent to which a pregnant woman has autonomy over healthcare decisions that may affect the continued existence of the fetus, including the decision to refuse treatment through an advance directive. This exception means that only a medical proxy can refuse treatment for an incompetent woman who is pregnant.

A substantive directive is not a medical order to which physicians and other clinicians can be held accountable, which is why some clinicians, often fearing lawsuits from patients' families, ignore patients' expressed wishes in favor of more aggressive treatment. So, a substantive directive should be accompanied by a **portable medical order,** such as a Do Not Resuscitate/Do Not Attempt Resuscitation (DNR/DNAR) or Allow Natural Death (AND) order, or Physician (or Portable) Orders for Life-Sustaining Treatment (POLST). These orders are applicable to any healthcare professional, including emergency medical technicians (EMTs), regardless of where they originated. These instructions must be signed by a physician (or, in some places, a physician assistant or nurse practitioner), and they become part of the patient's medical record. They may also be initiated by a medical proxy, unlike the substantive advance directive. Whereas advance directives set out patients' preferences in a range of hypothetical scenarios, DNR and POLST forms articulate which treatments patients do and do not want, given their current medical situation. EMTs will default to aggressive treatment to stabilize a patient unless a medical order says otherwise, but they will not follow an advance directive as a medical instruction. Medical organizations recommend that everyone complete an advance directive regardless of current health status, but portable medical orders are most relevant for people who are frail or seriously ill. Even these orders are sometimes not communicated at a critical moment or are willfully disregarded (Raphael 2024).

The second type of advance directive, a **proxy directive,** allows patients to designate in advance who will serve as their surrogate. These directives are often called durable power of attorney for healthcare or medical power of attorney. Rather than recording the decisions a person makes now in anticipation of a hypothetical medical situation in the future, these instructions designate a surrogate—typically, a spouse, sibling, or adult child—to make decisions in real time. A proxy may consult a substantive directive, if one exists, or interpret what the patient would want based on less formal evidence, such as prior conversations or medical decisions.

In response to levels of medical illiteracy among the general public and pervasive cultural aversion to discussing end-of-life issues, some clinicians and bioethicists have proposed simplifying advance directives down to two key questions: (1) "If you cannot, or choose not to participate in health care decisions, with whom should we speak?" and (2) "If you cannot, or choose not to participate in decision making, what should we consider when making decisions about your care?" (Mahon 2011, 805). These questions address the "what" (substantive directive) and the "who" (proxy directive): what a person wants for themselves and who should make medical decisions on their behalf. Both forms of advance directives are intended to be the tangible result of robust, substantive communication while the patient is still capable of expressing their values and priorities so that respect for autonomy is preserved in some form.

Advance directives are used when patients do not fully meet the criteria for capacity. If patients are capable of informed consent, their decisions will override whatever is recorded in an advance directive. If patients have designated a medical proxy, in some states their judgments will also override whatever is recorded in a substantive directive if they can show that they are acting in the best interests of the patient (Potter and Lee 2020). Some bioethicists have referred to the moral principle underlying this flexibility as **limited familial autonomy**: the people most likely to understand the patient's wishes and interests, and to apply them to the current situation, should have some discretion in following a substantive directive as long as they are not clearly acting against the best interests of the patient or demanding futile medical treatments (Arras 1988, 943–44). Clinicians are not obligated to provide futile treatment, regardless of what is said by a substantive directive or proxy. Unlike medical orders, then, advance directives are interpreted and judged by clinicians.

Once advance directives are created, as legal documents they carry authority indefinitely unless retracted by the patient themselves. However, they carry that authority only when a patient is taken to be at the end of life, or what the Washington state law, for example, calls "an incurable and irreversible condition" (RCW 70.122.030 [1979]). Patients are usually advised to update advance directives with major life changes (such as divorce or the death of a spouse), a new diagnosis, or if their existing directive is more than ten years old.

## Problems with Substantive Directives

Although advance directives have clear legal authority, both substantive and proxy directives raise moral issues when applied in healthcare settings. One major issue with substantive directives is that they may not be communicated to clinicians or family members and may be ignored in treatment decisions. As legal documents rather than medical orders, physicians and other clinicians may not be aware of them, especially in emergency situations or if there are multiple specialists involved in treatment. Clinicians may also ignore a directive if they morally or medically disagree with it or if it violates the healthcare organization's policies. In these cases, the patient or their family is legally entitled to transfer to a different clinician or facility.

Even when clinicians are aware of substantive directives and attempt to follow them, their usefulness can be limited. Ambiguous directives may be misinterpreted. Absent a specific diagnosis and prognosis, people find it difficult to predict the medical situations they will confront in some indefinite future. Angela Fagerlin and Carl Schneider note that

> even patients making contemporary decisions about contemporary illnesses are regularly daunted by the decisions' difficulty. . . . We humans falter in gathering information, misunderstand and ignore what we gather, lack well-considered preferences to guide decisions, and rush headlong to choice. How much harder, then, is it to conjure up preferences for an unspecifiable future confronted with unidentifiable maladies with unpredictable treatments? (2004, 33)

Substantive directives may easily capture people's wishes about treatment at the extreme ends of the spectrum—on the one hand, when they are in persistent vegetative states or have severe cognitive impairments from which there is no reasonable prospect of recovery; or, on the other hand, when they have minimal impairment and a strong chance of recovering. But those are not the cases that generate the most decisional turmoil. Our cultural images of life and death tend to be relatively binary, and it is challenging to draw a sharp line between an acceptable and an unacceptable quality of life before a medical crisis happens.

For example, those without medical training tend to be influenced by popular representations of the success rate of cardiopulmonary resuscitation (CPR), which sharply contrast with the reality that patients experiencing cardiac arrest are successfully resuscitated only 7.6 percent of the time outside of a hospital and only 17 percent of the time inside of a hospital. Furthermore, people who survive through resuscitation are likely to suffer from broken ribs, and they may have experienced brain injury, leading to questions about the quality of the life that has been saved (Dalton 2023). People may also be influenced by how healthcare practitioners present treatments. Are risks and failure rates highlighted, or do they emphasize success rates? Are short- and long-term outcomes shared? Are clinicians or family members being honest in their conversations with the patient about their prognosis, or are those conversations shaped by a cultural antipathy toward acknowledging mortality? Especially if they are not healthcare professionals, people are likely to have difficulty predicting their quality of life following treatment. All these factors may hinder people's ability to form and clearly articulate their healthcare preferences.

A second problem emerges directly from what is also the great advantage of substantive directives: their preservation of the patient's wishes over time. If an advance directive was recorded several decades ago or in much different circumstances, the patient's preferences may have changed radically. Younger people may find the prospect of being physically dependent on others for their care intolerable, whereas older adults may be willing to accept various impairments in exchange for a longer life with experiences they continue to value. A 2006 study found that patients' choices regarding life-sustaining treatment depended heavily on whether they were asked prior to hospitalization, immediately after recovering from being hospitalized, or several months later: "Preferences for life-sustaining treatment are dependent on the context in which they are made, and thus individuals may express different treatment preferences when they are healthy than when they are ill" (Ditto et al. 2006). Recent research has revealed that sometimes patient preferences remain stable over time, and sometimes they do not (Auriemma et al. 2014; Jabbarian et al. 2019). We could also put this issue of legitimacy over time in terms of informed consent: Can substantive directives substitute for autonomous decision-making, given how little information people can have about their future conditions?

Complex philosophical issues arise around the concept of prospective autonomy. Should the "former self" be able to have decision-making authority over the "current self"? Has there been enough of a change in the patient's cognitive capacities that they should no longer be seen as the same person, in which case the advance directive of the "former self" would have no bearing on decisions made for the "current self"? Dementia presents a particularly thorny version of this question. Should a patient who had signed an advance directive refusing medical intervention if they become cognitively incompetent, and who now (suffering from Alzheimer's disease) requires artificial hydration, be deprived of that intervention? What if that patient seems otherwise physically comfortable and able to enjoy having their hair brushed or having people read to them? Does personal identity persist through these cognitive changes? Norman Cantor (who has long advocated for the use of advance directives) also raises the scenario of a person who desires life-sustaining medical interventions but who, for religious reasons, is opposed to analgesics and sedatives. If the patient becomes incompetent and experiences significant pain, are clinicians justified in following the advance directive or in mitigating the patient's pain (Cantor 1993, 101)?

The various problems with extending autonomy through substantive directives have led some scholars to advocate for using the best interests approach with incapacitated or incompetent patients instead of substituted judgment. Notably, Rebecca Dresser and John Robertson argue that proxies should determine what is objectively in the best interests of current (incompetent) patients, because treating them as if they were competent patients refusing treatment, only prospectively rather than contemporaneously, is likely to harm them (1989, 234). They claim that autonomous decision-making requires more information than people writing substantive directives can possibly have and that patients' present interests, now that they are incompetent, are unlikely to mirror what their interests were while competent:

> With their reduced mental and physical capacities, what was once of extreme importance to them no longer matters, while things that were previously of little moment assume much greater significance.... It is difficult, if not impossible, for competent individuals to predict their interests in future treatment situations when they are incompetent because their needs and interests will have so radically changed. (236)

Substantive directives therefore are unlikely to capture what is currently best for patients. Dresser and Robertson worry about undertreatment—that competent patients may not be able to predict and therefore leave instructions to preserve what is in fact valuable to them even in a diminished state, and that families may have some psychological or financial incentive not to prolong that diminished state (238–39). Substantive directives, in support of substituted judgment, may also result in overtreatment, in which clinicians maintain an existence that is painful or otherwise not beneficial to the patient.

According to Dresser and Robertson, using the best interests approach for all incompetent patients allows caregivers to assess their quality of life and what they value in objective terms. The question is "whether treatment actually serves the incompetent patient's best interests" in the present and future (Dresser and Robertson 1989, 239–40). They note that this approach can more transparently consider the family's burdens or the just distribution of healthcare resources. It means that the person's current situation becomes the foundation for decision-making, rather than (possibly disputed or inferred) substantive directives: "The ethical commitment to a patient-centered approach requires a focus on the patient as she now is, and not on the desires that she previously had when her interests were quite different" (240). Respecting the person who is currently being treated might mean not respecting the anticipatory instructions made while competent and attending instead to the preferences and values expressed through the behavior of the incompetent patient in the present.

A third issue is generated by the fact that an advance directive has legal status only when the person is dying. Specifically, it takes effect when the patient has "an incurable and irreversible condition caused by injury, disease, or illness, that would within reasonable medical judgment cause death within a reasonable period of time in accordance with accepted medical standards, and where the application of life-sustaining treatment would serve only to prolong the process of dying" (RCW 70.122.030 [1979]). Families and clinicians are often reluctant to recognize that this stage has been reached. Fagerlin and Schneider note that even the day before people die, doctors, on average, predict that patients with heart failure have a 50 percent chance of living for another six months (2004, 36). In a study of terminally ill patients referred to hospice care, physicians' survival estimates were 5.3 times longer than the actual length of survival (Christakis and Lamont 2000). Atul Gawande (2014) notes a general tendency among physicians to minimize a patient's mortality risk and avoid conversations about end-of-life care. If patients are only recognized as being at the end of life immediately before they die, advance directives serve little purpose.

Finally, in many U.S. states, an advance directive may be overridden by the decision of a designated healthcare proxy, whose judgments may or may not be guided by those recorded preferences. In a 2001 study, people designated as medical proxies (mostly spouses or adult children) were asked to predict patients' wishes, and those were compared with what the patients themselves indicated. Proxies who were unable to see the patients' own substantive directives were able to predict the patients' wishes with 72 percent accuracy overall, which is somewhat reassuring. However, the proxies who read the patients' directives or discussed them with the patients were not significantly more accurate in predicting their specific healthcare directives or valued life activities directives—between 69 and 75 percent (Ditto et al. 2001, 426).

## Problems with Proxy Directives

The great advantage of designating a healthcare proxy is that the proxy will (presumably) have the patient's best interests and wishes in mind as well as information about the specific medical situation that they confront, including the ability to ask clinicians about the potential risks and benefits of different treatment options. But proxy directives raise their own set of logistical and moral concerns. First, as we discussed above, even a proxy who has indications of a patient's wishes—through conversation or by reading a substantive directive—can misinterpret those wishes. Sometimes this is deliberate, when they intentionally override the patient's judgment with their own. But even when a proxy tries to reconstruct a patient's stance, in the substituted judgment approach, bias may be more subtle and unintentional, with the surrogate projecting onto the patient their own moral or religious values (Fagerlin et al. 2001; Marks and Arkes 2008). A proxy may be struggling with grief, anxiety, or guilt as they try to make medical decisions, which may distort the outcome of that process in cases where the patient may see their options more clearheadedly if they were making the decision themselves. Someone with close emotional attachments to the patient may be more invested in prolonging their life than the patient themselves. Although a durable power of attorney for healthcare typically designates just one person as a proxy (or a succession of people, in the case of that person's death or unavailability), that person may encounter a jumble of different views from family members and friends. Frequently, adult children or siblings who have not experienced a patient's decline on a daily basis may advocate for more aggressive life-sustaining treatment than regular caregivers. Such conflicts may delay or impede the proxy's ability to effectively make decisions using either the best interests or substituted judgment approach. Clinicians also have some incentive to overtreat when the proxy demands it rather than following an advance directive that refuses care because the proxy is in a position to complain or bring legal proceedings against the clinician and their employer.

When proxies use substituted judgment, they may question whether the patient's prior judgments are applicable in the current situation. This uncertainty replicates a problem in substantive directives: the previously capable patient may have left instructions that would not serve the interests of the current patient (with diminished capacity) or align with the preferences they are able to express now. Debates among medical ethicists on the relative weight of past patient autonomy and present beneficence raise these specific issues in the context of broader philosophical questions such as what defines personal identity, how to distinguish persons from nonpersons, and what constitutes the minimum threshold for autonomy.

However, when proxies use the best interests approach, the patient's incapacity (the very reason a proxy is needed) obscures judgments about what benefits them. They often cannot express their interests clearly and consistently. Caregivers—both clinicians and family members—thus have to interpret behavior, such as facial expressions or verbalizations, to establish what the patient finds valuable. And those interpretations may be even more susceptible to bias and other sources of inaccuracy than are interpretations of substantive directives. Even if patients demonstrate preferences for one type of music over another or seem to enjoy social interactions, their incapacity precludes the possibility of conversations about whether these pleasurable experiences amount to a life that they find worth living. If a patient seems to be experiencing unmanageable, constant pain and not much else, that seems objectively to be a life not worth prolonging. If a patient has diminished cognitive capacity but otherwise appears to be contented by various small pleasures, then medical treatments may preserve their current, positive quality of life. However, between these two poles lies a lot of uncertain ground. Even determining how much pain a noncommunicative patient is experiencing or how much a minimally conscious patient is aware of is not a purely objective judgment. In other words, the simplest forms of autonomy—what does this person want, and how are they subjectively experiencing reality?—are still relevant.

Applying the principle of beneficence to incapacitated patients, deciding for someone whether they live or die, opens up broader moral issues. Who has the authority to judge when a life is worth living? Will those judgments reflect cultural prejudices that devalue the lives of marginalized populations such as people with disabilities, people living in poverty, incarcerated people, and migrants? Objections to the arbitrariness of human judgments resonate with the arguments from Catholic philosophers and disability rights activists against withdrawing treatment from Terri Schiavo and other PVS patients. The judgment of whether another person's life is worth living should raise profound moral concern, given the history of eugenics, which explicitly associated euthanasia and sterilization with treating the present or future person with compassion by extinguishing their future existence and thereby protecting the health of the wider society. That is, beneficence has been used to rationalize violence, sometimes with the complicity of medical professionals. Substantive directives attempt to ensure that the person's own sense of when and whether life is worthwhile will guide future medical decisions. Focusing exclusively on current well-being leaves open the risk that a third-person assessment of a patient's interests will not reflect their own judgments.

## Conclusion: What Advance Directives Can and Cannot Do

The purpose of advance directives (both proxy and substantive) is to extend the patient's autonomy past the temporal range of their own cognitive or communicative capacity and to prevent, as much as possible, medical decision-making from escalating into a legal dispute. Clinicians, social workers, and hospital ethics boards can facilitate decision-making and conflict resolution, especially when multiple family members are involved. But advance directives function most effectively when they are completed in the broader context of conversations with those who will be responsible for following them: medical proxies, primary care physicians, hospice care workers, or other caregivers. Substantive directives will also be most effective when they take into account the patient's specific, predictable medical circumstances—for example, if they are revised after a patient is diagnosed with a terminal illness. The limitations of advance directives sketched out in this chapter present significant challenges, but the complete absence of an advance directive creates even more uncertainty and moral turmoil: as Linda Emanuel (2005) puts it, "living wills are for everyone. They are analogous in many ways to a safety belt. They don't solve everything, but they certainly minimize the damage." Encouraging patients to complete advance directives and encouraging clinicians to follow their instructions also need to be part of a larger cultural conversation about what it means to respect autonomy within the real limitations of aging and mortality.

# References

"Advance Directive." n.d. AdvanceDirectives.com. Accessed January 15, 2025. https://advancedirectives.com/wp-content/uploads/2020/11/Advance-Directive.pdf.

Arras, John D. 1988. "The Severely Demented, Minimally Functional Patient: An Ethical Analysis." *Journal of the American Geriatrics Society* 36, no. 10 (October): 938–44. doi:10.1111/j.1532-5415.1988.tb05788.x.

Auriemma, Catherine L., Christina A. Nguyen, Rachel Bronheim, Saida Kent, Shrivatsa Nadiger, Dustin Pardo, and Scott D. Halpern. 2014. "Stability of End-of-Life Preferences: A Systematic Review of the Evidence." *JAMA Internal Medicine* 174, no. 7 (July): 1085–92. doi:10.1001/jamainternmed.2014.1183.

Cantor, Norman L. 1993. *Advance Directives and the Pursuit of Death with Dignity.* Bloomington: Indiana University Press.

———. 2005. "The Bane of Surrogate Decision-Making: Defining the Best Interests of Never-Competent Persons." *Journal of Legal Medicine* 26, no. 2: 155–205. doi:10.1080/01947640590949922.

Charatan, Fred. 2005. "Autopsy Supports Claim That Schiavo Was in a Persistent Vegetative State." *BMJ* 330, no. 7506 (June 25): 1467. doi:10.1136/bmj.330.7506.1467-a.

Christakis, Nicholas A., and Elizabeth B. Lamont. 2000. "Extent and Determinants of Error in Physicians' Prognoses in Terminally Ill Patients." *Western Journal of Medicine* 172, no. 5 (May): 310–13. doi:10.1136/ewjm.172.5.310.

Committee for Pro-Life Activities, National Conference of Catholic Bishops. 1992. "Nutrition and Hydration: Moral and Pastoral Reflections." *Linacre Quarterly* 59, no. 4 (November): 33–49. doi:10.1080/00243639.1992.1187817.

Dalton, Clayton. 2023. "For Many, a 'Natural Death' May Be Preferable to Enduring CPR." *NPR.* May 29. https://www.npr.org/sections/health-shots/2023/05/29/1177914622/a-natural-death-may-be-preferable-for-many-than-enduring-cpr.

Ditto, Peter H., Joseph H. Danks, William D. Smucker, Jamila Bookwala, Kristen M. Coppola, Rebecca Dresser, et al. 2001. "Advance Directives as Acts of Communication: A Randomized Controlled Trial." *Archives of Internal Medicine* 161, no. 3 (February 12): 421–30. doi:10.1001/archinte.161.3.421.

Ditto, Peter H., Jill A. Jacobson, William D. Smucker, Joseph H. Danks, and Angela Fagerlin. 2006. "Context Changes Choices: A Prospective Study of the Effects of Hospitalization on Life-Sustaining Treatment Preferences." *Medical Decision Making* 26, no. 4 (July–August): 313–22. doi:10.1177/0272989X06290494.

Dresser, Rebecca S., and John A. Robertson. 1989. "Quality of Life and Non-treatment Decisions for Incompetent Patients." *Law, Medicine & Health Care* 17, no. 3 (September): 234–44. doi:10.1111/j.1748-720x.1989.tb01101.x.

Emanuel, Linda. 2005. "Living Wills." Interview by Jim Lehrer. *NewsHour with Jim Lehrer*, PBS (television broadcast). March 22. https://americanarchive.org/catalog/cpb-aacip_507-959c53fn6t.

Fagerlin, Angela, Peter H. Ditto, Joseph H. Danks, and Renate M. Houts. 2001. "Projection in Surrogate Decisions about Life-Sustaining Medical Treatments." *Health Psychology* 20, no. 3 (May): 166–75. doi:10.1037/0278-6133.20.3.166.

Fagerlin, Angela, and Carl E. Schneider. 2004. "Enough: The Failure of the Living Will." *Hastings Center Report* 34, no. 2 (March–April): 30–42. doi:10.2307/3527683.

Gawande, Atul. 2014. *Being Mortal: Illness, Medicine, and What Matters in the End*. New York: Henry Holt.

Grisso, Thomas, and Paul S. Appelbaum. 1998. *Assessing Competence to Consent to Treatment: A Guide for Physicians and Other Health Professionals*. New York: Oxford University Press. doi:10.1093/oso/9780195103724.001.0001.

Hegde, Soumya, and Ratnavalli Ellajosyula. 2016. "Capacity Issues and Decision-Making in Dementia." In "Medicolegal Issues in Neurology," edited by Subhash Kaul and Suvarna Alladi. Supplement, *Annals of Indian Academy of Neurology* 19, no. S1 (October): S34–39. doi:10.4103/0972-2327.192890.

Jabbarian, Lea J., Renee C. Maciejewski, Paul K. Maciejewski, Judith A. C. Rietjens, Ida J. Korfage, Agnes van der Heide, Johannes J. M. van Delden, and Holly G. Prigerson. 2019. "The Stability of Treatment Preferences among Patients with Advanced Cancer." *Journal of Pain and Symptom Management* 57, no. 6 (June): 1071–79. doi:10.1016/j.jpainsymman.2019.01.016.

Jennett, Bryan, and Fred Plum. 1972. "Persistent Vegetative State after Brain Damage: A Syndrome in Search of a Name." *Lancet* 299, no. 7753 (April 1): 734–37. doi:10.1016/s0140-6736(72)90242-5.

Kutner, Luis. 1969. "Due Process of Euthanasia: The Living Will, a Proposal." *Indiana Law Journal* 44, no. 4 (Summer): 539–54. https://www.repository.law.indiana.edu/ilj/vol44/iss4/2/.

Mahon, Margaret M. 2011. "An Advance Directive in Two Questions." *Journal of Pain and Symptom Management* 41, no. 4 (April): 801–7. doi:10.1016/j.jpainsymman.2011.01.002.

Marks, Melissa A. Z., and Hal R. Arkes. 2008. "Patient and Surrogate Disagreement in End-of-Life Decisions: Can Surrogates Accurately Predict Patients' Preferences?" *Medical Decision Making* 28, no. 4 (July–August): 524–31. doi:10.1177/0272989X08315244.

McCloskey, Elizabeth Leibold. 1991. "The Patient Self-Determination Act." *Kennedy Institute of Ethics Journal* 1, no. 2 (June): 163–69. doi:10.1353/ken.0.0062.

McMahan, Jeff. 1995. "The Metaphysics of Brain Death." *Bioethics* 9, no. 2 (April): 91–126. doi:10.1111/j.1467-8519.1995.tb00305.x.

Potter, Jordan, and Susannah W. Lee. 2020. "When Advance Directives Collide." *Journal of General Internal Medicine* 35, no. 7 (July): 2191–92. doi:10.1007/s11606-020-05680-x.

Raphael, Kate. 2024. "Doctors Saved Her Life. She Didn't Want Them To." *New York Times*. August 26. https://www.nytimes.com/2024/08/26/well/patients-dnr-orders-ignored.html.

Weijer, Charles. 2005. "A Death in the Family: Reflections on the Terri Schiavo Case." *Canadian Medical Association Journal* 172, no. 9 (April 26): 1197–98. doi:10.1503/cmaj.050348.

Yadav, Kuldeep N., Nicole B. Gabler, Elizabeth Cooney, Saida Kent, Jennifer Kim, Nicole Herbst, Adjoa Mante, Scott D. Halpern, and Katherine R. Courtright. 2017. "Approximately One in Three US Adults Completes Any Type of Advance Directive for End-Of-Life Care." *Health Affairs* 36, no. 7 (July 1): 1244–51. doi:10.1377/hlthaff.2017.0175.

## FURTHER READING

Buchanan, Allen E., and Dan W. Brock. 1990. *Deciding for Others: The Ethics of Surrogate Decision Making*. Cambridge: Cambridge University Press. doi:10.1017/CBO9781139171946.

> Sets out a theoretical framework for making decisions on behalf of incompetent patients. Buchanan and Brock first discuss what competence and incompetence mean in healthcare settings. They then discuss the use of advance directives, substituted judgment, and the best interests standard with incompetent patients, and they consider a range of scenarios, including minors, people diagnosed with psychiatric disorders, and people at the end of life.

DeGrazia, David. 1999. "Advance Directives, Dementia, and 'the Someone Else Problem.'" *Bioethics* 13, no. 5 (October): 373–91. doi:10.1111/1467-8519.00166.

> A consideration of whether advance directives remain legitimate across time, especially in the situation of a patient with dementia. DeGrazia examines the basic philosophical assumptions around personal identity that ground this problem: Has the patient become "someone else"? He argues that the philosophical focus on personal identity is unhelpful in such situations and considers an alternative, that personhood is "inessential."

Dresser, Rebecca. 1986. "Life, Death, and Incompetent Patients: Conceptual Infirmities and Hidden Values in the Law." *Arizona Law Review* 28, no. 3: 373–405.

    A review of the legal framework governing advance directives. Dresser argues that protecting the self-determination of incompetent patients is unjustified, and she criticizes the legal authority of advance directives and the substituted judgment doctrine. As an alternative, she supports the present best interests approach to proxy decision-making, which allows families' interests to be legally recognized.

Jaworska, Agnieszka. 1999. "Respecting the Margins of Agency: Alzheimer's Patients and the Capacity to Value." *Philosophy & Public Affairs* 28, no. 2 (Spring): 105–38. doi:10.1111/j.1088-4963.1999.00105.x.

    Applies respect for autonomy to patients diagnosed with Alzheimer's. Jaworska considers Rebecca Dresser's argument in favor of the best interests standard and Ronald Dworkin's argument in favor of respecting advance directives or other stated wishes. She then develops a third alternative for Alzheimer's patients in which respecting their (limited) autonomy means asking, "Does this patient still value?" and then acting in accordance with what they value.

Kushner, Thomasine, and Steve Heilig, eds. 1992. "The Patient Self-Determination Act." Special section, *Cambridge Quarterly of Healthcare Ethics* 1, no. 2 (Spring): 97–126. https://www.cambridge.org/core/journals/cambridge-quarterly-of-healthcare-ethics/issue/AFF35EA414FCB783E3FEF84CCCB3AE9A.

    The Patient Self-Determination Act of 1990 is the U.S. legislation that requires every hospital, hospice, and other healthcare institution that accepts federal funds (Medicare and Medicaid) to recognize advance directives. Contributors explain what the act requires, consider its benefits and challenges (both legal and moral), and describe how it is being implemented in select states.

Lack, Peter, Nikola Biller-Andorno, and Susanne Brauer, eds. 2014. *Advance Directives*. Dordrecht: Springer. doi:10.1007/978-94-007-7377-6.

    A review of the moral and legal issues related to advance directives in various national and cultural contexts. Contributors cover the history of advance directives, how advance directives apply to psychiatric care, the difficulties clinicians experience in trying to adhere to patients' written wishes, and some of the conflicts between legal requirements and ethical considerations.

Olick, Robert S. 2001. *Taking Advance Directives Seriously: Prospective Autonomy and Decisions near the End of Life*. Washington, DC: Georgetown University Press.

A bioethical analysis of end-of-life decision-making, including the use of advance directives. Olick argues that respect for patient autonomy entails giving patients and families control over such decisions. He surveys the history of advance directives, considers the underlying concepts of autonomy and personal identity, and discusses how advance directives work in actual clinical settings.

Schneiderman, Lawrence J. 2008. *Embracing Our Mortality: Hard Choices in an Age of Medical Miracles*. New York: Oxford University Press.

A critique of the medicalization of mortality and technological attempts to extend life. Written for the general public, this text by a physician and bioethicist attempts to overcome the denial of mortality pervasive in Western cultures. Schneiderman uses stories of his own patients and other case studies to illustrate the consequences of these attitudes. He then offers practical advice on how to avoid such consequences, including writing clear and effective advance directives.

Weller, Penelope. 2013. *New Law and Ethics in Mental Health Advance Directives: The Convention on the Rights of Persons with Disabilities and the Right to Choose*. New York: Routledge.

Examines how advance directives can be used by patients with psychiatric diagnoses in a range of different countries. Starting from legislation asserting rights for people with disabilities, Weller considers how psychiatric patients can not only refuse treatment but also have positive rights that need to be recognized (including the right to demand treatment). She analyzes a number of legal cases as well as the enforceability of advance directives for patients with mental health conditions.

Wolfson, Jay. 2006. "Defined by Her Dying, Not by Her Death: The Guardian Ad Litem's View of Schiavo." *Death Studies* 30, no. 2 (March): 113–20. doi:10.1080/07481180500455590.

An account of the Terri Schiavo controversy from the perspective of the guardian ad litem appointed by the court to safeguard her interests. Wolfson describes his experiences and observations trying to ascertain her cognitive capacities and potential for recovery. He explains the steps in the legal battle and the public debate over whether her artificial hydration and nutrition should have been removed, and he reflects on why the case became so politicized.

# CHAPTER 8
# Medical Aid in Dying

**Key topics in this chapter:**

- The difference between medical aid in dying, passive euthanasia, and active euthanasia
- The legal landscape governing these practices in the U.S. and elsewhere
- Moral arguments against medical aid in dying based on concerns about the physician's role and slippery slopes
- Moral arguments for medical aid in dying based on the principles of respect for autonomy and beneficence

## Introduction

Many central issues in medical ethics intersect in the discussion of medical aid in dying, including the purpose of medicine, the value of life, and the limits of patient autonomy. Is there a morally significant difference between killing and letting die? Is death always an evil to be fended off by clinicians? Does recognizing patient self-determination mean honoring requests to end their lives and, if so, under what circumstances should those requests be honored? Alternatively, does respect for autonomy demand that vulnerable groups be protected against coercive social pressures to devalue their lives? The charged moral debate and fractured legal landscape of medical aid in dying in the United States and elsewhere stem from profoundly different answers to these questions.

## Terminology

Names carry moral implications, and there are several synonymous terms for having a medical professional help a patient end their own life. Although calling it physician-assisted suicide was once commonplace—the American

Medical Association (AMA) still uses the phrase—advocates for medical aid in dying often avoid the term due to the social stigma associated with suicide, and also to highlight the difference between wanting not to live and wanting to control the way that one's life inevitably ends. Several professional medical associations reject the phrase "assisted suicide," including the British Medical Association, the American Academy of Hospice and Palliative Medicine, the American College of Legal Medicine, the American College of Family Physicians, and the American Public Health Association. Instead, they call it medical aid in dying, physician-aided dying, or death with dignity. The American Association of Suicidology, which advocates for suicide prevention, also distinguishes suicide from physician aid in dying (Battin 2019). This distinction is reflected in most state laws. For example, the Washington Death with Dignity Act (RCW 70.245 [2008]) specifies that "state reports shall not refer to practice under this chapter as 'suicide' or 'assisted suicide'" (70.245.180). In this chapter, we call it medical aid in dying because it is the term increasingly used by bioethicists. Most states that have legalized medical aid in dying require that a physician write the prescription for life-ending medication, although some states (such as Washington) also count physician assistants and advanced registered nurse practitioners as "qualified medical providers" (70.245.010).

Furthermore, although the terms "euthanasia" and "medical aid in dying" are often used interchangeably in ordinary language, they refer to different practices. **Euthanasia**, from the Greek roots *eu* (good) and *thanatos* (death), is deliberately ending a person's life in order to spare them unnecessary suffering. It is sometimes called mercy killing. We use the same term to describe ending the life of a nonhuman animal when it has this purpose of preventing suffering—euthanizing pets with terminal conditions, injured horses, or chickens to prevent the spread of avian flu.

Bioethicists distinguish between active and passive euthanasia. **Active euthanasia** directly ends another person's life, for example, by administering an overdose of sedatives; **passive euthanasia** is an act of withholding or withdrawing life-supporting treatment, such as refusing to treat a deadly injury or removing someone from a ventilator when they cannot breathe on their own. They also distinguish between **voluntary, nonvoluntary,** and **involuntary euthanasia**: respectively, when the patient consents to it, is incapable of consenting to it (e.g., because they are unconscious), or opposes it. Typically, when nonphilosophers use the term "euthanasia," they mean active euthanasia, which is illegal in all fifty states, prohibited by state medical boards, and disallowed in institutions that accept federal funds (Pub. L. 105-12 [1997]). For this reason, many clinicians do not refer to withholding or withdrawing treatment as a form of euthanasia at all. When requested by a competent patient or a designated proxy, refusing treatment, even life-sustaining treatment, is legal everywhere in the United States—as established in *Cruzan v. Director, Missouri Department of Health* (497 U.S. 261 [1990]) and codified in the Patient Self-Determination Act (HR 4449 [1990])—and in many other countries. Although active euthanasia is illegal everywhere in the United States, it is legal under certain conditions in the Netherlands, Belgium, Luxembourg, Canada, New Zealand, and Spain. In addition, active euthanasia was decriminalized (but not legalized) in Colombia by a 1997 court ruling.

As opposed to euthanasia, **medical aid in dying** means that the patient directly brings about their own death with the assistance of a physician. Where it is legal in the United States, the patient must be able to give themselves life-ending medication, typically by swallowing pills. The medication does not need to be taken under direct medical supervision, but it must be prescribed by a physician or other prescribing clinician. This requirement means not only that a patient must be medically capable of making their own decisions when they request it but also physically capable of taking it—a requirement that excludes people who are paralyzed or otherwise dependent on others to administer their medication. In 2014, Brittany Maynard experienced a recurrence of a brain tumor that was deemed to be inoperable. At the time, her home state of California did not permit medical aid in dying, so she established residency in Oregon. Her goal was to live as long as she could but to "die on her own terms" rather than extend her suffering (Maynard 2014). The brain tumor caused progressively stronger seizures, and the risk she took was that any one of those seizures might have impaired her ability to swallow the life-ending medication (Diaz 2017). Such calculations are necessary with medical aid in dying but not passive or active euthanasia.

In addition to self-administration, U.S. death with dignity laws have the following eligibility requirements: the patient must be (1) at least eighteen years old; (2) a resident of the state (although Vermont and Oregon no longer require residency); (3) diagnosed with a terminal condition (expected to die of their condition within six months); and (4) capable of making and communicating medical decisions. The attending physician's terminal diagnosis must be confirmed by a consulting physician. Both physicians must agree that the patient is cognitively capable and not suffering from depression or a mental illness that impairs their judgment; either physician may refer the patient for psychiatric evaluation. In terms of process, the patient must voluntarily make a verbal request to their physician for a prescription of life-ending medication; the doctor cannot initiate it. They must wait at least fifteen days before making a second verbal request (although in Oregon, patients with less than fifteen days to live are exempt from this waiting period). The clinician must tell the patient that they can rescind the request. The patient then makes a written request, signed in the presence of two witnesses, at least one of whom cannot be related to the patient or work for the clinician or healthcare facility responsible for the patient's care. No less than forty-eight hours must elapse between the written request and writing the prescription. The physician must inform the patient of alternatives to medical aid in dying, such as hospice care and treatment options, and they must recommend (but not require) that the patient discuss the decision with their family. The patient, the attending physician, or an agent of the patient must obtain the medication from a pharmacist (or from the physician themselves, if they are a dispensing physician), and the patient must take the medication themselves (Oregon Death with Dignity Act, ORS 127.800-897 [1997]). Physicians and pharmacists morally opposed to medical aid in dying have the right to refuse to participate. These provisions jointly attempt to ensure that medical aid in dying is an autonomous decision on the part of each patient rather than resulting from lack of information, psychiatric disorder, or external coercion. They also recognize physicians' and pharmacists' autonomy in deciding whether to be part of the process. Whether the patient uses the life-ending medication or not, the cause of death on their death certificate will be listed as the underlying terminal condition (e.g., cancer, amyotrophic lateral sclerosis, or heart disease).

Oregon was the first U.S. state to legally allow medical aid in dying, and its Death with Dignity Act (1997) has been the model for other state legislation. Empirical data collected since its legalization give a snapshot of who is taking advantage of the law. In 2023, 560 patients requested life-ending medication, 367 died after taking the medication (including 30 who requested the medication in previous years), 82 died of natural causes, and it is unknown whether the remaining people took the medication or not. Medical aid in dying accounted for 0.8 percent of all deaths in Oregon in 2023. Medically assisted deaths have been gradually increasing over the last two and a half decades—from 16 people in 1998, to 60 people in 2008, and 367 in 2023. Between 1997, when the law was passed, and 2023, 4,274 people received prescriptions under Oregon's Death with Dignity Act, and 2,847 people (66.6 percent) died by taking the medications. Most patients were sixty-five or older (77 percent), and the most common underlying diagnoses were cancer (70.7 percent), neurological disorder (10.9 percent), and heart disease (7.2 percent). Patients most commonly gave the following reasons for requesting life-ending medication: loss of autonomy (90.4 percent), decreasing ability to participate in activities that made life enjoyable (89.6 percent), and loss of dignity (70.3 percent). Inadequate pain control (28.8 percent) and financial burdens of treatment (5.5 percent) were the least frequent reasons cited (Center for Health Statistics 2024). The percentage of patients motivated by financial concerns has trended upward, however, as has the ratio of patients who rely on government-supported healthcare (Regnard, Worthington, and Finlay 2023). Most patients were enrolled in hospice care (91 percent), and most died at home (92 percent). Very few (2.6 percent) reported complications, such as regurgitating the medication. The median time to unconsciousness after ingesting the medication was five minutes, and the median time to death was thirty-five minutes (Center for Health Statistics 2024).

## The History of Medical Aid in Dying Legislation in the U.S.

The legal debate about whether people have the **right to die** (the right to choose the circumstances of their death) hinges primarily on a constitutional question, but it is rooted in an underlying moral question about the extent to which individual autonomy around end-of-life decisions should be respected. In "The Philosophers' Brief," an amicus curiae brief submitted to the U.S. Supreme Court in *Washington v. Glucksberg* (521 U.S. 702 [1997]) and *Vacco v. Quill* (521 U.S. 793 [1997]), Ronald Dworkin et al. (1997) claim that the right to die is derived from the Due Process Clause of the Fourteenth Amendment: people have a liberty right to do with themselves whatever they wish unless the state has some compelling reason why that right should be limited. In *Planned Parenthood v. Casey*

(505 U.S. 833 [1992]), the Supreme Court reaffirmed the right to abortion, based in the right to privacy, and asserted that people can make their own decisions, without state interference, about matters "involving the most intimate and personal choices a person may make in a lifetime, choices central to personal dignity and autonomy" (851; quoted in Dworkin et al. 1997, 43). The choice of when and how to die is a personal matter that reflects someone's deep moral and religious convictions. Liberty of conscience requires that people be allowed to make this important decision for themselves. The state can promote the value of human life, which is a legitimate state interest, by limiting medical aid in dying to the terminally ill and regulating it so that people who receive such aid are of sound mind. However, proscribing the practice would amount to imposing a particular conception of the value of life onto everyone: "Just as a blanket prohibition on abortion would involve the improper imposition of one conception of the meaning and value of human existence on all individuals, so too would a blanket prohibition on assisted suicide" (Dworkin et al. 1997, 44).

The Supreme Court ruled unanimously that state prohibitions on physician-assisted suicide, including Washington's Natural Death Act (1979), could stand; the right to die is "not a fundamental liberty interest protected by the Due Process Clause" because it is not "deeply rooted in this Nation's history and tradition," as evidenced by the fact that the majority of states at the time banned assisted suicide (*Washington v. Glucksberg*, 521 U.S. 702 [1997], at 728, 721). The Justices also held that the line between refusing life-sustaining treatment and requesting medical aid in dying is a significant one. The latter practice raises legitimate concerns about "maintaining physicians' role as their patients' healers; protecting vulnerable people from indifference, prejudice, and psychological and financial pressure to end their lives; and avoiding a possible slide toward euthanasia" (704). That June 1997 decision left it to individual states to decide whether medical aid in dying would be allowed or prohibited by statute.

Oregon voters had approved the Death with Dignity Act as a citizens' initiative in 1994. There was a court challenge, and the U.S. District Court in Oregon struck down the law, reasoning that people who have suicidal impulses need to be protected from committing that act, whether they have terminal illnesses or not. The Ninth Circuit Court of Appeals reversed this decision, and the U.S. Supreme Court declined to hear an appeal. The Death with Dignity Act was allowed to stand. There was an attempt by the Oregon state legislature to repeal the law in 1997 (Ballot

Measure 51), but the voters rejected it. The law therefore went into effect in November 1997, making Oregon the first state to legalize medical aid in dying. It was challenged in court again in 2001 under the federal Controlled Substances Act (1970), which restricts prescribing drugs that are likely to lead to abuse or dependence, especially if those drugs have little or no "legitimate medical purpose." The U.S. attorney general claimed that the drugs being prescribed under the Death with Dignity Act did not serve a legitimate medical purpose because they contravened the goal of medical treatment, which is to save and prolong life.

*Gonzales v. Oregon* (546 U.S. 243 [2006]) was appealed to the U.S. Supreme Court, where, in a 6–3 decision, the Justices ruled that individual states could determine what constitutes the appropriate use of medications. The Oregon law was again allowed to stand, and since that time, eight other states—Washington (2008), Vermont (2013), California (2016), Colorado (2016), Hawai'i (2018), Maine (2019), New Jersey (2019), and New Mexico (2021)—and the District of Columbia (2016) have passed legislation almost identical to Oregon's. Montana also legalized medical aid in dying as the result of a 2009 state Supreme Court decision (*Baxter v. Montana*, 354 Mont. 234, 224 P.3d 1211) that has been challenged unsuccessfully in every subsequent legislative session. This tangled history has resulted in a patchwork of laws, with advocates working to expand medical aid in dying and opponents working to recriminalize the practice.

## Global Comparisons

Beyond the United States, ten countries have legalized medical aid in dying and/or euthanasia under certain conditions. This legal landscape is continually shifting. For instance, in December 2024 the United Kingdom passed preliminary legislation allowing medical aid in dying. One of the first countries to allow the practice was Switzerland (in 1942), which stipulates that the person assisting the patient must not be motivated by self-interest. The law limits its use to people competent to make medical decisions and who have "ownership [*Tatherrschaft*]" of their death—the latter condition meaning that patients must swallow their own medication or push a button to activate an intravenous injection. Swiss doctors have sometimes been reluctant to write prescriptions in cases where the person is not terminally ill (Bondolfi 2020). Unlike most other countries where medical aid in dying and euthanasia are legal, Switzerland does not have a citizenship or residency requirement, and assisted deaths at voluntary assisted death organizations such as Dignitas have increased in recent decades.

In 2002, Belgium and the Netherlands legalized medical aid in dying and euthanasia for both terminal conditions and nonterminal ones that cause a patient "unbearable suffering with no prospect of improvement" (Government of the Netherlands, n.d.). Physicians must prescribe the medication at the patient's request, but that request may be made as part of an advance directive. Physicians are responsible for ensuring that the patient's request is "voluntary and well-considered." In the Netherlands, children who are at least twelve years old may request euthanasia or medical aid in dying, but they need their parents' permission until the age of sixteen. Parents must be involved in some way in the decision-making process until the patient turns eighteen. Finally, newborn infants may be euthanized under the same conditions—when their suffering is unbearable, with no prospect of improvement, at the parents' request. In this case, a second physician must verify the prognosis. Belgium has no specific age minimum but stipulates that minors must be capable of making medical decisions for themselves (European Institute of Bioethics 2021).

Luxembourg (as of 2009), Colombia (2015), Canada (2016), and Spain (2021) have similar laws that allow for medical aid in dying and physician-administered euthanasia for people who have been diagnosed with terminal conditions or (like the Netherlands and Belgium) with conditions that (in the words of Canada's law) are "serious and incurable" and cause "enduring and intolerable physical or psychological suffering that cannot be alleviated under conditions that the person finds acceptable" (Government of Canada 2024). Age limits vary. In Canada, Luxembourg, and Spain, the patient must be eighteen; in Colombia, patients fourteen and older are eligible, and twelve- and thirteen-year-olds are eligible with their parents' permission.

As of 2022, Austria legalized medical aid in dying (but not euthanasia) for adults with terminal or "permanent, debilitating" conditions. The law specifically excludes people suffering from psychiatric disorders. After two doctors have confirmed the prognosis and the person's capacity, the waiting period after the request is twelve weeks, unless they suffer from a terminal disease, in which case it is two weeks ("New Law Allowing Assisted Suicide" 2022).

New Zealand (as of 2021) and the six states of Australia (2022) have legalized medical aid in dying and euthanasia for patients with terminal conditions. Under New Zealand's End of Life Choice Act (2019), the patient must be at least eighteen years old, a citizen or permanent resident, "in an advanced state of irreversible decline in physical capability," "experiencing unbearable suffering that cannot be relieved in a manner that the person considers tolerable," and legally competent. Mental disorders do not make a patient ineligible, but there must be an accompanying terminal condition and the patient must be capable of making autonomous decisions. Requests cannot be made as part of an advance directive. Diagnosis, prognosis, and competence must be verified by two physicians, with a referral for psychological evaluation if either physician deems it necessary (New Zealand Ministry of Health 2024; see also Go Gentle Australia, n.d.). Withdrawing or withholding treatment on a patient's request or sedating to unconsciousness as a form of pain management is legal in all these jurisdictions, as well as in the U.S., and it is not considered a form of medical aid in dying or euthanasia.

As we have seen, countries disagree about what kind of suffering or loss would justify state-sanctioned suicide. The conversation is ongoing. In Canada, for example, the law was amended in 2021 to expand eligibility to patients whose only medical condition is a mental illness, as long as they meet the other eligibility criteria. However, the Canadian government has repeatedly enacted temporary exclusions of such patients so they can establish a process to assess competence. The debate around this particular expansion of eligibility has raised some of the same concerns that have emerged in the U.S. context about medical aid in dying more generally: if it is legal, that vulnerable populations will be offered a chance to die rather than be appropriately supported and treated, thus generating a slippery slope to involuntary euthanasia; and if it is illegal, that people will suffer unnecessary pain and loss of dignity. But the debate about psychiatric disorders introduces new questions as well. For example, since the "irremediability" of a mental illness is what makes one eligible for medical aid in dying, how can a physician reliably measure whether it can be successfully treated (Honderich 2023)?

## Arguments against Medical Aid in Dying

These legal issues concern respect for autonomy, reduction of suffering, and the purpose of medicine. All three issues reemerge in moral arguments both for and against medical aid in dying. Two principal arguments have been made against it: (1) that helping to end someone's life conflicts with the physician's role as a healer; and (2) that accepting this practice (morally or legally) will lead to accepting voluntary and involuntary euthanasia that targets vulnerable groups, such as people with disabilities—a kind of slippery slope.

## 1. The physician's role as healer

The incompatibility between the goal of healing patients and the act of assisting them in dying is typically justified with reference to the Hippocratic Oath, which prohibits physicians from providing "a lethal drug to anyone, if I am asked" and from "advis[ing] such a plan" ("Hippocratic Oath" 2002). This seems to pose a relatively straightforward moral objection to medical aid in dying, and it is referenced repeatedly in the American Medical Association's statements opposing the practice (Bristow 1997; see also Kass 1989).

Appealing to the Hippocratic Oath is not as compelling as it initially seems, however. First, Anton van Hooff (2004) claims that this is a mistranslation of the Greek, which instead prohibits doctors from taking advantage of access to patients to secretly poison them on behalf of third parties. Moreover, as we noted in Chapter 5, the Hippocratic Oath represents only one perspective on the proper role of physicians. With many illustrative examples, Danielle Gourevitch shows that, in ancient Greece and Rome, "the intervention of physicians in rational suicides was common practice, particularly if motivated by reasons of health" (1969, 509). Many contemporary versions of the Hippocratic Oath, such as the one written by Louis Lasagna (1964), do not include a prohibition on medical aid in dying. A study of 141 U.S. medical schools in 2000 found that just 17.7 percent of the oaths taken by graduates include a prohibition on physician-assisted suicide or euthanasia. Only one used the ancient version of the Hippocratic Oath (Kao and Parsi 2004). The proper role of the physician with patients who no longer find their lives valuable is thus open to debate rather than unequivocally defined by the Hippocratic Oath. As J. M. Dieterle argues: "If PAS [physician-assisted suicide] is wrong, its wrongness cannot be *constituted* by its conflict with the Hippocratic Oath. After all, the Hippocratic Oath is just a bunch of words. Without moral reasons to back them up, those words cannot dictate medical ethics or physicians' duties" (2007, 138). In other words, even if the Hippocratic

Oath does prohibit medical aid in dying, why should clinicians follow it? Justifying that prohibition simply by referencing the Hippocratic Oath commits a fallacious appeal to authority.

Medical associations are split when it comes to medical aid in dying. Some, such as the British Medical Association, have adopted neutral positions; others, such as the American Academy of Family Physicians, have a policy of "engaged neutrality," providing advice to physicians in states where the practice is legal; and still others, such as the World Medical Association, have recently reiterated their opposition. The leading voice on this issue in the U.S. is the American Medical Association, which has staunchly opposed medical aid in dying since first articulating its views in 1973. Its most recent Code of Medical Ethics recognizes that "thoughtful, morally admirable individuals hold diverging, yet equally deeply held and well-considered perspectives about physician-assisted suicide" and that both those who advocate for and those who argue against it are motivated by the desire to support patient autonomy and diminish unnecessary suffering (American Medical Association, n.d., 5.7). However, the AMA draws the moral boundary at the point of a physician intending to bring about a patient's death: "The right of self-determination is a right to accept or refuse offered interventions, but not to decide what should be offered. The right to refuse life-sustaining treatment does not automatically entail a right to insist that others take action to bring on death" (1993, 264). The AMA maintains that "physician-assisted suicide is fundamentally incompatible with the physician's role as healer, would be difficult or impossible to control, and would pose serious societal risks" (n.d., 5.7; see also Bristow 1997). This position is echoed by the American College of Physicians: "Physician-assisted suicide . . . is problematic given the nature of the patient-physician relationship, affects trust in the relationship and in the profession, and fundamentally alters the medical profession's role in society" (Sulmasy and Mueller 2017, 578). On this view, because assisting in a suicide conflicts with the physician's role as healer—health, not death, is a legitimate aim for medical professionals—and because it could lead to involuntary euthanasia, it should not be among the treatments offered to patients (see also Kass 1989; Pellegrino 1992; Bok 1998, 107–39; Marcoux 2010; Randall and Downie 2010). The value of bodily self-determination comes up against the medical duty to protect patients' health, especially if their choice to die might be coerced by external or internal forces, such as family pressure or psychiatric illness.

## 2. *Theoretical and empirical slippery slopes*

The second class of arguments against medical aid in dying warns of a slippery slope, the "serious societal risks" invoked in the AMA Code of Medical Ethics. In a previous articulation of their position, the American Medical Association argued that

> permitting assisted suicide opens the door to policies that carry far greater risks. For example, if assisted suicide is permitted, then there is a strong argument for allowing euthanasia. It would be arbitrary to permit patients who have the physical ability to take a pill to end their lives, but not let similarly suffering patients die if they require the lethal drug to be administered by another person. Once euthanasia is permitted, however, there is a serious risk of involuntary deaths. (1993, 266)

The worry is that once medical aid in dying is morally or legally accepted, it will be difficult to sustain its current eligibility restrictions and other limitations. Why should eighteen-year-olds but not seventeen-year-olds be eligible? Why should people who are terminally ill be eligible but not people suffering from chronic and unbearable pain due to nonterminal conditions? Why are people legally prohibited from including medical aid in dying instructions in their advance directives?

John Arras (1998) calls this the **theoretical slippery slope**, also known as the legal or logical slippery slope, which would erode the legal restrictions on who is eligible for medical aid in dying (see also Keown 2002, 76–79). If the moral principles of autonomy and beneficence are taken to justify bringing about a patient's death under certain, highly circumscribed conditions (all the current eligibility requirements codified in death with dignity laws in the U.S., for instance), why would those same principles not apply to people who are not currently eligible? Arras argues that once medical aid in dying is legalized, excluding patients from using it and prohibiting active euthanasia would function as a form of discrimination (1998, 283–84). Thus, there would be social and legal pressure to expand medical aid in dying until active euthanasia is legalized (Walker 2001). If all these limitations are lifted, the concern is that people's lives will be ended without their consent or against their will. That is, medical aid in dying may lead to the moral and legal acceptance of active euthanasia or medical participation in the involuntary deaths of vulnerable people—people who are elderly, people who are disabled, and others who have been designated as unhealthy by their societies.

In addition, Arras (1998) worries about an **empirical slippery slope**, also known as the practical or psychological slippery slope, which would erode protections against abuse, even if the legal eligibility is not expanded, because of the difficulty of verifying that a patient's request is fully voluntary and autonomous (see also Kamisar 1958; Bok 1998, 107–27; Keown 2002, 72–76). A patient may be suffering from undiagnosed depression, coerced by family members, or pressured by poverty or forms of social discrimination, such as lack of access to affordable, effective palliative care. Outside of equity issues, Arras warns that physicians receive insufficient training in supporting patients at the end of life, both in terms of pain management and psychological needs, so they will be more prone to think that assisted suicide is the right option: "Instead of vigorously addressing the pharmacological and psychosocial needs of [terminal] patients, physicians no doubt will continue to ignore, undertreat or treat many of their patients in an impersonal manner" (1998, 285). Although medical aid in dying may be a morally justified option under ideal circumstances, the world that we actually inhabit is marked by various kinds of prejudice and discrimination, inadequate treatment for people at the end of life, and difficulty in identifying subtle forms of coercion. The language of autonomy (or liberty) can be used to justify providing people with fewer healthcare resources without offering the support people need to have meaningful options. The moral justification for medical aid in dying can be used to promote policies that serve the purposes of economic efficiency rather than supporting the health of patients (Pellegrino 1992). As John Keown (2002) puts it, medical aid in dying will end up being a more accepted and more frequent form of treatment rather than an option of last resort. In the Netherlands, for example, euthanasia and medical aid in dying accounted for 1.9 percent of all deaths in 1990 and grew to 4.2 percent in 2019 (Groenewoud et al. 2024).

The eugenicist history of euthanasia practices, especially in Nazi Germany, offers a cautionary tale. Appealing to the principle of beneficence, Adolf Hitler in 1939 authorized doctors to "grant a mercy death" to patients "suffering from illnesses judged to be incurable." This led to the creation of the T4 program, which killed approximately 250,000 people by the end of the war (United States Holocaust Memorial Museum 2020). The possibility of deliberately ending life (with the stated intent of sparing those people suffering) "divides populations into two classes of people: Those who are supposed to benefit from their own quick deaths and those who are supposed to benefit from others' quick deaths" (Francis and Silvers 2015, 488). In many discussions of euthanasia, the benefits to the second group are not explicitly delineated, but references to allocating resources such as equipment and staffing to other patients or alleviating the financial burden on families suggest this calculation. Eugenics attempts to benefit those who are designated as fundamentally healthy (and therefore deserving of resources to support that health) at the expense of those who are seen as "useless eaters" or "life unworthy of life" (Mostert 2002). The quasi-scientific character of eugenicist theory makes the distinction between healthy and unhealthy appear to be objective rather than culturally generated. The moral implications of this theory also violate the core intuition behind the principle of beneficence: that those who need medical care should receive it rather than being killed or expected to kill themselves.

Although medical euthanasia was not practiced regularly in the United States, eugenicist justifications of involuntary sterilization laws in the twentieth century—used against the poor, people with disabilities, people of color, and people who did not conform to gender and sexual norms—invoked these same medicalized arguments (Stern 2005). Ending the lives of those marginalized people may be framed as acts of compassion, in relieving them of the burden of experiencing an existence that is dominated by pathology, where pathology can be any condition seen as socially abnormal and then medicalized as disease or disability. Medical aid in dying would thus normalize a worldview in which life in general is treated as only instrumentally valuable and the lives of people in marginalized groups are judged to be illegitimately using resources (Dyck 2002).

Disability rights advocates have been particularly concerned about the legalization of medical aid in dying because of the social stigma surrounding disability. As Ron Amundson remarks, cultural stereotypes about physical and cognitive disabilities, as well as mental illness, may lead to judgments that no one can lead a dignified life if their impairments are severe:

> I began to notice that when assisted suicide advocates really wanted to scare their audience, they didn't use unremitting pain to do it. They used disability. . . . I began to see the smug slogan "Death with Dignity" in a new light: It hid the assumption that dignity was forever out of the reach of people who were disabled; "Better Dead than Disabled." (Amundson and Taira 2005, 54)

Physicians may reinforce this stigma by interpreting disability as chronic pathology rather than acknowledging how people with temporary or more enduring disabilities adjust to their circumstances and lead purposeful lives within them. As we discussed in relation to disability-selective abortion in Chapter 6, many critical disability theorists argue that the source of suffering or indignity is not the impairment itself but the significance that the impairment takes on in a social context—in a built environment that may not be hospitable to people with limited vision or people in wheelchairs, or in a cultural environment in which disability provokes infantilizing, pathologizing, or objectifying reactions. We must distinguish between disabilities from handicaps, the latter of which "represents socialization of an impairment or disability, and as such . . . reflects the consequences for the individual—cultural, social, economic, and environmental—that stem from the presence of impairment and disability" (World Health Organization 1980, 182). Someone new to a disability or level of impairment may experience the grief of losing abilities and may grapple with their own internalized ableism. However, Amundson and Taira (2005) argue that healthcare practitioners, as well as the legal landscape around people with disabilities, should not validate that reaction by presenting suicide as a legal option.

David Velleman (1992) makes a similar argument about the moral undesirability of social pressure, but he claims that some terminally ill patients experience harm just by being given the option of medical aid in dying, even if the slippery slope does not in fact occur. This sounds counterintuitive—more choices are presumably better, especially for patients who want to die—but Velleman claims that those who do not want to die are subjected to various harms. Such patients feel pressured to die from friends and family who incur the financial and emotional costs of prolonged medical care; they are told by society that, although suicide is legally proscribed in general because life is worth preserving, we are making an exception for them because it is not worth living with the pain and loss of dignity of a terminal illness; and having the option to die puts patients in the position of having to justify their continued existence.

As an alternative to medical aid in dying, opponents say that we should offer support so that patients can adapt to their current conditions. This means caring for a patient's needs at a physical, psychological, and social level, and respecting their autonomy up to the point of acceding to a request to end their lives. In order to avoid both forms of the slippery slope, Arras (1998) insists that physicians must focus on effectively treating patients at the end of life, giving them access to high-quality primary care, psychiatric care, pain management, and hospice care.

Those who reject medical aid in dying argue that patients can experience much that is valuable as they approach death. Bonnie Steinbock warns us that a "quick and painless death" is not always preferable:

> We must be cautious about attributing to defective children [children with incurable conditions at birth] *our* distress at seeing them linger. Waiting for them to die may be tough on parents, doctors, and nurses—it isn't necessarily tough on the child. The decision not to operate need not mean a decision to neglect, and it may be possible to make the remaining months of the child's life comfortable, pleasant, and filled with love. (1979, 63)

The compassion of clinicians and family members may be misapplied, in other words, to justify ending a life that may contain valuable elements for that patient, even if it also carries negative experiences (Pellegrino 1992; Francis and Silvers 2015, 487–89). Hence, opponents of medical aid in dying appeal primarily to the principle of beneficence and, in a secondary way, to the principle of respect for autonomy—the need to protect patients from coercion—to justify their position.

## Arguments for Medical Aid in Dying

Arguments for medical aid in dying tend to claim (1) that people should have control over their own health outcomes and may even have a right to die, or (2) that medical aid in dying will reduce suffering at the end of life. Thus, justifications of medical aid in dying, like criticisms of it, appeal to respect for autonomy and beneficence.

## 1. Respect for autonomy

One of the first well-publicized arguments in favor of medical aid in dying was Dr. Timothy Quill's moral reasoning in response to a terminally ill patient who requested life-ending medication, published in the *New England Journal of Medicine* in 1991. Diagnosed with acute myelomonocytic leukemia, the patient had refused chemotherapy and wanted to control the process of her dying. Prior to any death with dignity legislation, Quill followed much of its spirit. When his patient requested a prescription for barbiturates, he had a substantive conversation with her "to be sure that she was not in despair or overwhelmed in a way that might color her judgment" (1991, 693). Once he concluded that she was making this request freely, he gave her instructions on how to use the medication to aid in sleep and also to bring about death. His moral justification for this act centered on her autonomy: "I . . . felt strongly that I was setting her free to get the most out of the time she had left, and to maintain dignity and control on her own terms until her death" (693). Autonomy at a visceral level means bodily self-determination: the person controls what happens and does not happen to them. That respect for self-control undergirds the moral and legal commitment to informed consent and withholding or withdrawing treatment at a capable patient's request. Advocates of medical aid in dying see the practice as a natural extension of the principle of honoring a patient's wishes about their own health and life. Their values and judgments determine what they will and will not experience, at least as far as medicine can support those wishes.

Merely having access to life-ending medication, even if it remains unused, may be psychologically empowering. Oregon's Death with Dignity annual reports show that approximately one-third of patients who get such prescriptions do not use them, allowing themselves to die from their terminal conditions (Center for Health Statistics 2024). Anecdotally, patients have reported some level of comfort knowing that they can choose the circumstances of their deaths because it allows them to focus on what is valuable in their remaining time (Dieterle 2007, 134). The experience of terminal illness, above and beyond whatever pain a person endures, carries a sense of helplessness and loss of agency. Being able to control the timing and manner of one's death—having the option to avoid an existence that one would not find valuable, even if they do not use it—reclaims some of that loss.

Quill's patient was also concerned about the loss of autonomy and dignity that may come with the methods of pain management that would be necessary, given her condition—hence the language from the Canadian law that refers to suffering "that cannot be alleviated under conditions that the person finds acceptable" (Government of Canada 2024). If curing the underlying disease is not possible and medicine can only control symptoms or prolong an existence that the patient does not "find acceptable," medical aid in dying seems to honor the basic moral principles of beneficence and respect for autonomy. According to the **doctrine of double effect**, foreseeable but unintended harms are allowable if the intended effects of an action are good, the good and bad consequences are practically inseparable (the good cannot be accomplished without the bad), and the good consequences sufficiently outweigh the bad consequences. Just as sedating a patient to unconsciousness or withdrawing treatment in accordance with a patient's wishes should not be described as an act of killing them, so too (advocates of medical aid in dying claim) providing life-ending medication and instructions on how to use it effectively is a way to spare the patient unnecessary pain and support their bodily self-determination. Death is a consequence but not the purpose (Dieterle 2007, 138).

In a legal sense, respect for autonomy entails protecting the judgments of individuals from state coercion. Although critics worry about family or economic necessity influencing terminally ill patients, "the most serious pressure of all [is] the criminal law which tells them that they may not decide for death if they need the help of a doctor in dying, no matter how firmly they wish it" (Dworkin et al. 1997, 46). In emphasizing the parallels between constitutional protections for abortion and proposed death with dignity laws, Dworkin et al. (1997) defend the individual's right to make major life decisions for themselves, including the decision of whether to continue living. That is, respecting autonomy means allowing the individual to decide whether their own life has instrumental or intrinsic value, a question deeply tied to that singular person's religious and moral commitments. For a physician, a healthcare system, or a government to impose such value judgments on a patient would be an act of coercion:

> These cases do not invite or require the Court to make moral, ethical, or religious judgments about how people should approach or confront their death or about when it is ethically appropriate to hasten one's own death or to ask others for help in doing so. On the contrary, they ask

the Court to recognize that individuals have a constitutionally protected interest in making those grave judgments for themselves, free from the imposition of any religious or philosophical orthodoxy by court or legislature. . . . Denying that opportunity to terminally ill patients who are in agonizing pain or otherwise doomed to an existence they regard as intolerable could only be justified on the basis of a religious or ethical conviction about the value or meaning of life itself. Our Constitution forbids government to impose such convictions on its citizens. (43)

The six philosophers who contributed to "The Philosophers' Brief" suggest that the moral opposition to medical aid in dying is a vestige of religiously based prohibitions on suicide, or the idea that individual human beings must cede the decision of when they die to divine authority. But the value judgments of any particular religious tradition should not limit the legal exercise of individual freedoms. The U.S. Constitution protects the ability of individuals to make those moral judgments for themselves (Thomson 1999, 506–7).

## *2. Beneficence*

A second major justification for medical aid in dying is that it reduces suffering. Quill writes:

> Although I know we have measures to help control pain and lessen suffering, to think that people do not suffer in the process of dying is an illusion. Prolonged dying can occasionally be peaceful, but more often the role of the physician and family is limited to lessening but not eliminating severe suffering. (1991, 694)

When medicine can neither cure the underlying condition nor eliminate a patient's pain, allowing the patient to release themselves by ending their life can reasonably be interpreted as promoting their well-being. An easy death is preferable to prolonged and pointless suffering.

To be sure, a consequentialist approach such as this needs to consider not only the implications for the individual patient but the wider society. Does medical aid in dying cause a slippery slope leading to active euthanasia? In response to the theoretical slippery slope argument, advocates point to decades of legal medical aid in dying in Oregon and other U.S. states, which have not led to significantly expanded eligibility (Dieterle 2007,

129–32). Dworkin et al. (1997) claim that the state can justify restricting who is eligible for medical aid in dying precisely to protect autonomy and maximize beneficence. These restrictions function as a kind of soft paternalism: the state has a legitimate interest in ensuring that a person is acting autonomously (making an informed, deliberate, uncoerced decision). It can also exclude nonterminal patients because they have a much higher risk of cutting themselves off from a worthwhile future. Although the state can justifiably limit medical aid in dying, prohibiting it for everyone would amount to preventing competent people who have no good medical choices from deciding to end their lives with the aid of a physician. The state would be engaging in hard paternalism, substituting its judgment about the patient's well-being for the patient's own competent judgment and thus undermining their autonomy.

As for the empirical slippery slope argument, studies have shown that, at least in the U.S., existing death with dignity laws have not been abused. Although the number of patients and physicians participating in medical aid in dying has been increasing in Oregon, less than 1 percent of all deaths (367 out of 44,593) resulted from medical aid in dying in 2023; only about 2.6 percent of physicians participated (167 out of 6,386) (Center for Health Statistics 2024, 6, 9). Despite concerns that legalizing physician-assisted suicide would exert pressure on poor people as a cost-containment strategy (Marker 1997), there also has been no evidence of heightened risk for the poor or the chronically ill in Oregon (Battin et al. 2007). In fact, physicians were less likely to grant a request if a patient raised a concern about being a burden to others (Ganzini et al. 2000). Patients also tend to be relatively privileged in terms of educational attainment, race, and access to health insurance, which suggests that vulnerable groups have not been pressured into medical aid in dying (Center for Health Statistics 2024, 11–12). There is no evidence that large numbers of patients have been driven to give up hope or to devalue their lives because the option is available.

Furthermore, advocates argue that legalizing medical aid in dying allows it to be carefully regulated. If medical aid in dying were illegal, a certain proportion of physicians might be willing, as Dr. Quill was, to accede to a patient's request or even end a patient's life without their explicit request, out of benevolence. A 2003 European study found that 0.6 percent of all deaths in the Netherlands resulted from a physician ending a patient's life without their request (excluding deaths hastened by high levels of pain medication and by patient refusal of treatment), even though medical aid in dying is legal there. But other countries had similar or higher numbers prior to or without legalization: 0.67 percent in Denmark, 1.5 percent in Belgium, and 3.5 percent in Australia (Heide et al. 2003). Although this practice is not tracked in the United States, a small nationwide study of oncologists in 1998 (only a year after Oregon's Death with Dignity law came into effect) found that 15.8 percent self-reported participating in physician-assisted suicide or euthanasia, with some of those cases fitting the description of nonvoluntary euthanasia (Emanuel et al. 1998, 507). A separate study of more than 3,000 oncologists found that 56 percent of them received a patient request for medical aid in dying, and 38 percent received a request for euthanasia; 11 percent had in fact participated in physician-assisted suicide, while almost 4 percent had participated in euthanasia at least once (Emanuel et al. 2000, 529). At some level, these statistics indicate that some physicians have a strong moral intuition that they owe their patients release from life. But depending on individual physicians to make these moral judgments outside of a legal structure means that patients have inequitable access to medical aid in dying. The legal channel creates a more regulated process of decision-making in which eligibility requirements and the mandatory procedure protect patient autonomy. Without such options, patients may try to end their lives in more painful and less effective ways.

Defenders of medical aid in dying claim that, since doctors who write prescriptions for life-ending medication are supporting patients' well-being and autonomy, it does not corrupt the physician's role as healer (Gill 2005, 60–63). First, the doctor is only being asked to assist the patient in doing what they want. The doctor is not forcing a decision on the patient as they would in the case of involuntary euthanasia. Rather, they are deciding only whether the patient has a terminal illness and whether the patient is capable of making informed medical decisions, both of which are factual questions having to do with the doctor's professional opinion. The patient carries the moral burden of evaluating their continued existence and deciding whether to take the medication.

The phrase "life-ending medication" seems paradoxical because it runs against ingrained assumptions that the purpose of medicine is to protect health and prolong life. Medical aid in dying opens up a debate about how medical care fits into the broader priorities and values that patients have. Defenders of medical aid in dying insist that doctors are obligated not only to heal but also to reduce suffering. Terminal patients, by definition, cannot be healed, so in such cases, physicians' obligation to manage pain becomes most important. And one way to escape pain is to end one's life.

## Passive Euthanasia and Its Implications for Medical Aid in Dying

Although the American Medical Association opposes medical aid in dying, it supports the use of what bioethicists call passive euthanasia—withholding or withdrawing life-sustaining treatment to respect the autonomy of the patient, as expressed in real time, in an advance directive, or by a medical proxy; and avoiding medically ineffective interventions (n.d., 5). According to the AMA Code of Medical Ethics,

> a patient who has decision-making capacity appropriate to the decision at hand has the right to decline any medical intervention or ask that an intervention be stopped, even when that decision is expected to lead to his or her death and regardless of whether or not the individual is terminally ill. (5.3)

When interventions are ineffective in treating the underlying pathology, the AMA supports **palliative sedation** in order to manage symptoms, but not with the goal of ending a patient's life:

> The duty to relieve pain and suffering is central to the physician's role as healer and is an obligation physicians have to their patients. When a terminally ill patient experiences severe pain or other distressing clinical symptoms that do not respond to aggressive, symptom-specific palliation it can be appropriate to offer sedation to unconsciousness as an intervention of last resort. Sedation to unconsciousness must never be used to intentionally cause a patient's death. (5.6)

Since many painkillers cause depressed respiration, a secondary and foreseeable consequence of some palliative sedation is that it hastens a patient's death. Thus, the AMA is appealing to the doctrine of double effect: palliative sedation is justified as an attempt to control a patient's pain, even if it brings about death as an unintended consequence (see American Medical Association 1993, 264).

We mentioned earlier that bioethicists *typically* describe the refusal of life-sustaining treatment as passive euthanasia. Steinbock has challenged that identification by highlighting the importance of physician intent, in line with the doctrine of double effect (1979, 60–61). She argues that ceasing life-sustaining treatment has two legitimate medical purposes: either respecting a competent patient's autonomy or not imposing unnecessary suffering on them. If fulfilling those two obligations has the secondary effect of hastening the patient's death, that is morally irrelevant as long as the physician's goal is not to kill the person. It is not euthanasia of any variety because it does not intentionally cause a patient's death. This fine-grained focus on the physician's intent thus separates a morally justifiable act (ceasing life-sustaining treatment) from a morally unjustifiable one (passive euthanasia), even if what the physician does in each case is indistinguishable to an observer.

Some advocates for medical aid in dying argue that it is inconsistent to allow patients to refuse life-sustaining treatment without also endorsing medical aid in dying or even active euthanasia. Actively ending a competent patient's life, on their request, is likely to spare them unnecessary pain more effectively than allowing the disease to "take its natural course":

> If we simply withhold treatment, it will take [a terminal patient] *longer* to die, and so he will suffer *more*, than if we administered the lethal injection. Why, if we have already decided to shorten his life because of the pain, should we prefer the option that involves more suffering? (Rachels 1986, 108–9)

If, as part of humane treatment, healthcare professionals are morally obligated to reduce patients' suffering, then in certain circumstances, actively killing them or assisting them in ending their lives is better than letting them die.

Similarly, if respecting patient autonomy is a moral duty for clinicians, why would it be important to respect their refusal of life-sustaining treatment but not their desire for medical aid in dying—a controlled, willed form of death? The difference between actively killing a patient (or providing them with the means to kill themselves) and letting a patient die from natural causes may not be morally significant, because not treating a patient is still a deliberate action with consequences for their health. Judith Jarvis Thomson provides the following analogy: "If I knock out the main beam that is currently preventing the fall of a roof, I do not merely let gravity take its course and the roof therefore fall on those locked in the house. I intervene—I cause gravity to take its course" (1999, 501; see also Dworkin and Frey 1998; Doyal and Doyal 2001). Withdrawing treatment is a morally significant action that allows the disease to kill the patient. If a patient needed life-saving medical treatment (for instance, if they were suffering from dehydration or a burst appendix) and wanted to live, a physician's decision to let the disease take its natural course would be in a legal sense malpractice (and possibly manslaughter) and in a moral sense a violation of their obligation to respect the patient's autonomy and act beneficently toward them (Rachels 1986, 115). We hold people responsible for their decisions not to act as well as to act; the question is when action or inaction is morally justified. According to James Rachels (1986), what is important in moral assessment is the purpose that is being accomplished—whether the patient wants to live or not, whether their pain is being alleviated—and the motive of the person committing the act, not the method.

Withholding or withdrawing life-sustaining treatment (again, what most bioethicists call passive euthanasia) also puts patients at greater risk of coerced or nonvoluntary death than medical aid in dying does. In every state, medical aid in dying requires the patient's present, iterated, and witnessed desire to be articulated, and their capacity and terminal condition to be assessed by two physicians. By contrast, an advance directive or medical proxy's decision may authorize the refusal of treatment without any such constraints. An advance directive can be filled out in entirely unregulated circumstances, and its instructions stand as long as they are not contradicted by the patient. A medical proxy may make decisions based on their best interpretation of the patient's wishes (or what they say is their best interpretation) without any written directive. In short, they are less likely to track what a patient wants. Therefore, medical aid in dying more carefully protects patient autonomy than passive euthanasia as it is currently practiced. Yet the latter is taken to be morally uncontroversial.

## Conclusion: Normative Commitments within the Debate

Larger existential questions emerge when we consider medical aid in dying, such as the value of human life and whether patients can decide when it ends.

Recent cultural shifts have tended to emphasize individual control over oneself, including the right to die, as opposed to traditional views about owing one's life to a divine or political authority. Constitutional debates can only partially capture the deeply rooted religious and moral beliefs that define our sense of ourselves. Acknowledging these more fundamental commitments may help to explain our disparate positions on this issue and illuminate why medical aid in dying is so politically and emotionally charged.

## REFERENCES

American Medical Association. 1993. "Reports of Council on Ethical and Judicial Affairs: Report 8: Physician-Assisted Suicide." In *Proceedings of the House of Delegates*, 47th Interim Meeting, 263–67. New Orleans: American Medical Association.

———. n.d. "Code of Medical Ethics." Accessed January 15, 2025. https://code-medical-ethics.ama-assn.org/.

Amundson, Ron, and Gayle Taira. 2005. "Our Lives and Ideologies: The Effect of Life Experience on the Perceived Morality of the Policy of Physician-Assisted Suicide." *Journal of Disability Policy Studies* 16, no. 1 (Summer): 53–57. doi:10.1177/10442073050160010801.

Arras, John D. 1998. "Physician-Assisted Suicide: A Tragic View." In *Physician Assisted Suicide: Expanding the Debate*, edited by Margaret P. Battin, Anita Silvers, and Rosamond Rhodes, 279–300. New York: Routledge.

Battin, Margaret P. 2019. "Development of the AAS Statement on 'Suicide' and 'Physician Aid in Dying.'" *Suicide and Life-Threatening Behavior* 49, no. 3 (June): 774–76. doi:10.1111/sltb.12453.

Battin, Margaret P., Agnes van der Heide, Linda Ganzini, Gerrit van der Wal, and Bregje D. Onwuteaka-Philipsen. 2007. "Legal Physician-Assisted Dying in Oregon and the Netherlands: Evidence Concerning the Impact on Patients in 'Vulnerable' Groups." *Journal of Medical Ethics* 33, no. 10 (October): 591–97. doi:10.1136/jme.2007.022335.

Bok, Sissela. 1998. "Part Two." In *Euthanasia and Physician-Assisted Suicide—For and Against*, by Gerald Dworkin, R. G. Frey, and Sissela Bok, 81–139. Cambridge: Cambridge University Press.

Bondolfi, Sibilla. 2020. "Why Assisted Suicide Is 'Normal' in Switzerland." *SWI Swissinfo*. July 24. https://www.swissinfo.ch/eng/life-aging/why-assisted-suicide-is-normal-in-switzerland/45924614.

Bristow, Lonnie. 1997. "Physician's Role as Healer: American Medical Association's Opposition to Physician-Assisted Suicide." *St. John's Journal of Legal*

*Commentary* 12, no. 3 (Summer): 653–58. https://scholarship.law.stjohns.edu/jcred/vol12/iss3/8/.

Center for Health Statistics. 2024. *Oregon Death with Dignity Act: 2023 Data Summary.* March 20. https://www.oregon.gov/oha/PH/PROVIDERPARTNERRESOURCES/EVALUATIONRESEARCH/DEATHWITHDIGNITYACT/Documents/year26.pdf.

Diaz, Dan. 2017. "Endings Matter." Interview by Nora McInerny. *Terrible, Thanks for Asking* (podcast). September 6.

Dieterle, J. M. 2007. "Physician-Assisted Suicide: A New Look at the Arguments." *Bioethics* 21, no. 3 (March): 127–39. doi:10.1111/j.1467-8519.2007.00536.x.

Doyal, Len, and Lesley Doyal. 2001. "Why Active Euthanasia and Physician Assisted Suicide Should Be Legalised: If Death Is in a Patient's Best Interest Then Death Constitutes a Moral Good." *BMJ* 323, no. 7321 (November 10): 1079–80. doi:10.1136/bmj.323.7321.1079.

Dworkin, Gerald, and R. G. Frey. 1998. "Part One." In *Euthanasia and Physician-Assisted Suicide—For and Against*, by Gerald Dworkin, R. G. Frey, and Sissela Bok, 1–80. Cambridge: Cambridge University Press.

Dworkin, Ronald, Thomas Nagel, Robert Nozick, John Rawls, Thomas Scanlon, and Judith Jarvis Thomson. 1997. "Assisted Suicide: The Philosophers' Brief." *New York Review of Books*. March 27, 41–47.

Dyck, Arthur J. 2002. *Life's Worth: The Case against Assisted Suicide.* Grand Rapids, MI: Eerdmans.

Emanuel, Ezekiel J., Elisabeth R. Daniels, Diane L. Fairclough, and Brian R. Clarridge. 1998. "The Practice of Euthanasia and Physician-Assisted Suicide in the United States: Adherence to Proposed Safeguards and Effects on Physicians." *JAMA: Journal of the American Medical Association* 280, no. 6 (August 12): 507–13. doi:10.1001/jama.280.6.507.

Emanuel, Ezekiel J., Diane Fairclough, Brian C. Clarridge, Diane Blum, Eduardo Bruera, W. Charles Penley, Lowell E. Schnipper, and Robert J. Mayer. 2000. "Attitudes and Practices of U.S. Oncologists regarding Euthanasia and Physician-Assisted Suicide." *Annals of Internal Medicine* 133, no. 7 (October 3): 527–32. doi:10.7326/0003-4819-133-7-200010030-00011.

European Institute of Bioethics. 2021. "Belgium: Euthanasia of Newborns Practiced outside the Law." June 24. https://www.ieb-eib.org/en/news/end-of-life/euthanasia-and-assisted-suicide/belgium-euthanasia-of-new-borns-practiced-outside-the-law-2041.html.

Francis, Leslie P., and Anita Silvers. 2015. "Disability and Assisted Death." In *The Routledge Companion to Bioethics*, edited by John D. Arras, Elizabeth Fenton, and Rebecca Kukla, 486–99. New York: Routledge.

Ganzini, Linda, Heidi D. Nelson, Terri A. Schmidt, Dale F. Kraemer, Molly A. Delorit, and Melinda A. Lee. 2000. "Physicians' Experiences with the Oregon Death with Dignity Act." *New England Journal of Medicine* 342, no. 8 (February 24): 557–63. doi:10.1056/NEJM200002243420806.

Gill, Michael B. 2005. "A Moral Defense of Oregon's Physician-Assisted Suicide Law." *Mortality* 10, no. 1 (February): 53–67. doi:10.1080/13576270500031055.

Go Gentle Australia. n.d. "Voluntary Assisted Dying in Australia." Accessed January 15, 2025. https://www.gogentleaustralia.org.au/vad_in_australia.

Gourevitch, Danielle. 1969. "Suicide among the Sick in Classical Antiquity." *Bulletin of the History of Medicine* 43, no. 6 (November–December): 501–18. https://www.jstor.org/stable/44449274.

Government of Canada. 2024. "Canada's Medical Assistance in Dying (MAID) Law." Last modified July 31, 2024. https://www.justice.gc.ca/eng/cj-jp/ad-am/bk-di.html.

Government of the Netherlands. n.d. "Euthanasia." Accessed January 15, 2025. https://www.government.nl/topics/euthanasia.

Groenewoud, A. Stef, Femke Atsma, Mina Arvin, Gert P. Westert, and Theo A. Boer. 2024. "Euthanasia in the Netherlands: A Claims Data Cross-Sectional Study of Geographical Variation." *BMJ Supportive & Palliative Care* 14: e867–77. doi:10.1136/bmjspcare-2020-002573.

Heide, Agnes van der, Luc Deliens, Karin Faisst, Tore Nilstun, Michael Norup, Eugenio Paci, Gerrit van der Wal, and Paul J. van der Maas. 2003. "End-of-Life Decision-Making in Six European Countries: Descriptive Study." *Lancet* 362, no. 9381 (August 2): 345–50. doi:10.1016/S0140-6736(03)14019-6.

"Hippocratic Oath." 2002. Translated by Michael North. National Library of Medicine, National Institutes of Health. https://www.nlm.nih.gov/hmd/topics/greek-medicine/index.html.

Honderich, Holly. 2023. "Who Can Die? Canada Wrestles with Euthanasia for the Mentally Ill." *BBC.* January 14. https://www.bbc.com/news/world-us-canada-64004329.

Hooff, Anton J. L. van. 2004. "Ancient Euthanasia: 'Good Death' and the Doctor in the Graeco-Roman World." *Social Science & Medicine* 58, no. 5 (March): 975–85. doi:10.1016/j.socscimed.2003.10.036.

Kamisar, Yale. 1958. "Some Non-Religious Views against Proposed 'Mercy-Killing' Legislation." *Minnesota Law Review* 42, no. 6 (May): 969–1042. https://scholarship.law.umn.edu/mlr/2588.

Kao, Audiey C., and Kayhan P. Parsi. 2004. "Content Analyses of Oaths Administered at U.S. Medical Schools in 2000." *Academic Medicine* 79, no. 9 (September): 882–87. doi:10.1097/00001888-200409000-00015.

Kass, Leon R. 1989. "Neither for Love nor Money: Why Doctors Must Not Kill." *Public Interest* 94 (Winter): 25–46. https://www.nationalaffairs.com/public_interest/detail/neither-for-love-nor-money-why-doctors-must-not-kill.

Keown, John. 2002. *Euthanasia, Ethics and Public Policy: An Argument against Legalisation*. Cambridge: Cambridge University Press. doi:10.1017/CBO9780511495335.

Lasagna, Louis. 1964. "The Hippocratic Oath: Modern Version." https://www.pbs.org/wgbh/nova/doctors/oath_modern.html.

Marcoux, Hubert. 2010. "Should Physicians Be Open to Euthanasia? No." *Canadian Family Physician/Médecin de Famille Canadien* 56, no. 4 (April): 321–23. https://www.cfp.ca/content/56/4/321.

Marker, Rita L. 1997. "Assisted Suicide: Legal, Medical & Ethical Considerations for the Future." *St. John's Journal of Legal Commentary* 12, no. 3 (Summer): 670–79. https://scholarship.law.stjohns.edu/jcred/vol12/iss3/10/.

Maynard, Brittany. 2014. "My Right to Death with Dignity at 29." *CNN*. November 2. https://www.cnn.com/2014/10/07/opinion/maynard-assisted-suicide-cancer-dignity/index.html.

Mostert, Mark P. 2002. "Useless Eaters: Disability as Genocidal Marker in Nazi Germany." *Journal of Special Education* 36, no. 3 (November): 157–70. doi:10.1177/00224669020360030601.

"New Law Allowing Assisted Suicide Takes Effect in Austria." 2022. *BBC*. January 1. https://www.bbc.com/news/world-europe-59847371.

New Zealand Ministry of Health. 2024. "Assisted Dying Eligibility and Access." Last modified September 11, 2024. https://www.tewhatuora.govt.nz/for-the-health-sector/assisted-dying-service/assisted-dying-information-for-the-public/assisted-dying-eligibility-and-access/.

Pellegrino, Edmund D. 1992. "Doctors Must Not Kill." *Journal of Clinical Ethics* 3, no. 2 (Summer): 95–102. doi:10.1086/JCE199203202.

Quill, Timothy E. 1991. "Death and Dignity: A Case of Individualized Decision Making." *New England Journal of Medicine* 324, no. 10 (March 7): 691–94. doi:10.1056/NEJM199103073241010.

Rachels, James. 1986. *The End of Life: Euthanasia and Morality*. New York: Oxford University Press.

Randall, Fiona, and Robin Downie. 2010. "Assisted Suicide and Voluntary Euthanasia: Role Contradictions for Physicians." *Clinical Medicine* 10, no. 4 (August): 323–25. doi:10.7861/clinmedicine.10-4-323.

Regnard, Claud, Ana Worthington, and Ilora Finlay. 2023. "Oregon Death with Dignity Act Access: 25 Year Analysis." *BMJ Supportive & Palliative Care* 14, no. 4 (December): 455–61. doi:10.1136/spcare-2023-004292.

Steinbock, Bonnie. 1979. "The Intentional Termination of Life." *Ethics in Science and Medicine* 6, no. 1: 59–64.

Stern, Alexandra Minna. 2005. *Eugenic Nation: Faults and Frontiers of Better Breeding in Modern America.* Berkeley: University of California Press.

Sulmasy, Lois Snyder, and Paul S. Mueller. 2017. "Ethics and the Legalization of Physician-Assisted Suicide: An American College of Physicians Position Paper." *Annals of Internal Medicine* 167, no. 8 (October 17): 576–78. doi:10.7326/M17-0938.

Thomson, Judith Jarvis. 1999. "Physician-Assisted Suicide: Two Moral Arguments." *Ethics* 109, no. 3 (April): 497–518. doi:10.1086/233919.

United States Holocaust Memorial Museum. 2020. "Euthanasia Program and Aktion T4." October 7. https://encyclopedia.ushmm.org/content/en/article/euthanasia-program.

Velleman, J. David. 1992. "Against the Right to Die." *Journal of Medicine and Philosophy* 17, no. 6 (December): 665–81. doi:10.1093/jmp/17.6.665.

Walker, Robert M. 2001. "Physician-Assisted Suicide: The Legal Slippery Slope." *Cancer Control* 8, no. 1 (January–February): 25–31. doi:10.1177/107327480100800104.

World Health Organization. 1980. *International Classification of Impairments, Disabilities, and Handicaps.* Geneva: World Health Organization.

## Further Reading

Battin, Margaret P., Rosamond Rhodes, and Anita Silvers, eds. 2015. *Physician Assisted Suicide: Expanding the Debate.* New York: Routledge.

> An anthology exploring various perspectives on medical aid in dying, including advocates and opponents, but also elaborating the philosophical significance of relevant issues—on the meaning of death, the moral considerations of specific vulnerable groups, religious approaches, and the legal landscape. Different chapters cover the significance of medical aid in dying for various populations: the elderly, people with disabilities, Black Americans, and women.

Bloom, Amy. 2022. *In Love: A Memoir of Love and Loss.* New York: Random House.

> A memoir detailing the author's husband's diagnosis with Alzheimer's disease in his sixties. He refuses "the long goodbye" of a gradual decline and investigates ways to end his life when he finds that his existence is no longer meaningful or tolerable to him. Finding few legal options in the United States, he decides to end his life through active euthanasia

in Switzerland. Bloom considers the psychological implications of the restrictions on medical aid in dying in the U.S.

*Commission on the Study of Medical Practice concerning Euthanasia: Medical Decisions concerning the End of Life.* 1991. The Hague: SdU.
Known as the Remmelink Report after the Dutch attorney general who led the 1991 commission, this was the first comprehensive study of end-of-life decisions in the Netherlands. There have been two further studies, in 1995 and 2001. It contains qualitative interviews with physicians, quantitative results of surveys completed by the physicians of people who have died, and a prospective survey to track changes in their attitudes. Like the Death with Dignity reports in U.S. states, it contains statistics about who has taken advantage of medical aid in dying.

Dembo, Justine, Udo Schuklenk, and Jonathan Reggler. 2018. "'For Their Own Good': A Response to Popular Arguments against Permitting Medical Assistance in Dying (MAID) Where Mental Illness Is the Sole Underlying Condition." *Canadian Journal of Psychiatry* 63, no. 7 (July): 451–56. doi:10.1177/0706743718766055.
Discusses the extension of the Canadian medical aid in dying law to psychiatric patients without a separate, nonpsychiatric diagnosis. The authors argue that the principle of patient autonomy means that medical aid in dying should not be categorically denied to such patients. However, they acknowledge the difficulties in establishing competence.

Dunson, James A. 2018. *Sedation, Suicide, and the Limits of Ethics.* Lanham, MD: Lexington.
A moral argument for legalizing medical aid in dying based on the subjective experience of end-of-life care, which typically involves significant sedation. The book includes a discussion of how the doctrine of double effect is not only theoretically debated but also applied in hospital and hospice settings. Dunson argues that medical aid in dying is justified, paradoxically, by the right to life.

Emanuel, Linda L., ed. 1998. *Regulating How We Die: The Ethical, Medical, and Legal Issues Surrounding Physician-Assisted Suicide.* Cambridge, MA: Harvard University Press.
An anthology gathering arguments from major medical ethicists, organized into chapters advocating for and against medical aid in dying. A third section provides perspectives on the debate itself: a history of euthanasia and medical aid in dying, empirical studies relevant to end-of-life care, and suggestions about how the debate could constructively move forward.

Quill, Timothy. 1986. *Death and Dignity: Making Choices and Taking Charge*. New York: Norton.

> Written for the general public, this text offers an argument for medical aid in dying by a physician who later publicized his assistance in helping a terminal patient to die. Published prior to the legalization of medical aid in dying in any U.S. state, it gives practical advice to patients and families about how to preserve autonomy through advance directives and other forms of medical advocacy.

Warnock, Mary, and Elisabeth Macdonald. 2008. *Easeful Death: Is There a Case for Assisted Suicide?* Oxford: Oxford University Press. doi:10.1093/oso/9780199539901.001.0001.

> Argues in favor of medical aid in dying, primarily based on compassion for those at the end of life. Warnock and Macdonald consider a range of positions on this issue, including the current legal landscape in the United States, the Netherlands, and Belgium. They criticize the traditional debate between the abstract principles of autonomy and the sanctity of life, and instead focus our attention on addressing unnecessary suffering while also protecting those who do not wish to die.

Wolf, Susan. 1996. "Gender, Feminism, and Death: Physician-Assisted Suicide and Euthanasia." In *Feminism and Bioethics: Beyond Reproduction*, edited by Susan Wolf, 282–317. New York: Oxford University Press. doi:10.1093/oso/9780195085686.003.0011.

> A feminist critique of legalizing medical aid in dying. Wolf argues that the cultural training imposed on women makes them unfairly vulnerable to being coerced into ending their lives, and any attempts to regulate the practice cannot effectively guard against this risk. Patients should not be treated as generic individuals but as people located in specific social identities that impact their ability to resist subtle forms of coercion.

Woodward, Paul A., ed. 2001. *The Doctrine of Double Effect: Philosophers Debate a Controversial Moral Principle*. Notre Dame, IN: University of Notre Dame Press.

> An anthology of works by prominent philosophers discussing the meaning, legitimacy, and scope of the doctrine of double effect. The book opens with an introduction to the concept and a consideration of the historical origins of the doctrine in the Catholic natural law tradition. Later chapters focus on the applications of the doctrine and the debate around it in recent moral philosophy.

# CHAPTER 9
# Healthcare and Social Justice

**Key topics in this chapter:**

- How healthcare policy is a form of allocation
- Three models of healthcare distribution—single-payer, free market, and multi-payer—and how they function in the U.S. and other countries
- The moral commitments that underlie each of these models, including justice and the right to healthcare
- How much healthcare we deserve

## Introduction

There is a limited supply of medical resources—the services, medical expertise, equipment, and pharmaceuticals needed to diagnose and treat adverse physical and mental conditions—yet it often seems that there is limitless demand. During times of scarcity, such as a mass casualty incident, some patients must be prioritized over others. In normal times, some treatments must be prioritized over others. Not every healthcare expense is worth it when it would redirect funding from other things we value. An aging population, longer life expectancy, new medical technologies, and rising drug prices are some of the pressures leading to increasing healthcare costs. In 2023, healthcare spending in the U.S. rose to $4.9 trillion, 17.6 percent of gross domestic product (GDP), more than the total GDP of nearly every other country in the world (Centers for Medicare and Medicaid Services, n.d.). But cost is not the only issue. The Association of American Medical Colleges (2024) anticipates that, by 2036, the United States will have between 13,500 and 86,000 fewer physicians than it needs. Healthcare policy must take these pressures into account while meeting existing healthcare needs as best it can within the constraints of justice.

## Allocation versus Rationing

The **allocation** or distribution of medical resources does not by itself imply that anyone is deprived of needed or wanted care. For example, a country may have enough influenza vaccine for every eligible resident. Allowing every resident to get the vaccine at no cost is an allocation scheme. But we sometimes have to allocate resources under conditions of scarcity, when the supply cannot meet the demand. This is called **rationing**. When there are not enough resources, some people are selected to receive them and others are not, even though they need, want, or would otherwise benefit from them. For example, when COVID-19 vaccines were initially being produced, an allocation system had to be developed to prioritize some people over others, even though everyone was at risk of infection.

**Macroallocation** refers to general policies concerning hypothetical lives. For example, during the height of the COVID-19 pandemic, states developed guidelines for triage committees to use: Which characteristics—prognosis, comorbidities, age, and so on—would give one patient priority over another patient if there was only one remaining spot in the intensive care unit (ICU)? **Microallocation** applies such a policy to actual patients. Some triage committees were given anonymized data about patients who had come to hospitals needing treatment (for COVID or other ailments), and they had to decide which patients would be given beds in the ICU, since there were not enough spots for all of them. Although every patient who could benefit was considered for treatment, only some received it.

Healthcare policy, which is the focus of this chapter, is also a form of rationing. With a finite amount of resources, no society can cover every desired medical service for its people without diverting money from other valued services such as education, public safety, and infrastructure. A rationing mechanism prevents overutilization and controls healthcare costs by determining who has access to a given service—for example, people who can afford to pay, all citizens, or all residents—as well as what is covered—often, a class of "basic" or "essential" services, however that is defined. For example, in the United States, nonurgent primary care is limited to those who can pay out of pocket or carry public or private insurance—none of which covers every possible medical intervention. Thus, some patients are prioritized over others, and not all treatments are funded. On the other hand, emergency medical care is guaranteed for everyone, regardless of ability to pay, insurance coverage, or citizenship status. Each of these decisions about healthcare policy reflects judgments about our obligations to one another and thus what counts as social justice in healthcare.

## Types of Healthcare Systems

We can distinguish different allocation schemes based on who is responsible for providing healthcare and under what conditions. For example, under a single-payer system, the government provides health insurance for all the country's residents; under a free-market system, each individual covers the cost of needed services for themselves. This taxonomy is complicated by the fact that "providing" healthcare is ambiguous: it could mean paying for medical services, owning the facilities and employing the clinicians who treat patients, or both.

### *1. Single-payer*

In a **single-payer system**, a public or quasi-public agency covers the cost of basic healthcare services for all residents. There is a lot contained in this brief description. First, insurance is mandatory for the whole population, which finances their coverage with tax revenues. By bringing the whole population under a single risk pool, the country can reduce and stabilize insurance costs and ensure access even for people who would, in a free market, be uninsurable or face high premiums because of their medical conditions. Their healthcare costs are subsidized by the taxes of relatively healthy people, thus mitigating the risk of losses. Second, every resident gets uniform coverage of essential services. Third, a single purchaser (the state) sets rules for which healthcare services are essential and which are supplementary, quality standards for clinicians who are eligible for reimbursement, and reimbursement rates.

In a single-payer model, the government may employ its own physicians in facilities that it operates—a system of **socialized medicine**—or it may negotiate with and pay for services from independent physicians and privately owned facilities. In the U.S., the Veterans Health Administration is an example of the former, and Medicare is an example of the latter. There are different versions of the single-payer model. In Canada, for example, under Canadian Medicare, healthcare is funded and administered by the provinces and territories, subsidized by the federal government. Physicians are employed by their provincial/territorial government, which contracts with delegated, nonprofit health authorities (such as Alberta Health Services) to operate the healthcare system, including hospitals, long-term care, and public health services. Citizens and permanent residents receive medically necessary hospital services and basic physician services for free at the point of service. This is known as a **National Health Insurance Model**. Another example of socialized medicine is the United Kingdom's National Health Service (NHS). The NHS is funded through general taxation, and it provides free public healthcare, including hospital, physician, and mental healthcare. The government owns the hospitals and clinics, and it employs the clinicians. This is known as the **Beveridge Model**.

Even in countries with publicly funded healthcare, people may supplement their coverage with private insurance. In Canada, for example, about two-thirds of the population carries private insurance to pay for services not covered under Canadian Medicare, including outpatient prescription drugs, dental care, and vision care. These plans are often paid for by one's employer or union. For specific groups without employer-sponsored insurance, the government provides a public plan. Ontario, for example, funds a universal prescription drug program for seniors, children without private insurance, and the poor. On a single-payer model, justice means giving every resident or citizen access to basic health services, regardless of ability to pay or preexisting conditions.

### *2. Free market*

On the other side of the spectrum is a **free-market system** or out-of-pocket model, where individual patients/customers pay for their own healthcare as they would any other private service. This kind of healthcare system, like any other free-market system, is predicated on free entry into the market, unregulated competition among producers of goods and services, and consumer choice. According to free-market economists such as Milton Friedman, one reason for the high cost of healthcare in the U.S. is that the supply of physicians is tightly controlled by the American Medical Association, which exerts monopoly power to restrict competition through the licensure process. Friedman suggests that we do away with the licensing of physicians altogether in order to make the healthcare industry truly a free market (2002, 147–55). Consumers would then make informed choices among available providers for needed services, paying attention to both cost and quality of care. In principle, this would lead to more competition, thus driving down prices and increasing innovation, just like in any other industry. In the U.S., this is one of the impetuses behind the Centers for Medicare and Medicaid Services (CMS) Price Transparency Rule (45 CFR Part 180), which requires hospitals to post their charges online for "shoppable services" that healthcare consumers can schedule in advance.

Proponents of a free-market healthcare system usually defend their view with two different kinds of arguments (e.g., Sade 2008). First, for the government to cover the cost of healthcare for those in need, it has to forcibly confiscate property from richer, healthier people and redistribute it to the sick and the poor. Assuming that taxpayers rightfully earned their wealth, the government is violating their individual property rights in order to promote the common good. Using the language of Robert Nozick (1974), the government is treating wealth like manna from heaven rather than realizing that it rightfully belongs to someone as a result of just acquisition and transfer. It engineers what it takes to be a just end result (using a patterned principle) rather than recognizing that what you deserve depends on how you came to possess it (a historical principle of justice in holdings). Just because someone needs something does not entitle them to another person's property: a hungry person is not entitled to my sandwich, I do not owe a homeless person a room in my house, and a sick person has no right against me to pay their medical bill. This is a libertarian theory of justice: I have a right to what I own (Engelhardt 1996).

A second reason given in support of free-market healthcare is utilitarian. In a free market, consumers determine acceptable trade-offs through prices. The invisible hand ensures that needed services are available at minimal cost, achieving a state of equilibrium in which consumers and producers both benefit. But in a centrally planned healthcare system, the government does not know which trade-offs to make. Government control (as in a single-payer system), government regulation, or other forms of interference in the free market introduce inefficiency and risk the overprovision of services. In the U.S., for example, employers get tax breaks when they supply private insurance to their employees, which incentivizes more generous benefits. Patients who only make small co-payments for office visits are more likely to see doctors for minor ailments than if they had to pay the true cost. And doctors are disincentivized from preventing illness and encouraged to order unnecessary tests for which they will be reimbursed. This drives up prices and makes healthcare less available to some consumers.

### 3. Arguments against a purely free market

There are several arguments against the libertarian approach. Among other things, there is evidence that the invisible hand does not work to maximize efficiency and lower prices in the healthcare market. First, consumers do not treat healthcare like other commodities, since they base their decisions on need and what their clinicians recommend rather than on cost (Melecki, Burack, and Quincy 2014). There is also information asymmetry: patients cannot always evaluate the effectiveness of medical treatments, not only because medicine is so complex—with different clinicians proposing alternative treatments with different likelihoods of success, possible side effects, and variable costs—but also because as an illness progresses, they often have to make such decisions with little time to collect and evaluate information (Arrow 1963). We do not consume healthcare in the same way that we consume major household appliances or groceries. Furthermore, consolidated hospital and insurance markets lead to a lack of options, especially in rural areas, thus reducing competition and raising prices. In this context, the only way to control prices is through government regulation, such as an administered pricing system like Medicare (Gaynor and Town 2012).

Perhaps the best response to a proposed free-market system is that we are committed to the so-called **rule of rescue** (Jonsen 1986). One interpretation of this rule is that people generally experience a sense of obligation—either an actual ethical duty or a psychological impulse—to save identifiable people whose lives are at risk. Thus, moral attention is not an abstract rule but a response to singular persons whom we encounter and who need our help. In the United States, this imperative is codified statutorily with the **Emergency Medical Treatment and Labor Act (EMTALA)** (1986). Under EMTALA, emergency departments have to give medical screenings to anyone who comes to the hospital for emergency care, stabilize patients with emergency medical conditions (including active labor), and transfer or accept such patients for treatment, regardless of their ability to pay.

Paul Menzel (2011) argues that this basic commitment—something that both Democrats and Republicans in the U.S. support—has important implications. When someone has no insurance but requires emergency treatment, the hospital has to cover it with funding from insured patients, taxpayers (through government reimbursement), or charitable foundations. This poses a free rider problem: the uninsured are getting benefits they are not paying for, which is unfair. It is also inefficient. Because primary care clinics can turn away the uninsured, such patients are forced to go to the emergency room for everyday ailments that could be treated more cheaply in a doctor's office, or they forego preventive care and are only treated for serious, more costly medical conditions down the line. To correct the free rider problem, Menzel says that we should require people to buy insurance so those who get benefits pay into the system. Because not everyone can afford insurance, though, we should both regulate insurance companies—so, for example, they cannot turn away people with preexisting conditions—and provide subsidies so poorer people can afford it. This not only addresses the free rider problem but also makes it possible for private insurance companies to function, since everyone, including healthier people, is sharing the financial burdens of medical care. Following three principles that Menzel thinks we all accept—the duty of rescue (codified in the form of the EMTALA), avoidance of free riding (when the uninsured are treated without any cost to them), and "just sharing between well and ill" (which justifies subsidies) (2011, 108)—we have arrived at something like the Affordable Care Act.

### *4. Multi-payer*

Between these two extremes—single-payer and free-market systems—are **multi-payer systems** that combine elements of free and regulated markets in unique ways. In France and Germany, for example, healthcare is funded by public and private contributions, with employees and employers paying money into nonprofit sickness funds, which are nongovernmental insurance plans. Healthcare facilities are privately owned. This is the so-called **Bismarck Model**, a national health plan that covers all legal residents, with private supplemental insurance available for those who can afford it.

However, not all multi-payer systems guarantee universal coverage. The **Affordable Care Act (ACA)** (2010), which currently regulates healthcare in the United States, is also a multi-payer model. It has three main provisions. First, private insurance companies are heavily regulated by the government. They are allowed to operate only if they do several things, including:

- not turning people away for preexisting conditions;
- charging women and men the same rates;
- letting children be covered as dependents under their parents' policy until they are twenty-six years old; and
- keeping costs down by minimizing administrative overhead and contributing a high percentage of people's premium payments to patient care. Specifically, insurance companies must return 80–85 percent of premiums back to consumers in the form of benefits. They can only spend 15–20 percent on overhead.

If these were the only regulations in place, private health insurance companies would not be financially viable. Only the smaller group of people who needed high-cost medical care would buy insurance, and they would pay for the policies only when they needed the coverage, while the majority of people, who are generally healthy, would opt out. The second main provision of the ACA addresses this problem. The **individual mandate** requires everyone to have basic health insurance or pay a tax penalty. Premiums from healthy people subsidize care for unhealthy people, and premiums paid while someone is healthy defray the cost of care when they have health problems. However, because not everyone can afford insurance, the third main provision of the ACA is that the government subsidizes the cost for low-income people and families, and gives tax credits to small businesses that provide insurance for their employees. People can also purchase coverage through **health insurance marketplaces** (or exchanges), where the state or federal government helps customers compare plans that meet certain coverage and rate requirements.

The individual mandate faced several court challenges and was eventually repealed by Congress in 2019 when it dropped the penalty for not getting insurance to $0. However, the Supreme Court upheld the constitutionality of the ACA, saying that the entire act was not nullified by the repeal of that one provision. Although the number of newly uninsured rose after the loss of the individual mandate (Soni 2022), many people continue to sign up for insurance coverage through ACA marketplaces, including a record 21.3 million people in 2024 (Centers for Medicare and Medicaid Services 2024). This has allowed the system to persist.

The ACA aims to achieve universal healthcare but maintains a network of regulated private insurers, so it is not a single-payer system. It is clearly not a free-market system, but neither was a free market in place prior to the legislation's passage. Throughout most of the twentieth century and now, the Department of Defense provides civilian health benefits, called Tricare, for members of the military, veterans, and their dependents, with the Veterans Health Administration funding it, administering services, and employing clinicians—a form of socialized medicine like the U.K.'s National Health Service. People over sixty-five get federally funded health insurance (Medicare), like in Canada. The federal government and the states provide health insurance for people with low income (Medicaid) and for children from families with modest incomes who do not qualify for Medicaid (State Children's Health Insurance Program [SCHIP]). CMS creates health and safety guidelines for hospitals and other healthcare facilities, and the Food and Drug Administration (FDA) regulates medical devices and pharmaceuticals. These programs, along with EMTALA, are hardly laissez-faire. To be sure, over half the U.S. population has private insurance through their employers. But, as mentioned earlier, this is incentivized in the form of tax credits: employer-paid health insurance premiums are exempt from federal income and payroll taxes. For working Americans who get healthcare through their employers, the U.S. is like Germany. Furthermore, although there are many private, for-profit healthcare systems, the majority of systems in the U.S. are nonprofit, either owned by charitable organizations or controlled by state, county, or city governments and paid for in part by special levies (for example, community hospitals). It is an enormously complex system, composed of government facilities and both for-profit and nonprofit organizations, all tightly regulated and largely publicly funded.

## The Right to Healthcare

The different healthcare systems are based on different conceptions of society's moral or legal obligations to its people. The single-payer model presupposes either that there is a human **right to healthcare** and that the government ought to protect that right, or that healthcare is an entitlement, with guaranteed access based on legally established rights or social custom. The free-market system conceives of healthcare as a privilege, meaning that the government will not restrict someone's purchase of healthcare but will not provide it either. One must qualify for a privilege, or it must otherwise be earned—in this case, by being able to pay for one's own healthcare.

The **right to health**, along with the right to healthcare and the right to have social determinants of health addressed, is acknowledged by many countries and by several international organizations. The World Health Organization's Constitution (1946) states: "The enjoyment of the highest attainable standard of health is one of the fundamental rights of every human being without distinction of race, religion, political belief, economic or social condition" (Preamble). The United Nations' Universal Declaration of Human Rights (1948)—to which the U.S. is a signatory—states in part: "Everyone has the right to a standard of living adequate for the health and well-being of himself and of his family, including food, clothing, housing and medical care and necessary social services" (Article 25). The U.N.'s International Covenant on Economic, Social and Cultural Rights (1966) recognizes "the right of everyone to the enjoyment of the highest attainable standard of physical and mental health" (Article 12). Sixty-nine countries have a right to health embedded in their constitutions, with another twenty-four listing it as an aim or objective; seventy-three countries recognize a right to medical care services, with twenty-seven more aspiring to provide such services (Heymann et al. 2013).

Philosophers attempting to justify this right often appeal to justice, specifically John Rawls's theory of justice as fairness (discussed in Chapter 1). Rawls claims that we establish the principles of justice from a fair starting point. In the original position, behind a veil of ignorance, we would commit ourselves to the liberty principle and the distribution principle: "Each person is to have an equal right to the most extensive basic liberty compatible with a similar liberty for others," and "social and economic inequalities are to be arranged so that they are both (a) reasonably expected to be to everyone's advantage, and (b) attached to positions and offices open to all" (1999, 53). To take advantage of their freedom and have the means to pursue what they value, people must have primary goods, including natural goods such as health and intelligence, and social goods such as rights and liberties, income and wealth, and the social bases of self-respect. Furthermore, not all health problems are the result of bad choices; many are undeserved. Because diseases, disorders, and injuries are unfairly distributed, addressing them attempts to correct unfairness. Providing healthcare to everyone gets us closer to fair equality of opportunity.

Norman Daniels (1985, 1998, 2007) especially has drawn on Rawls's theory of justice to argue that everyone has a right to basic healthcare. His argument is straightforward: Health is important so that people can have options and take advantage of opportunities to pursue the good life. All people deserve a level of physical and mental functioning that would allow them to have a "normal opportunity range." Healthcare is a social primary good because it helps people to achieve a level of normal (species-typical) functioning. Therefore, everyone deserves a basic level of healthcare. Inequalities are allowed—some people may afford private coverage for care that is extraordinary (expensive care that provides little additional benefit) or that satisfies mere preferences (such as cosmetic surgeries)—as long as everyone has coverage for basic things such as physician services, preventive medicine, inpatient and outpatient hospital visits, emergency treatment, and so on.

Other approaches emphasize the ability to achieve valued outcomes (capability theory) or the core facets of human welfare (well-being theory). On these views, people have a right to health, not only healthcare (Ruger 2006). Capability theory is represented by Amartya Sen (1980, 1999) and Martha Nussbaum (2003, 2013), who claim that we ought to promote human flourishing (what Aristotle called *eudaimonia*), that people need certain capabilities to have the actual opportunity to live well (that is, to pursue what they have reason to value) in their particular social circumstances, and that a just social arrangement would provide people with those capabilities. A society is more just the more that it helps people to develop their capabilities across its population, and the world is more just the more that we assist the global poor in developing their capabilities, thus reducing inequalities both within and between societies. Nussbaum's list of ten central human capabilities includes life—living a complete and satisfying life (not dying prematurely or suffering so much that life is not worth living)—and bodily health—being in decent physical condition and having adequate nutrition and shelter (2013, 33). Since, as a matter of justice, these capabilities should be socially sustained, we are obligated to provide healthcare (and food, housing, etc.) when necessary so that everyone can live a long, healthy life and thus have a chance to flourish.

The well-being theory proposed by Madison Powers and Ruth Faden (2006, 2019) is a form of consequentialism that, like utilitarianism, values an end state in which everyone flourishes and values justice insofar as it promotes that state of affairs. However, unlike something like preference utilitarianism, according to which the value of health is a function of our collective preferences, Powers and Faden claim that we ought to do what justice requires, a standard separate from our accumulated preferences. The six core elements of well-being—health, personal security, knowledge and understanding, equal respect, personal attachments, and self-determination—are interconnected (2006, 16–29). For example, places with greater economic inequality have lower life expectancy and lower average health. Therefore, societies must not only provide healthcare but must also address systemic inequalities in order to promote overall well-being.

In its report to the U.S. Congress, the President's Commission for the Study of Ethical Problems in Medicine and Biomedical and Behavioral Research adopted as "an ethical standard: access for all to an adequate level of care without the imposition of excessive burdens" (1983, 1). It gave four reasons for the importance of healthcare that justify its equitable distribution. First, health is essential to a person's well-being. As John Stuart Mill says, it is not only a means to happiness but is also desired for its own sake as part of happiness (1979, 35–36). As the President's Commission puts it, people want to avoid pain and suffering "both because of the intrinsic quality of the experience and because of their effects on the capacity to pursue and achieve other goals and purposes" (1983, 16). Since health is a good, we ought to maximize it, promoting individual well-being and thus increasing happiness in the aggregate—a utilitarian view. Second, insofar as health can "broaden a person's range of opportunities," healthcare promotes fair equality of opportunity by helping to "maintain or restore normal functioning" (17), a line of argument much like Daniels's (who himself reported to the Commission). Third, getting information about one's health condition (diagnosis) and being informed about possible treatments (prognosis) can relieve a person's worry. Not only does this promote happiness, but it is also crucial to supporting patient autonomy, since an informed patient can take more control over their treatment decisions. Fourth, the President's Commission says that healthcare "expresses and nurtures bonds of empathy and compassion" (17). Not only is this reminiscent of care ethics, but it also describes a special entitlement that people have by being part of a community. If we conceive of society as formed by a social contract, the whole takes on obligations to individual members to protect them from suffering and death, not only from external enemies but from illness. Although a prior commission, the

President's Commission on the Health Needs of the Nation, had asserted that "access to the means for the attainment and preservation of health is a basic human right" (1952, 3), the Commission for the Study of Ethical Problems in Medicine and Biomedical and Behavioral Research stopped short of asserting that there is a right to healthcare, concluding only that "society has an ethical obligation to ensure equitable access to health care for all" (1983, 4; see also 32–35).

Although some discussions of healthcare allocation focus on the provision of health insurance and access to medical practitioners, all the philosophers who write about justice—including Daniels, Sen, Nussbaum, Powers, and Faden—claim that our obligation to maintain people's health extends to the social conditions that affect it (see, e.g., Daniels 2001). In fact, although healthcare is important to maintain and restore proper functioning, it is not the primary driver of healthcare outcomes. There is evidence that variation in health outcomes is primarily due to **social determinants of health**—the conditions under which people are born, grow, work, and live—rather than access to medical care. According to Carlyn Hood et al. (2016), socioeconomic factors account for 47 percent of health outcomes, while health behaviors, clinical care, and the physical environment account for 34 percent, 16 percent, and 3 percent, respectively. Such nonmedical factors as housing instability and homelessness, food insecurity, lower educational achievement, economic and employment instability, transportation issues, discrimination and social exclusion, and interpersonal violence have an outsized negative impact on the health of individuals and communities. So, for example, the capability approach has been used to call attention to food and housing insecurity (e.g., Nicholls 2010; Burchi and De Muro 2012; Lawson 2020; Miller and Thomas 2020), and Thomas Pogge (2002, 2004) extends Rawlsian principles beyond the borders of nation-states to argue that more affluent nations have a duty to alleviate global poverty, in part, to improve the health of the global poor. Domestically, many U.S. hospitals have been actively promoting affordable housing in their communities, offering on-site food pantries, providing transportation to medical appointments, and screening patients for domestic violence. If there is a right to health or a duty to promote normal human functioning, the just allocation of healthcare involves not only access to medical facilities but also a more just distribution of food, housing, education, and employment.

## How Much Healthcare Do We Deserve?

The social obligation to ensure equitable access to healthcare raises other important questions. If we grant that the government should provide healthcare, how much healthcare is it obligated to provide? What counts as "basic," "adequate," or "equitable" care, or what level of care would ensure that people have a "normal" opportunity range? Answering these questions delineates the extent of our social obligations regarding health (assuming there is such an obligation).

The President's Commission for the Study of Ethical Problems in Medicine and Biomedical and Behavioral Research (1983) rejected two proposed definitions of "equitable access." First, it rejected equity as equality of care. If everyone must have the same level of healthcare, then if the level of care were set too high—if we must do everything we can to prevent the loss of life—it would drain our resources from other social goods such as education and public safety. However, if the expected level of care were set too low, people who needed more care and could afford it themselves would be prohibited from doing so. We would have to restrict people's freedom to purchase additional services based on their needs or preferences, which not only violates their autonomy (a deontological concern) but would also result in a black market for healthcare (a consequentialist concern) (18–19). Second, the President's Commission rejected the idea that equity means giving people all the care that they need or that would benefit them. Again, this excessively prioritizes health by treating it as the only good, thus diverting all necessary resources to that end and depriving us of other things we value. "Need" is also an ambiguous standard. If needed treatment is whatever confers a benefit, then the level of care is still set too high. If needed treatment is whatever is necessary to prevent death, then the level of care is set too low (19). As an alternative to these formulations, the Commission concluded that everyone ought to have access to an "adequate level of care," "enough care to achieve sufficient welfare, opportunity, information, and evidence of interpersonal concern to facilitate a reasonably full and satisfying life" (20). It recognized that such a standard is vague, in part because it is "society-relative," depending on "societal resources" and "a consensus of expectations about what is adequate in a particular society at a particular time" (20). Rather than setting out specific recommendations for adequate care in the United States in the 1980s, it purported to provide a framework for policymakers at different times and places.

Ronald Dworkin (2000) is among the many philosophers who have proposed ways to ration healthcare in order to provide "necessary and appropriate" medical treatment. Dworkin rejects the rescue principle, which he characterizes as the view that life and health are the chief goods and that healthcare should be distributed equally, based on need. Although health is important, it is not the only thing we value, and because we only have a finite amount of resources, we have to make trade-offs. How do we decide which trade-offs to make? Dworkin has us imagine that we each have to pay for our own insurance, and we have to decide what kind of coverage to get. Imagine that healthcare coverage is not a benefit of employment, and the costs of care are not hidden behind co-payments and deductibles. What would we do?

In the actual world, the kind of coverage we get depends on how much money we have, how well we estimate the costs and benefits of potential treatments, and how our rates are affected by our preexisting conditions, our gender or race, or even where we live. So, to determine the standard level of care we ought to have, Dworkin comes up with a hypothetical scenario, what he calls the **prudent insurance test** (2000, 317–18): If we each had average income, we knew what we were buying, and we were not priced out of the market because of preexisting conditions, what would we buy? We would not spend money that we would otherwise spend on food and housing to cover plastic surgery, which is purely cosmetic, nor to cover extraordinarily expensive things such as organ transplants, which we are unlikely to need. However, we would give up a trip to Europe so our kids can be immunized, get preventive care, and get emergency services when necessary. Dworkin says that whatever level of coverage we *would* get in this scenario is the coverage that everyone *should* get. We should judge what is necessary and appropriate against that standard:

> If most prudent people would buy a certain level of medical coverage in a free market if they had average means—if nearly everyone would buy insurance covering ordinary medical care, hospitalization when necessary, prenatal and pediatric care, and regular checkups and other preventative medicine, for example—then the unfairness of our society is almost certainly the reason some people do not have such coverage now. A universal health-care system should make sure, in all justice, that everyone does have it. (Dworkin 2000, 315)

The only reason any actual person does not have this coverage is because they are poor and cannot afford it, due to "the unfairness of our society." According to Dworkin, society is obligated to provide this standard level of healthcare to everyone to correct this injustice. We should be mindful, of course, that these moral considerations arise in an economic reality of aging populations worldwide and rising healthcare costs. Actual social and economic conditions affect the trade-offs we would be willing to make.

## Conclusion: Who Controls Healthcare?

Evaluating healthcare policy is not merely an academic exercise. It has real-world implications for patient care in the clinical setting. The way that we structure and regulate health insurance markets has a profound impact on price, quality, and safety. For example, David Goldhill (2013) makes the case that in the U.S. private insurers, Medicare, and Medicaid are the "true customers" who act as "surrogates" in dictating the choice of doctors, which services are covered, and how much hospitals and clinics are reimbursed. With the consumer out of the decision-making, there is little incentive to drive down costs to patients (since insurers want to drive up premiums) or to improve quality and safety to attract patients (since clinicians do not have to compete for patients, who are not deciding what kind of care should be compensated) (esp. 64–93). In recent years, insurance companies have used artificial intelligence programs to approve or (more often) deny pre-authorization requests or claims, effectively taking treatment decisions away from clinicians and patients (Napolitano 2023). Understanding the corporate structure around healthcare is crucial to understanding how medicine functions in an everyday sense—the pressures on "providers" and "healthcare consumers."

Furthermore, in the U.S., many healthcare facilities are so economically dependent on government programs—Medicare and Medicaid account for over 40 percent of a typical hospital's revenue and cover the majority of inpatient days (American Hospital Association 2024; Definitive Healthcare 2024)—that changes to payment policies pose an existential threat. The debate in Congress over expanding **site-neutral payments** is a good example. Under site-neutral payment policies, hospital outpatient departments are reimbursed at the same Medicare rate as independent physician offices and ambulatory surgery centers (ASCs).

Defenders of site-neutrality claim that it disincentivizes hospitals from acquiring outpatient offices, thus protecting independent practices; substantially reduces Medicare spending by the federal government; and lowers commercial prices for private insurers whose prices move in parallel with Medicare's fee schedule. Critics of site-neutral payments claim that differential reimbursement is justified because hospitals have more licensing, accreditation, and regulatory requirements than physicians' offices and ASCs; unlike independent practices, nonprofit hospitals must take all patients regardless of their insurance status, including vulnerable populations, resulting in a lot of uncompensated care; and hospitals treat more complex cases and provide more complex procedures, which adds to cost. What seems like an esoteric economic policy debated at the federal level has an impact especially on struggling rural hospitals and urban hospitals that serve poorer populations, thus affecting the distribution of healthcare services.

Questions about justice and healthcare are practical issues for clinicians, healthcare administrators, and patients but raise theoretical problems for medical ethicists and political philosophers. How we allocate healthcare at a policy level expresses a sense of our collective obligations. What kinds of healthcare resources does each person deserve? What can be taken from others in a society to support that standard of medical care? Do we have special obligations to our fellow citizens or residents, or do our obligations extend to all persons, even beyond our borders? How we answer these questions has wide-ranging implications not only for individual well-being but also for autonomy—so that people can pursue their own purposes without being hindered by preventable forms of ill-health—and justice—whether benefits and burdens are equitably distributed in our society.

## REFERENCES

American Hospital Association. 2024. "Fact Sheet: Majority of Hospital Payments Dependent on Medicare or Medicaid." Last modified May 6, 2024. https://www.aha.org/fact-sheets/2022-05-25-fact-sheet-majority-hospital-payments-dependent-medicare-or-medicaid.

Arrow, Kenneth J. 1963. "Uncertainty and the Welfare Economics of Medical Care." *American Economic Review* 53, no. 5 (December): 941–73. https://www.jstor.org/stable/1812044.

Association of American Medical Colleges. 2024. *The Complexities of Physician Supply and Demand: Projections from 2019 to 2036*. Washington, DC: Association of American Medical Colleges. https://www.aamc.org/media/75236/download.

Burchi, Francesco, and Pasquale De Muro. 2012. "A Human Development and Capability Approach to Food Security: Conceptual Framework and Informational Basis." United Nations Development Programme, Working Paper 2012-009. February. https://www.undp.org/sites/g/files/zskgke326/files/migration/africa/Capability-Approach-Food-Security.pdf.

Centers for Medicare and Medicaid Services. 2024. "Historic 21.3 Million People Choose ACA Marketplace Coverage." January 24. https://www.cms.gov/newsroom/press-releases/historic-213-million-people-choose-aca-marketplace-coverage.

———. n.d. "National Health Expenditures 2023 Highlights." Accessed January 15, 2025. https://www.cms.gov/files/document/highlights.pdf.

Daniels, Norman. 1985. *Just Health Care*. Cambridge: Cambridge University Press. doi:10.1017/CBO9780511624971.

———. 1998. "Is There a Right to Health Care and, If So, What Does It Encompass?" In *A Companion to Bioethics*, edited by Helga Kuhse and Peter Singer, 362–72. Oxford: Blackwell. doi:10.1002/9781444307818.ch31.

———. 2001. "Justice, Health, and Healthcare." *American Journal of Bioethics* 1, no. 2 (Spring): 2–16. doi:10.1162/152651601300168834.

———. 2007. *Just Health: Meeting Health Needs Fairly*. Cambridge: Cambridge University Press. doi:10.1017/CBO9780511809514.

Definitive Healthcare. 2024. "Breaking Down U.S. Hospital Payor Mixes." Last modified July 12, 2024. https://www.definitivehc.com/resources/healthcare-insights/breaking-down-us-hospital-payor-mixes.

Dworkin, Ronald. 2000. "Justice and the High Cost of Health." In *Sovereign Virtue: The Theory and Practice of Equality*, 307–19. Cambridge, MA: Harvard University Press.

Engelhardt, H. Tristram. 1996. "Rights to Health Care, Social Justice, and Fairness in Health Care Allocations: Frustrations in the Face of Finitude." In *The Foundations of Bioethics*, 2nd ed., 375–410. New York: Oxford University Press. doi:10.1093/oso/9780195057362.003.0008.

Friedman, Milton. 2002. *Capitalism and Freedom*. 40th anniversary ed. Chicago: University of Chicago Press.

Gaynor, Martin, and Robert Town. 2012. "The Impact of Hospital Consolidation—Update." Robert Wood Johnson Foundation, Synthesis Project. June. doi:10.13140/RG.2.1.4294.0882.

Goldhill, David. 2013. *Catastrophic Care: Why Everything We Think We Know about Health Care Is Wrong*. New York: Vintage.

Heymann, Jody, Adèle Cassolab, Amy Rauba, and Lipi Mishrab. 2013. "Constitutional Rights to Health, Public Health and Medical Care: The Status of Health Protections in 191 Countries." *Global Public Health* 8, no. 6 (July): 639–53. doi:10.1080/17441692.2013.810765.

Hood, Carlyn M., Keith P. Gennuso, Geoffrey R. Swain, and Bridget B. Catlin. 2016. "County Health Rankings: Relationships between Determinant Factors and Health Outcomes." *American Journal of Preventive Medicine* 50, no. 2 (February): 129–35. doi:10.1016/j.amepre.2015.08.024.

Jonsen, Albert R. 1986. "Bentham in a Box: Technology Assessment and Health Care Allocation." *Law, Medicine & Health Care* 14, nos. 3–4 (September): 172–74. doi:10.1111/j.1748-720x.1986.tb00974.x.

Lawson, Julie, ed. 2020. "The Application of the Capabilities Approach to the Field of Housing." Special issue, *Housing, Theory and Society* 37, no. 3.

Melecki, Sarah, Victoria Burack, and Lynn Quincy. 2014. "Consumer Attitudes toward Health Care Costs, Value and System Reforms: A Review of the Literature." Consumers Union. October. https://advocacy.consumerreports.org/wp-content/uploads/2014/10/ConsumersAndHealthCostsLiteratureReview-Oct-2014.pdf.

Menzel, Paul T. 2011. "The Cultural Moral Right to a Basic Minimum of Accessible Health Care." *Kennedy Institute of Ethics Journal* 21, no. 1 (March): 79–119. doi:10.1353/ken.2011.0003.

Mill, John Stuart. 1979. *Utilitarianism*. Edited by George Sher. Indianapolis: Hackett.

Miller, Daniel P., and Margaret M. C. Thomas. 2020. "Policies to Reduce Food Insecurity: An Ethical Imperative." *Physiology & Behavior* 222 (August 1): article no. 112943. doi:10.1016/j.physbeh.2020.112943.

Napolitano, Elizabeth. 2023. "Lawsuits Take Aim at Use of AI Tool by Health Insurance Companies to Process Claims." *CBS News*. December 18. https://www.cbsnews.com/news/health-insurance-humana-united-health-ai-algorithm/.

Nicholls, Carol McNaughton. 2010. "Housing, Homelessness and Capabilities." *Housing, Theory and Society* 27, no. 1: 23–41. doi:10.1080/14036090902764588.

Nozick, Robert. 1974. *Anarchy, State, and Utopia*. New York: Basic.

Nussbaum, Martha C. 2003. "Capabilities as Fundamental Entitlements: Sen and Global Justice." *Feminist Economics* 9, nos. 2–3: 33–59. doi:10.1080/1354570022000077926.

———. 2013. *Creating Capabilities: The Human Development Approach*. Cambridge, MA: Belknap.

Pogge, Thomas. 2002. *World Poverty and Human Rights: Cosmopolitan Responsibilities and Reforms*. Cambridge: Polity.

———. 2004. "Relational Conceptions of Justice: Responsibilities for Health Outcomes." In *Public Health, Ethics, and Equity*, edited by Sudhir Anand, Fabienne Peter, and Amartya Sen, 135–61. Oxford: Clarendon. doi:10.1093/oso/9780199276363.003.0008.

Powers, Madison, and Ruth Faden. 2006. *Social Justice: The Moral Foundations of Public Health and Health Policy*. Oxford: Oxford University Press. doi:10.1093/oso/9780195375138.001.0001.

———. 2019. *Structural Injustice: Power, Advantage, and Human Rights*. Oxford: Oxford University Press. doi:10.1093/oso/9780190053987.001.0001.

President's Commission for the Study of Ethical Problems in Medicine and Biomedical and Behavioral Research. 1983. *Securing Access to Health Care: The Ethical Implications of Differences in the Availability of Health Services*. Vol. 1, *Report*. Washington, DC: U.S. Government Printing Office. https://repository.library.georgetown.edu/bitstream/handle/10822/559375/securing_access.pdf?sequence=1&isAllowed=y.

President's Commission on the Health Needs of the Nation. 1952. *Building America's Health: A Report to the President by the President's Commission on the Health Needs of the Nation*. Vol. 1, *Findings and Recommendations*. Washington, DC: U.S. Government Printing Office.

Rawls, John. 1999. *A Theory of Justice*. Rev. ed. Cambridge, MA: Belknap.

Ruger, Jennifer Prah. 2006. "Toward a Theory of a Right to Health: Capability and Incompletely Theorized Agreements." *Yale Journal of Law & the Humanities* 18, no. 2: 273–326. http://hdl.handle.net/20.500.13051/7382.

Sade, Robert M. 2008. "Foundational Ethics of the Health Care System: The Moral and Practical Superiority of Free Market Reforms." *Journal of Medicine and Philosophy* 33, no. 5 (October): 461–97. doi:10.1093/jmp/jhn023.

Sen, Amartya. 1980. "Equality of What?" In *Tanner Lectures on Human Values*, edited by Sterling M. McMurrin, 195–220. Cambridge: Cambridge University Press.

———. 1999. *Development as Freedom*. Oxford: Oxford University Press.

Soni, Aparna. 2022. "The Impact of the Repeal of the Federal Individual Insurance Mandate on Uninsurance." *International Journal of Health Economics and Management* 22, no. 4 (December): 423–41. doi:10.1007/s10754-022-09324-x.

## Further Reading

Bognar, Greg, and Iwao Hirose. 2022. *The Ethics of Health Care Rationing: An Introduction*. 2nd ed. London: Routledge. doi:10.4324/9781003050216.

Accessible survey of the ethical issues that arise in healthcare rationing, including various proposed distribution principles, cost-effectiveness analysis, whether to penalize people for unhealthy behaviors, and the potential to discriminate against the disabled and the elderly. Bognar and Hirose illustrate their discussion with examples from healthcare systems in the United States, the United Kingdom, and other countries.

Brody, Baruch A. 1991. "Why the Right to Health Care Is Not a Useful Concept for Policy Debates." In *Rights to Health Care*, edited by T. J. Bole II and W. B. Bondeson, 113–31. Dordrecht: Kluwer. doi:10.1007/978-0-585 -28295-4_6.

Asserts that appealing to the right to healthcare does not productively advance discussions about health policies. Such appeals tend to understand the right to healthcare only as the provision of medical interventions, even though social determinants of health have a greater impact on health outcomes. We also need to invoke other reasons to justify providing care to the indigent, such as reverence for the value of life, producing greater overall utility, and responding compassionately to our fellow citizens.

Buchanan, Allen. 2009. *Justice and Health Care: Selected Essays*. Oxford: Oxford University Press. doi:10.1093/oso/9780195394061.001.0001.

Collects ten previously published essays in which Buchanan considers the right to healthcare, trust in physicians and managed care organizations, rationing and resource allocation, the moral responsibilities of healthcare services in the public and private sectors, and our responsibility for global health. Buchanan argues that all citizens are obligated to address people's lack of access to basic healthcare, offering a pluralistic defense of public health rights that relies on principles of rectification, compensation, equal protection, and coordination, among others.

Daniels, Norman, Donald W. Light, and Ronald L. Caplan. 1996. *Benchmarks of Fairness for Health Care Reform*. New York: Oxford University Press. doi:10.1093/oso/9780195102376.001.0001.

Applies Daniels's theory of justice in healthcare to evaluate the fairness of four proposed healthcare reforms in the United States: the Jim McDermott-Paul Wellstone single-payer proposal (American Health Security Act of 1993), President Bill Clinton's managed competition strategy (Health Security Act of 1993), Jim Cooper's "Clinton lite" (Managed Competition Act of 1993), and Bob Michel's market-based reforms (Action Now Health Care Reform Act of 1993). The authors use ten benchmarks: universal access in coverage, minimizing nonfinancial barriers, comprehensiveness of benefits, equitable financing in terms of community rating and ability to pay, value for money in terms of clinical efficiency and financial efficiency, public accountability, comparability, and degree of consumer choice.

Gutmann, Amy. 1981. "For and against Equal Access to Health Care." *Milbank Quarterly* 59, no. 4 (December): 542–60. doi:10.2307/3349740.

> Examines arguments regarding equal access to healthcare and the implications of that principle for actual institutions in an inegalitarian society. The values of equality of opportunity, equal efforts to relieve pain, and equal respect seem to entail that there should be a one-class system in which everyone has access to the healthcare goods and services that they need. Gutmann considers challenges to applying that principle as well as challenges to the principle itself from proponents of free-market healthcare, among others.

McGee, Glenn, ed. 2001. *American Journal of Bioethics* 1, no. 2 (Spring).

> Begins with a target article by Daniels in which he explains his position, extends it to social determinants of health, and suggests a way to fairly ration care. The special issue also collects thirteen open peer commentaries on the article and on Daniels's overall approach, including contributions from Frances Kamm, Mary Mahowald, and Rosamond Rhodes.

Menzel, Paul T. 1990. *Strong Medicine: The Ethical Rationing of Health Care.* New York: Oxford University Press. doi:10.1093/oso/9780195057102.001.0001.

> Develops a rationing scheme based on presumed prior consent to risk. What kind of trade-offs would a rational person make over the course of a life when considering the risks of certain medical problems against the costs to address them? Menzel defends his account against objections, including the worry that lives must be given a price, and he applies it to several controversial cases such as perinatal care, organ transplantation, and end-of-life care.

Rhodes, Rosamond, Margaret Battin, and Anita Silvers, eds. 2012. *Medicine and Social Justice: Essays on the Distribution of Health Care.* 2nd ed. Oxford: Oxford University Press. doi:10.1093/acprof:osobl/9780199744206.001.0001.

> A comprehensive collection of forty-two chapters that cover a variety of theoretical approaches to justice in healthcare; how to prioritize and ration access to care; justice as it relates to traditionally underserved populations such as the poor, racial minorities, and the disabled; and specific applications to preexisting conditions, personalized medicine, and medical malpractice, among other topics.

Tikkanen, Roosa, Robin Osborn, Elias Mossialos, Ana Djordjevic, and George Wharton, eds. 2020. *International Health Care System Profiles.* Commonwealth Fund. December. https://www.commonwealthfund.org/international-health-policy-center/system-profiles.

A detailed description and analysis of the healthcare systems of twenty countries, including India, New Zealand, Brazil, Norway, Japan, and the United States. The report discusses how those systems are funded and governed, reform and cost containment efforts, and programs to improve quality of care, among other topics.

Ubel, Peter A. 2000. *Pricing Life: Why It's Time for Health Care Rationing*. Cambridge, MA: MIT Press. doi:10.7551/mitpress/5533.001.0001.

Claims that healthcare rationing is widespread in everyday medical practice and recommends cost-effectiveness analysis (CEA) as the best rationing tool. CEA allows us to compare the costs of different interventions and eliminate only marginally beneficial services. Ubel also argues that more rationing decisions should be made by physicians at the bedside, who can, on financial grounds, decide whether to withhold or withdraw services that are in patients' best interests.

# CHAPTER 10
# Allocating Scarce Medical Resources

**Key topics in this chapter:**
- Historical approaches to distributing scarce medical resources
- Possible allocation principles and their strengths and weaknesses
- How to measure cost-effectiveness using QALYs and DALYs
- Application to the U.S. organ transplant system and to triage and vaccine distribution during the COVID-19 pandemic

## Introduction

There is no one simple moral theory that drives public policy decisions around healthcare. Such decisions are informed by an amalgam of ethical values that sometimes conflict. When medical resources are sufficient, we tend to focus on duties to individual patients, including respecting their autonomy, promoting their well-being, and giving them equitable access to basic medical care. Although the duty of care persists in times of scarcity, the primary goal changes. Healthcare professionals have a duty to steward public resources responsibly and in accordance with distributive justice.

When resources are insufficient, we need to prioritize some patients over others. This is true during public health emergencies such as infectious disease outbreaks and bioterrorism events, and during mass casualty incidents such as natural disasters and plane crashes. It is also a persistent condition for specific populations. For example, more people need organ transplants than there are available organs.

In this chapter, we consider medical resources (such as organs) and medical interventions (such as treatment for COVID-19), and how they should be allocated when the demand outstrips the supply. We survey a range of proposed principles to guide triage decisions and show how those principles function in practice. Specifically, we consider the use of quality- and disability-adjusted life years, the United Network for Organ Sharing points system, and triage and vaccine distribution during the COVID-19 pandemic. It becomes clear that only a complex combination of principles with different weights can justify life-altering clinical and public health decisions.

## Case Study: The "God Committee"

From the French *trier* ("to sort" or "separate out"), **triage** has been practiced in the military for centuries. In World War I, for example, casualties were sorted into one of three categories: people who were likely to live without treatment, people who were likely to die even with treatment, and people for whom treatment would dramatically affect the outcome (for example, saving a life or preventing an amputation). Medical attention and resources were primarily directed toward patients in the third category.

One of the earliest uses of explicitly formulated allocation principles in a civilian context occurred at the nation's first freestanding outpatient dialysis facility, the Seattle Artificial Kidney Center, in the early 1960s. With the successful development of hemodialysis to provide long-term treatment of chronic renal failure, yet with limited funding for it, the clinic had to decide which patients to prioritize. An ethics committee was tasked with creating selection criteria, effectively deciding which patients with this otherwise fatal disease would live and which would die. A Medical Advisory Committee first screened patients using medical criteria to determine whether they would benefit from treatment. An Admissions Advisory Committee, nicknamed the "**God Committee**," then prioritized patients based on their importance to their family and community, especially whether other people depended on them. The original criteria thus included both physical prognosis and social value:

- a stable, emotionally mature, responsible citizen disabled by the symptoms of uraemia [waste products in the blood due to worsening renal function];
- absence of long-standing hypertension and its permanent complications, particularly coronary artery disease and cerebrovascular disease;
- demonstrated willingness to cooperate in carrying out the prescribed treatment, especially the dietary restrictions;

- age 25–45 years;
- slow deterioration of renal function (serum creatinine 8–12 mg/dl), since any residual function simplified the therapeutic problem;
- six months residence in the area (Washington, Alaska, Idaho, Montana and Oregon);
- financial support;
- value to the community;
- potential for rehabilitation;
- psychological and psychiatric compatibility; and
- children and young adults who were not potentially self-supporting were excluded. (Blagg 1998, 236)

The committee had considered other selection criteria, including first-come, first-served and choice by lottery, but neither approach would maximize benefit of the new technology, both for the patients themselves and for the broader community. The treatment would have been wasted on patients with poor chances of recovery, while those who would benefit from the treatment would have been left to die. And suffering would radiate out to families and communities if parents and essential workers (for example, a rural community's only primary care physician) were ranked below the childless and the unemployed.

The committee's existence and selection criteria were brought to the public's attention by a *Life* magazine article in November 1962 (Alexander 1962), which helped to initiate the field of medical ethics. Both its author and subsequent critics questioned the committee's appeal to a patient's "social value," which included their marital status, number of children, occupation, income, net worth, and educational background. Critics have claimed that these criteria reflected the committee members' cultural biases and reinforced racial, economic, and gender discrimination.

## Principles of Allocation

To understand the advantages and disadvantages of different allocation schemes, Govind Persad, Alan Wertheimer, and Ezekiel Emanuel (2009) set out what they take to be an exhaustive list of simple allocation principles. They identify eight principles, classified into four categories:

Category one: Treating people equally

1. Lottery
2. First-come, first-served

Category two: Favoring the worst-off (prioritarianism)

3. Sickest first
4. Youngest first

Category three: Maximizing total benefits (utilitarianism)

5. Save the most lives
6. Prognosis or life years

Category four: Promoting and rewarding social usefulness

7. Instrumental value
8. Reciprocity

Because all actual allocation schemes combine some of these principles and rank them in different ways, Persad, Wertheimer, and Emanuel provide us with a template to understand the values that are being emphasized in any given decision about treatment priorities in times of limited medical resources.

The first two principles—lottery and first-come, first-served—enjoin us to treat people equally rather than ranking their value or need. This class of principles is rooted in both duty-based and rights-based ethical theories. Immanuel Kant says that we ought to respect the humanity in every person, which entails that we should never treat someone merely as a means for the production of happiness. We should always treat people as ends in themselves, with intrinsic rather than instrumental value (1996, 4:427–29). John Locke (1980) says that each person has a natural right to life, liberty, and property, which entails that we have corresponding obligations to respect those rights. Human beings do not earn those rights; they have them simply by virtue of their humanity, so all human beings have equal rights. More recently, John Taurek has argued against the aggregating tendency of views such as utilitarianism, according to which we can add up the value of lives or experiences: "The discomfort of each of a large number of individuals experiencing a minor headache does not add up to anyone's experiencing a migraine" (1977, 308). We can only make sense of value judgments in relation *to* someone, not of value *in itself*. By not privileging a greater number of people over an individual, we acknowledge that the individual's loss is just as great as the loss that each member of the group would experience. According to Taurek, flipping a coin is the best way to determine whether to save the individual or the group because that shows everyone equal moral consideration. The refusal to maximize happiness by aggregating individual experience highlights the intrinsic value of each person, regardless of their relationship with or impact on others.

One way of treating patients equally is to select patients by **lottery**. If the names of people who need treatment are (metaphorically) thrown into a hat, then each person has an equal chance of being chosen. None of the morally irrelevant things that distinguish us—such as one's ability to pay or one's age, race, gender, religion, or sexuality—come into play. Everyone wants to live. Someone whose name was not chosen could not claim that they were unfairly disadvantaged in the process. Another way of treating patients equally is to give medical resources to the first people who demand them—**first-come, first-served**. This provides fair equality of opportunity: as long as treatment is available, anyone who needs it and shows up gets treated. If all the treatments are being used—for example, there are no ventilators left—then you need to wait your turn. On this view, a hospital is like a deli counter.

The initial intuition to treat patients equally gets complicated by competing intuitions, however, about morally significant inequalities—that is, features of patients' situation or character that should be taken into account. The third and fourth principles—sickest first and youngest first—seek to correct such inequalities. A key principle in John Rawls's theory of justice is that the unequal distribution of goods can only be justified if the least advantaged are better off than they would be under a system of equality (1999, 13, 72–73, 132–34). The least well-off in this case are the people who have the worst prospects if they are left untreated (**sickest first**) and the people who have had the fewest years of life and thus are at risk of being deprived of a supreme good—life itself and the chance to pursue their life plans—that adults have already had (**youngest first**). The sickest first principle is consistent with classic rules of triage: if someone will die without treatment, they should be prioritized over someone else who can walk off the battlefield. It is also consistent with a basic commitment of medicine: to care for those who are most vulnerable or experiencing the most suffering.

The sickest first criterion aligns with the rule of rescue. Albert Jonsen (1986) coined the phrase to describe our inclination to save the lives of identifiable individuals facing avoidable death instead of unidentified individuals. In the case of sickest first, the rule of rescue is conceived as a form of distributive justice, since the sickest are thought to be more deserving of treatment because their lives are more at risk. This has prompted debates in the secondary literature about whether someone should be deprioritized if they are responsible for their condition. For example, should alcoholics with end-stage liver disease receive lower priority for liver transplants than nonalcoholics? Are they less deserving of the organ than someone suffering from primary biliary cholangitis because the alcoholics caused their cirrhosis with their own bad choices? Moss and Siegler (1991) say yes; Cohen and Benjamin (1991) say no.

Some powerful moral intuitions support the youngest first principle. When an elderly person succumbs to cancer, it is sad, but when a child succumbs to cancer, it is tragic. The difference is that the child's potential is cut short, disappointing our hopes for their future. As bioethicists often put it, dying children have not had their **fair innings**. However, Persad, Wertheimer, and Emanuel (2009) themselves argue that youngest first allocation grates against our moral intuitions. The death of an adolescent or young adult is worse than the death of an infant, they say, because the adolescent or young adult "has drawn upon the investment of others," such as education and parental care, "to begin as-yet-unfulfilled projects" (425); they also have "a developed personality capable of forming and valuing long-term plans whose fulfillment requires a complete life" (428). Unlike infants, adolescents and young adults are pursuing goals of their own. Extending their lives would allow their and the community's investment in their projects to be realized.

The fifth and sixth principles—**saving the most whole lives** and **saving the most life years**—seek to distribute limited resources efficiently to produce the greatest benefit. The former view treats all people equally: since each individual values their own life, we maximize value by maximizing individual lives. According to the latter view, living itself is valuable, so more life years are better than fewer life years. If transplanting a heart into a person whose other organs are failing would gain them one more year of life, that is worse (on the life years model) than giving the same organ to a younger, otherwise healthy person who may live an additional fifty years. On the whole lives model, by contrast, people have value, not years, so the two options are equivalent.

The seventh and eighth principles—instrumental value and reciprocity—look beyond the people who need treatment to the effects of any treatment decision on society as a whole. **Instrumental value** allocation is contrary to Kant's moral theory and is consistent with utilitarianism because it considers people as means to promote social goods. As Persad, Wertheimer, and Emanuel note, this principle is "necessarily insufficient" because we must identify the good that treated patients would be instrumental in promoting, which introduces another principle (2009, 426). For example, whether instrumental value allocation would prioritize vaccinating pediatric respiratory therapists during the COVID-19 pandemic depends on whether we want to save the most lives or save the youngest first.

In contrast to the forward-looking instrumental view, **reciprocity** is backward-looking. In his deontological theory, W. D. Ross identifies three prima facie duties that "rest on previous acts": fidelity, reparation, and gratitude (2002, 21). Reciprocity allocation rests on claims of desert: To whom does society owe treatment, given their past sacrifices or service? There is a reason why budget-cutting politicians in the U.S. often target Medicare and Medicaid but not funding for VA hospitals. This commitment may be grounded in a promise we made to take care of our soldiers (fidelity), an attempt to make up for putting their lives at risk (reparation), or a way of thanking them for devoting their lives to their country (gratitude).

As we mentioned, none of these eight principles is sufficient on its own to justify an allocation scheme. One principle often has drawbacks that are only corrected by another principle. For example, by excluding prognosis when considering whom to treat, a lottery approach does not use medical resources efficiently to produce the best overall outcome; but focusing on prognosis or life years often reinforces social inequalities, since people of color (especially in the U.S.) often suffer from more comorbidities than white patients. Promoting instrumental value prioritizes the rich, the powerful, and people who have already lived full lives; favoring young people ignores how society as a whole is negatively affected by the loss of medical professionals, soldiers, police officers, and other essential workers. Despite its attempt at equal consideration, first-come, first-served may reinforce social hierarchies as well, because people who are socially privileged are more likely to be aware of the available resources and to have the opportunity to obtain them.

## Principlism

Philosophers and public health organizations have drawn on the simple principles in Persad, Wertheimer, and Emanuel's list to formulate different, complex allocation models. For example, Tom Beauchamp and James Childress (2019, 308–13) say that the just distribution of scarce medical treatments should consider both patients' health prospects (medical utility) and their future contributions to society (social utility). Medical utility considers both a patient's need—will they die without treatment?—and the probability of success—will the treatment benefit them, and for how long? Social utility considers how (and how much) others will benefit from a patient's continued existence. For example, whether clinicians are prioritized in a given triage scheme depends on whether we believe that treating them would keep them healthy enough to continue providing medical services to the community.

For Beauchamp and Childress, the just distribution of scarce medical resources is explicitly utilitarian. Once everyone's equal worth is recognized and they are all given fair opportunity, we ought to adopt "a utilitarian strategy that emphasizes overall maximum benefit for both patients and society" (2019, 308). Consider a case where an older patient with comorbidities on a ventilator is stable but not improving. Under crisis standards of care, triage committees should recommend taking the patient off the ventilator and giving it to a younger, healthier patient who is at risk of dying because they are more likely to benefit and benefit more quickly, thus saving the patient's life and perhaps the lives of others (who would have access to the ventilator after the younger patient has recovered). In the absence of some great social value that the older patient would provide, Beauchamp and Childress would prioritize the younger patient because they have more years and better quality of life ahead of them and because the older patient has already had a full life while the younger person has not had their fair innings (310).

## QALYs and DALYs

As mentioned in Chapter 1, a widely used measure for allocating resources, and one discussed at length by medical ethicists, is cost-effectiveness analysis (CEA), and specifically cost-utility analysis (CUA), which uses quality-adjusted life years (QALYs) as its basic unit of value. Richard Zeckhauser and Donald Shepard devised the QALY in 1976 as a measure that considers both the duration and quality of a person's life, and it is now widely used by many federal agencies and researchers to compare the value of alternative healthcare interventions and policies. In the United Kingdom, the National Institute for Health and Care Excellence (NICE) uses QALYs to determine which treatments the National Health Service (NHS) will cover. In the United States, the Centers for Disease Control and Prevention (CDC) and the National Institutes of Health (NIH) use QALYs to determine which public health interventions the federal government should fund.

Jeremy Bentham claims that we could calculate the right action with mathematical precision by considering several variables regarding pleasures and pains, such as their intensity (how strong?), duration (how long?), certainty or uncertainty (how likely?), and extent (how many people are affected?) (1970, 38–39). A QALY is similar to Bentham's hedons and dolors. On the QALY measure, one year of healthy life is worth one (1) and being dead is worth zero (0). One year of life with reduced health is worth less than one (< 1), with the number reduced for how much worse the quality of life is. Time is a known quantity, but quality of life is more difficult to measure. Some researchers determine quality of life by means of a health-related quality of life (HRQoL) survey such as the EQ-5D questionnaire, which assigns weights (or utility scores) based on a person's physical, occupational, and psychological function; social interaction; and somatic sensations. Researchers may also determine how much worse it is to be in a diminished state compared to perfect health by asking time trade-off questions—how many years of living with ailment X would you trade for a shorter number of years in perfect health?—or standard gamble questions—would you accept a treatment for ailment X if there were, say, a 50 percent chance it would return you to perfect health and a 20 percent chance it would kill you?

Cost-effectiveness analyses using QALYs are often done to determine if a new treatment works better or is a good value for the money. Here are some illustrative examples:

- Imagine someone who suffers from chronic pain due to severe arthritis, which reduces their quality of life to 50 percent of a fully healthy person. Five years of healthy life (5 years × 1 quality of life = 5 QALYs) is equivalent to ten years with severe arthritis (10 years × 0.5 quality of life = 5 QALYs). If researchers developed a drug (Y) that would eliminate the arthritis, thus restoring the person to full health, but the drug would reduce the person's lifespan by 30 percent, it would be worth it for the person to take the drug: ten years without drug Y is equivalent to five (5) QALYs, and seven years with drug Y is equivalent to seven (7) QALYs. On the other hand, if a new drug (Z) would only slightly improve their symptoms (from, say, 0.5 to 0.7 quality of life) and pose significant enough risks to, on average, reduce lifespan by half, it would not be worth it for the patient: five years with drug Z × 0.7 quality of life = 3.5 QALYs, versus ten years without drug Z × 0.5 quality of life = 5 QALYs.

- Annually in the U.S., about twenty-eight million people experience flu symptoms, and about thirty-five thousand die from the flu. Flu vaccines are typically 40–60 percent effective at preventing people from getting the flu as well as reducing the severity of the illness, flu-associated hospitalization, and risk of death (Centers for Disease Control and Prevention 2023). Some people experience slight aches or fever for a couple of days after getting the vaccine. About one in a million recipients of the vaccine develops Guillain-Barré Syndrome, which causes weakness and paralysis. Although they are complex equations, since not all flu patients experience the same level of suffering and not every year's vaccine is equally good, a cost-utility analysis was done to determine that vaccination yielded an incremental cost-effectiveness ratio of $95,000 per QALY for all age and risk groups, ranging from $194,000 per QALY for non-high-risk adults (eighteen to forty-nine years old) to actual cost savings for adults over fifty years old who are at high risk for influenza-related complications (DeLuca et al. 2023). At this cost-effectiveness ratio, private and public insurers usually provide flu vaccines at no cost.

- QALY calculations can also explain some people's decision to use medical aid in dying. If six more months with a terminal illness would subject a person to intense suffering, either because the pain could not be managed or because of the loss of control over one's body (0.5 years × -0.2 quality of life = -0.1 QALY), they may decide that a quick and painless death is preferable (0 years × 0 quality of life = 0 QALYs). Negative QALYs reflect health states that are worse than death.

To determine the distribution of scarce medical resources using a cost-effectiveness analysis, one would calculate the cost per QALY for alternative courses of action, compare the results, and choose the alternative that maximizes the good produced by the available resources. Tallying QALYs and comparing outcomes thus function much like a traditional utilitarian calculus. It provides a common denominator (cost/QALY) when comparing the efficiency of different health interventions. For example, imagine that, as production was ramping up, the government only had a thousand doses of flu vaccine. Who should receive them? For the high-risk subgroup of children ages two to four, the incremental cost-effectiveness ratio is $1,500/QALY; for low-risk adults ages eighteen to forty-nine, it is $194,000/QALY (DeLuca et al. 2023). The high-risk children should be prioritized ahead of the low-risk adults.

As an alternative to the QALY, the World Health Organization (WHO) and some other public health organizations have adopted the **disability-adjusted life year (DALY)**. QALY calculations only measure the benefits and burdens of medical interventions. By contrast, DALYs quantify overall disease burden, with the number determined by adding both the years lived with disability (YLD) and the years of life lost (YLL) to disability, with the former number adjusted based on the disability weight (with more severe disabilities getting a higher number). One DALY is equivalent to one year of healthy life lost. The goal is to reduce DALYs, and different public health options can be compared to determine the most efficient way to do that. For example, using the DALY measure, studies have found that in sub-Saharan Africa, prevention of mother-to-child transmission ($191/DALY averted) and voluntary medical male circumcision ($-388/

DALY averted [cost savings]) are the most cost-effective ways to reduce HIV transmission, compared to other interventions such as microbicides and condom distribution ($392/DALY averted) (Sarkar et al. 2019).

A common objection to QALYs and DALYs is that they are discriminatory. If a life is worth less when it falls short of an ideal standard of health, then, systemically, cost-effectiveness analyses will undervalue people who have more health problems and less mobility, such as the elderly, people of color (who tend to have more comorbidities), and disabled people. Extending the lives of people with underlying health conditions gains fewer QALYs and averts fewer DALYs than extending the lives of healthier people. The National Council on Disability (2019) officially opposes the use of QALYs by the federal government, its agencies, and public and private insurers, and Representative Cathy McMorris Rodgers has introduced a bill in the U.S. Congress (HR 485, the Protecting Health Care for All Patients Act) that would ban the use of QALYs in all federal programs because, she says, "The 'quality-adjusted life years' measurement is used to discriminate against people with chronic illnesses and disabilities" ("McMorris Rodgers Leads Legislation" 2023; see also Arnesen and Nord 1999; Brock 2000, 2009).

## Organ Transplants: UNOS Points System

As mentioned earlier, medical resources are often stretched thin during mass casualty incidents and public health emergencies. These events are unusual and often unexpected. But the distribution of organs for patients in need of transplants happens on a daily basis. The demand greatly outstrips the supply of transplantable organs: in the U.S. alone, 4,875 people died waiting for transplants in 2024 (Organ Procurement and Transplantation Network, n.d.). Because the current system of **voluntary consent** to donate ("opt in") produces not nearly enough transplantable organs, medical ethicists have proposed alternatives that they say would increase the number. Alternatives include **mandated choice**, where everyone must choose to either donate or not donate; **presumed consent**, where one must remove oneself from the donor list to avoid donating ("opt out"); and a **free market for organs**, where the buying and selling of organs would be allowed. It is unclear whether any of these alternatives would address the relative scarcity of transplantable organs, and they may face other moral problems (such as exploiting the poor in a free market). Two promising advancements that may alleviate the current organ shortage are xenotransplantation (the use of organs from nonhuman animals) and 3D-bioprinted organs. Until we can figure out how to secure an adequate supply of transplantable organs, however, organizations responsible for assigning organs to those in need must formulate guidelines for rationing.

In the United States, the National Organ Transplant Act of 1984 established the nation's transplant system, the Organ Procurement and Transplantation Network (OPTN), which is administered by a private, nonprofit organization, the United Network for Organ Sharing (UNOS). Following the principles of the Belmont Report, regulatory requirements set out in the OPTN Final Rule set the minimal requirements for allocation policies: they must maximize overall good (utility), ensure the fair distribution of benefits (justice), and respect people's right to refuse to donate or to direct a donation (respect for persons) (Organ Procurement and Transplantation Network 2015).

UNOS regularly refines its allocation policies to best reflect these basic moral principles. Their current policy regarding hearts was adopted in 2018, livers in 2019, kidneys and pancreases in 2021, and lungs in 2023. The lung allocation policy is the first to utilize an approach known as continuous distribution, which uses a single weighted score for each candidate that is recalculated with each new donor rather than ranking patients using a single criterion such as medical urgency or likelihood of post-transplant survival, which is what now happens with other organs. This allows UNOS to compare all candidates against one another on a single scale at the same time. Each candidate is assigned a number of points out of a possible 100, with the higher numbers more likely to receive transplants. The points are assigned as follows:

- Candidate medical urgency (maximum 25 points)

This measures the candidate's expected waitlist survival, or how long the person can live without a transplant. It prioritizes the sickest first.

- Likelihood of recipient survival over five years post-transplant (maximum 25 points)

This measures the candidate's prognosis. If one person would survive for less than a year (because, say, they also have terminal cancer), then it would be better to give the organ to another person who would live a longer, healthier life. The criterion of "survival over five years" is not, strictly speaking, a maximizing principle, since it makes no distinction between someone who will live five years and someone who will live fifty years. As we will see in the later discussion of COVID-19 triage, this attempts to guard against ageism and racism and to facilitate more equitable distribution. Justice thus serves as a side-constraint on the utilitarian impulse.

- Potential biological challenges in matching, such as the candidate's blood type, height or immune sensitivity (maximum 15 points)

This is a form of prognosis since it considers whether the benefits in the first two categories—saving the life of someone at risk of dying and increasing life years—are more or less likely (what Bentham calls certainty/uncertainty). These points will vary for the donor depending on the available organ. An adult's lungs are not usable by a small child. Since most donated organs are from people age eighteen to sixty-four (Statista 2023), young children are likely to be disadvantaged by this.

- Whether the candidate was younger than age 18 when listed for a transplant (20 points)

This is youngest first allocation in one sense but not in another. A sixteen-year-old is prioritized over a sixty-year-old, but no distinction is made between a sixteen-year-old and a six-year-old.

- Whether the candidate was a prior living organ donor (5 points)

This is a form of reciprocity allocation. The candidate deserves the organ because of their past sacrifice: having previously donated one of their own organs.

- Logistical considerations such as whether the lungs can be successfully preserved and transported to the candidate's hospital (maximum 10 points) (United Network for Organ Sharing 2023)

Like the "biological challenges" category, this is another measure of the likelihood of success, a different dimension of prognosis.

This theoretical model, which attempts to allocate organs fairly, has often been circumvented in recent years. Procurement organizations take shortcuts that allow people to skip ahead in line, purportedly to increase efficiency—to transplant organs before they degrade (Rosenthal, Hansen, and White 2025). In its ideal functioning, however, the UNOS points system illustrates many important things about resource allocation, especially its complexity. The simple principles that are listed by Persad, Wertheimer, and Emanuel (2009) can be combined in a variety of ways in a single system, the different principles can be given different weights in the calculation (in this case, points), the principles can be qualified or constrained by other principles (e.g., prognosis without maximization), and each principle is complex enough to include different kinds of considerations (e.g., prognosis is not only about a patient's life years but also the likelihood that the procedure will succeed). Because it is so complicated, public health organizations often revisit their allocation schemes. UNOS has changed its principles and the weights given to them many times, and the number of points a candidate has is adjusted over time through the continuous distribution process.

## Triage during the COVID-19 Pandemic

The public health crisis brought on by COVID-19 forced many countries to develop allocation plans and to update them as conditions on the ground changed. First, public health officials had to decide how to distribute treatment for those who contracted the disease (triage). Some healthcare systems did not have enough space, staff, or stuff—beds in the intensive care unit (ICU); qualified medical personnel, such as respiratory therapists and ICU nurses; or personal protective equipment (PPE), oxygen, and ventilators—to handle the influx of infected patients in addition to other, non-COVID patients. Early in the pandemic, there was a shortage of PPE, such as high-filtration N-95 masks, which had to be distributed to healthcare workers. After vaccines were developed, officials had to decide which people to inoculate first (vaccine distribution).

Although U.S. states and other countries had different standards, common themes ran through the allocation principles and procedures used during the pandemic. Most standards included a list of guiding ethical principles:

- Lee Daugherty Biddison et al. (2019) emphasized transparency and inclusivity.

- The University of Pittsburgh's Department of Critical Care Medicine (hereafter "Pittsburgh") emphasized "the duty to care, duty to steward resources to optimize population health, distributive and procedural justice, and transparency" (2020a, 1; 2020b, 1).

- The New York State Department of Health (hereafter "New York") emphasized the duty to care, the duty to steward resources, the duty to plan, distributive justice, and transparency (2015, 12).

- The Washington State Department of Health (hereafter "Washington") emphasized fairness, the duty to care, the duty to steward resources, transparency, consistency, proportionality, and accountability (2020a, 3; 2020b, 3; 2021, 3).

All the guidelines claimed to have been based on input from community stakeholders and consultation with medical professionals so that the standards reflected "community values" (Daugherty Biddison et al. 2019, 849).

Public health officials first considered a patient's desire for treatment and their advance directive, thus respecting patient autonomy. In addition, they strove to avoid bias and to treat all patients equally, regardless of age, race, gender, sexual orientation, or disability, thus promoting justice. Most guidelines then attempted to maximize benefits, understood as saving the most lives and the most life years. That is, they wanted to maximize the number of people who would survive in the short term (whole lives, defined as survival to discharge) and the number of people who would survive in the long term (life years, usually defined as survival one to five years post-discharge).

Different criteria were used to determine short-term prospects for surviving the treatment as well as long-term prospects post-discharge. With regard to adult triage, once a patient was admitted to the ICU, the likelihood of survival was measured by different groups in similar ways, with some variation:

- Daugherty Biddison et al. (2019) determined the prospects for survival by measuring the likelihood of organ dysfunction using the Sequential Organ Failure Assessment (SOFA) and considering comorbid conditions, such as severe congestive heart failure and severe chronic lung disease.

- Pittsburgh (2020a, 2020 b) also measured the degree of organ dysfunction using SOFA and considered comorbid conditions.

- New York focused only on "the short-term likelihood of survival of the acute medical episode and [was] not focused on whether a patient may survive a given illness or disease in the long-term (e.g., years later)" (2015, 236). It also used SOFA to determine a patient's mortality risk.

- Washington (2020a, 2020b) measured the degree of organ dysfunction using the Modified Sequential Organ Failure Assessment

(MSOFA), considered comorbid conditions, assessed how severely the patient was affected by COVID-19, and estimated how long the patient would need the critical care resources. Interestingly, the state of Washington later prohibited the use of *any* scoring systems because they "contain biased information" and "are oftentimes derived from patient populations not reflective or inclusive of historically oppressed communities" (2021, 48). Justice again serves as a side-constraint on the maximization of positive outcomes.

All four sets of guidelines placed patients into different triage categories, using a points system or color-coding system that assigned them a higher or lower priority for treatment—in the case of COVID-19, typically a bed in the ICU and/or use of a ventilator—compared with other patients. A patient's response to the treatment was occasionally reassessed: at 24, 48, and 120 hours for Daugherty Biddison et al. (2019, 852); "periodic[ally]" for Pittsburgh (2020a, 9; 2020b, 9); at 48 and 120 hours for New York (2015, 61–67); and every 24 hours for Washington (2020a, 36; 2020b, 37). If there was no improvement or the patient's response to the treatment was so slow that they would use ICU resources for a long time, this would place a burden on the system and might provide less benefit, understood in terms of progress per day, than if the resources were given to others. Treatment could then be redirected to patients with better chances of short- and long-term survival. First-come, first-served did not apply.

Washington struggled with an additional criterion, and it is unclear whether it was a measure of short-term survival, long-term survival, or quality of life after treatment. It was initially described as "baseline functional status (consider loss of reserves in energy, physical ability, cognition and general health)" (Washington 2020a, 34–35), but that was thought to discriminate against the disabled. By including baseline physical ability and cognition, it seemed to be saying that disabilities make life less worth living. The criterion was then changed to "prognostically relevant decompensation from a person's baseline health status, such as degree of frailty that impacts survival given the current circumstances that make crisis capacity triage necessary," with frailty defined as follows: "A syndrome of physiological decline in life, characterized by marked vulnerability to adverse health outcomes" (Washington 2020b, 35–37). There are many different scoring systems to determine frailty, such as the Clinical Frailty Scale (see Rockwood and Theou 2020), but none was mentioned in the guidelines.

With regard to triage decisions, a thirty-year-old with prospects equivalent to a forty-year-old would be prioritized by the utilitarian simply because they are younger and (probably) have more years to live. Young people tend to have more QALYs ahead of them. The early recommendation by the Italian Society of Anesthesia, Analgesia, Reanimation and Intensive Care (SIAARTI) that there be an age limit for admission to intensive care, regardless of comorbidities or likelihood of survival (Vergano et al. 2020), reflects this commitment to maximizing impact in terms of both life years and quality of life. However, SIAARTI's recommendation was viewed by many as unjust because it did not treat all people's lives as equally valuable (see Cesari and Proietti 2020). Health officials in the U.S. carefully tried to avoid decisions informed by ageism. In many state guidelines, age was only considered as a tiebreaker when two patients were otherwise identical in terms of likelihood of survival to discharge.

To guard against discrimination, Daugherty Biddison et al. defined long-term survival as survival one year or more after treatment (2019, 850). They made this cutoff to avoid giving lower priority to groups of people who, in the aggregate and individually, have shorter lifespans. For example, people of color are more likely to suffer from comorbidities such as diabetes and hypertension, but if they are not so severe as to cause death within one year, they do not affect a patient's score. New York did not consider long-term survival at all, stating that "advanced age was rejected as a triage criterion because it discriminates against the elderly" (2015, 5, 13; see also 45, 83, 104). Pittsburgh took a middle position: patients with less than one year to live (described as "severely life-limiting conditions" in Pittsburgh 2020a) got the lowest priority, while patients with less than five years to live (described as "major comorbidities [associated with significantly decreased long-term survival]" in Pittsburgh 2020a) got a lower priority than otherwise healthy patients, but a higher one than those who were likely to live for less than one year (2020a, 6; 2020b, 6). Washington considered "relevant comorbid conditions that impact survival," a vague standard, in determining admission to the ICU and in reevaluation (2020a, 36–37; 2020b, 36–37). It did not specify frailty in terms of life years but seemed to leave the determination of who counted as frail to individual hospitals and their triage committees.

Of course, an apparently race- and age-neutral prioritization system may still result in discriminatory outcomes. If comorbidities affect a patient's prognosis and people of color suffer from more comorbidities, then people of color are less likely to receive treatment under a system that attempts to save the most lives and the most life years. In an effort to promote equity, Washington included in a late version of its guidelines (2021) a tiebreaker that attempted to address structural forms of oppression in healthcare. In the case of a tie—meaning that facilities had fewer resources than patients in a given category, so they had to choose among them—triage committees were instructed to leave the resource with the patient who already had it. Absent this situation, they gave it to whichever of them was pregnant. If a tie remained, they assigned each patient in that category a number pegged to a **Social Vulnerability Index (SVI)**, which measures "the demographic and socioeconomic factors (such as poverty, lack of access to transportation, and crowded housing) that adversely affect communities that encounter hazards and other community-level stressors" (Agency for Toxic Substances and Disease Registry 2024). An SVI typically helps public health officials plan responses to public health emergencies by identifying which communities will need the most support. If two patients had the same likelihood of surviving to discharge, the patient with a higher SVI—meaning their access to healthcare was likely impeded due to poverty, unemployment, or discrimination—was given preference (Washington 2021, 7–10, 30–31). As Gary Jones (1985) argues, people who have experienced discrimination in the past should be prioritized in the allocation of scarce social goods, including healthcare resources, to correct past injustice (a backward-looking principle of allocation that, incidentally, Persad, Wertheimer, and Emanuel [2009] fail to mention).

At the height of the pandemic, triage committees were formed at local, regional, and state levels. Committees typically included two or more clinicians with experience in tertiary triage (e.g., emergency medicine) and at least one ethicist (with qualifications defined differently in different places). Some hospitals' standing ethics committees became de facto triage committees. Smaller healthcare systems without their own standing ethics committees, usually because of a lack of trained medical ethicists in the area, depended on regional and state committees. When crisis standards of care were activated and allocation decisions needed to be made, triage committees received anonymized, clinically relevant information about potential patients. In Washington, for example, patient data included the following:

- patient's preferences for ICU intervention, whether the patient meets ICU admission criteria, and indications for admission to ICU (e.g., requires ventilatory support, inability to protect or maintain airway);
- comorbidities and their severity (e.g., severe chronic lung disease, moderate coronary artery disease, mild diabetes);
- prognostically relevant decompensation from baseline health status, such as frailty, that impacts chance of survival;
- whether the patient is COVID positive and when the symptoms began;
- the patient's current level of respiratory support (e.g., CPAP, ventilator, low-flow oxygen) and degree of acute respiratory distress syndrome (ARDS);
- SOFA/MSOFA score; and
- the patient's response to current treatment and the estimated prognosis with ICU resources and without ICU resources. (Washington 2021)

Patients currently receiving treatment had no stronger claim on ICU resources—so it was not first-come, first-served (except as a tiebreaker). And triage committees prioritized patients relative to one another rather than giving specific treatment recommendations. That is, even if a patient's prognosis was bleak, no decision was made to forego treatment as long as the resources were available and the patient wanted it.

In applying the standards, committee members in Washington state raised important ethical questions that government agencies needed to address. For example:

- Should publicly funded community healthcare systems prioritize residents of their own state over residents of other states who cross the border? (The Department of Health said: No.)
- Should a vaccinated patient who is a resident of a state with a mask mandate be prioritized for treatment in that state over an

unvaccinated patient from a neighboring state with no mask mandate who must cross the border for treatment because their own hospitals are overrun? (No.)

- Should pregnant women be prioritized over nonpregnant women? (Washington used pregnancy as one of the tiebreakers [2021, 30]; some other states gave pregnant women additional "points" under their guidelines [Baker and Fink 2020].)

- What happens if members of the triage team disagree with the attending physician's determination of the patient's prognosis? (They should defer to the attending physician. The triage team is not a fact-finding body.)

Medical ethicists have already begun scrutinizing the policies developed during the COVID-19 pandemic, perhaps to prepare for the next crisis.

During the pandemic, medical ethicists were enlisted to help draft guidelines specifically geared toward COVID-19, ethics committees provided feedback to modify the standards, and triage committees were set up to apply the guidelines to patients. For some academics, it was the first time they had to draw on their theoretical background to make life-and-death decisions. Sometimes they had to be on call day and night in case crisis standards of care were put into effect. To avoid some of the mistakes made by the "God Committee," the actions of local and regional triage teams were strictly governed by policies transparently formulated at the state level. Still, it took judgment to apply those standards, and members of triage committees, although they eventually reached consensus, often began with different opinions. Under the circumstances, philosophically informed moral reasoning about the principles of allocation provided an important corrective to the unreflective intuitions of clinicians who came to realize that a medical prognosis alone does not settle any moral questions, even when triage guidelines have been established.

## Distribution of COVID-19 Vaccines

The second major class of decisions during the pandemic concerned how to distribute vaccines when there were not enough for the entire eligible population. Although healthcare systems are committed to the same moral principles in both vaccine distribution and triage, attempting to save the most lives and the most life years justifies different distribution patterns when it comes to prevention rather than treatment. Three main goals are to reduce transmission, protect people who are most likely to be exposed to the virus, and minimize serious illness and death.

In the United States, healthcare organizations followed the framework developed by the National Academies of Sciences, Engineering, and Medicine (2020). Guided by three ethical principles—maximum benefit, equal concern, and mitigation of health inequities—the allocation process included four (actually five) phases:

1. Phase 1
   a. Phase 1a: High-risk health workers, workers who support the healthcare system (transportation, environmental services, facility services), and first responders at risk of exposure

Three reasons were given in support of prioritizing these people above all others: "Their critical role in maintaining healthcare system functionality, their high risk of exposure to patients exhibiting symptoms of COVID-19, and their risk of then transmitting the virus to others, including family members" (National Academies 2020, 11). The idea was that this would have the biggest impact on reducing infections because (1) they maintain a system that can treat sick patients and administer vaccines; (2) their exposure puts them at special risk, especially compared to those who can shelter in place, so vaccinating them would lower the incidence of infection; and (3) they encounter a lot of sick people, including those who, because of age or comorbidities, are more likely to die if infected. Thus, protecting healthcare workers also prevents transmission to people who are most likely to have severe symptoms.

   b. Phase 1b: People with comorbid and other underlying health conditions that put them at high risk and older adults living in crowded settings

Research showed that people with comorbidities were more likely to get severe symptoms, be hospitalized, and die from COVID-19. Older people were also more at risk, and living in nursing homes or other group settings increased the potential for outbreaks.

2. Phase 2: K-12 teachers, school staff (such as administrators and support staff), and childcare workers; "critical workers" in high-risk

settings, such as those in the food supply system; people with comorbid or underlying conditions that put them at moderately higher risk; people in homeless shelters, group homes, prisons, and jails; and older adults not covered under Phase 1

Vaccinating school workers allowed them to continue providing an essential service to society while reducing transmission and minimizing their risks despite high exposure. People in homeless shelters and detention centers had high exposure and often could not follow social distancing directives, and they also often have "chronic healthcare needs." Older people and people with comorbidities are more likely to die if they are infected than younger, healthier people—indeed, age is a prognostically relevant indicator of surviving COVID-19 (Zhou et al. 2020)—so prioritizing the former over the latter minimizes harm by saving more lives. That is, younger people who have COVID are more likely to be asymptomatic or mildly symptomatic, so the overall effects of the disease will not be as bad if we focus our preventive measures on older people, for whom infection is more likely to be debilitating or fatal.

3. Phase 3: Children (under eighteen), young adults (ages eighteen to thirty), and workers in economically and socially important industries (such as universities and entertainment) who are at moderate risk of infection

Nowhere in the guidelines does it talk about fair innings. In fact, younger people are less likely to get severe symptoms. The reason for vaccinating young people was that they were vectors of transmission to adults and other, more vulnerable populations.

4. Phase 4: Anyone residing in the United States not covered by Phases 1–3.

Note that these standards make no distinction between citizens and non-citizens, including undocumented immigrants.

Early in the pandemic, Ezekiel Emanuel et al. (2020) put forward a different allocation plan called the **Fair Priority Model**, meant for international organizations such as the WHO. Rejecting national partiality—the tendency of a country to favor its own citizens—Emanuel et al. based their model on three basic moral values: benefiting people and limiting harm, prioritizing the disadvantaged, and equal moral concern (which they equated with nondiscrimination). They defined harm broadly to include death and organ damage from infection, rising mortality rates for non-COVID health problems that cannot be treated when health systems are strained, and economic and social deprivations. On their view, vaccines should be distributed in three phases to combat these harms in order of priority, with preventing death and organ failure as the most important goal. Their system prioritized the least well-off during all three phases:

1. Phase 1: They proposed using Standard Expected Years of Life Lost (SEYLL) to calculate life years lost against life expectancy and then determining how many lost years would be averted with the use of a vaccine. Since early deaths are more frequent in low-income countries, giving vaccines to the least well-off more effectively increases life years (Emanuel et al. 2020, 1310).

2. Phase 2: The economic impact was measured by how much each dose of vaccine would reduce the absolute size of the poverty gap, measured against a uniform poverty line. Since many developing countries already fall below the poverty line (certainly more than developed countries), the ratio of the mean income of the poor would be impacted more significantly by the administration of vaccines in developing countries.

3. Phase 3: Countries with higher transmission rates were prioritized. In terms of transmission, those with the highest rates are the worst off epidemiologically.

Emanuel et al. argued that this plan better aimed at global equity than the WHO's initial proposal in 2020, which called for distributing doses in proportion to a country's population. Although this treats people equally, Emanuel et al. claimed that the WHO "mistakenly assumes that equality requires treating differently situated countries identically rather than equitably responding to their different needs" (2020, 1311). The WHO's current guidelines, formulated in 2022, more closely follow these suggestions. The organization's main goal is to "sustain and enhance momentum to reduce mortality and morbidity, protect the health systems, and resume socio-economic activities with existing vaccines" (World Health Organization 2022, 6). They target the groups most at risk to reduce mortality and disease burden, followed by the remaining population, with the eventual goal of building population immunity.

## Conclusion: The Dialogue between Theory and Practice

Attempts to develop moral principles around resource allocation provide important insights into both theoretical and applied ethics. The typical introductory course in ethics presents students with the major moral theories: Kant says that we ought to respect rational agency in ourselves and others, Mill says that we ought to maximize happiness, Rawls says that we ought to form just social arrangements, and so on. Although philosophers such as R. M. Hare and Derek Parfit have tried to synthesize different approaches, the major moral theories are usually presented as alternatives. The reality of our moral deliberations is very different, however. All the live allocation schemes recognize the intrinsic value of persons, the value of maximizing positive future experiences, and the value of fair patterns of distribution, including nondiscrimination. As Persad, Wertheimer, and Emanuel say, "no single principle allocates interventions justly" (2009, 423). This lends support to pluralism in value theory.

When an organization such as UNOS revises its criteria over time, it exemplifies the effort to achieve reflective equilibrium. Sometimes we test principles against our moral intuitions: for example, equating a sixty-year-old's life year and a ten-year-old's life year contradicts a widely held preference to favor the young (Gu et al. 2015). Sometimes we should change our attitudes in response to well-argued principles: for example, perhaps an infant should not be prioritized over an eighteen-year-old who has a developed personality and unfulfilled projects. We are trying to reach a point where our allocation schemes make sense in light of both particular judgments and general principles. Therefore, medical ethics is not only a way of applying moral theories but of testing those theories and suggesting new ways forward in the philosophical study of normative ethics.

### References

Agency for Toxic Substances and Disease Registry. 2024. "CDC/ATSDR Social Vulnerability Index: Overview." Last modified June 14, 2024. https://www.atsdr.cdc.gov/placeandhealth/svi/index.html.

Alexander, Shana. 1962. "They Decide Who Lives, Who Dies: Medical Miracle Puts Moral Burden on Small Committee." *Life* 53, no. 19 (November 9): 102–25.

Arnesen, Trude, and Erik Nord. 1999. "The Value of DALY Life: Problems with Ethics and Validity of Disability Adjusted Life Years." *BMJ* 319, no. 7222 (November 27): 1423–25. doi:10.1136/bmj.319.7222.1423.

Baker, Mike, and Sheri Fink. 2020. "At the Top of the Covid-19 Curve, How Do Hospitals Decide Who Gets Treatment?" *New York Times*. March 31. https://www.nytimes.com/2020/03/31/us/coronavirus-covid-triage-rationing-ventilators.html.

Beauchamp, Tom L., and James F. Childress. 2019. *Principles of Biomedical Ethics*. 8th ed. New York: Oxford University Press.

Bentham, Jeremy. 1970. *An Introduction to the Principles of Morals and Legislation*. Edited by J. H. Burns and H. L. A. Hart. Oxford: Clarendon.

Blagg, C. R. 1998. "Development of Ethical Concepts in Dialysis: Seattle in the 1960s." *Nephrology* 4, no. 4 (August): 235–38. doi:10.1111/j.1440-1797.1998.tb00353.x.

Brock, Dan W. 2000. "Health Care Resource Prioritization and Discrimination against Persons with Disabilities." In *Americans with Disabilities: Exploring Implications of the Law for Individuals and Institutions*, edited by Leslie Pickering Francis and Anita Silvers, 223–35. New York: Routledge.

———. 2009. "Cost-Effectiveness and Disability Discrimination." *Economics and Philosophy* 25, no. 1 (March) 27–47. doi:10.1017/S0266267108002265.

Cesari, Matteo, and Marco Proietti. 2020. "COVID-19 in Italy: Ageism and Decision Making in a Pandemic." *Journal of the American Medical Directors Association* 21, no. 5 (May): 576–77. doi:10.1016/j.jamda.2020.03.025.

Cohen, Carl, and Martin Benjamin. 1991. "Alcoholics and Liver Transplantation." *JAMA: Journal of the American Medical Association* 265, no. 10 (March 13): 1299–301. doi:10.1001/jama.1991.03460100101033.

Daugherty Biddison, E. Lee, Ruth Faden, Howard S. Gwon, Darren P. Mareiniss, Alan C. Regenberg, Monica Schoch-Spana, Jack Schwartz, and Eric S. Toner. 2019. "Too Many Patients . . . a Framework to Guide Statewide Allocation of Scarce Mechanical Ventilation during Disasters." *CHEST* 155, no. 4 (April): 848–54. doi:10.1016/j.chest.2018.09.025.

DeLuca, Ellen Kim, Acham Gebremariam, Angela Rose, Matthew Biggerstaff, Martin I. Meltzer, and Lisa A. Prosser. 2023. "Cost-Effectiveness of Routine Annual Influenza Vaccination by Age and Risk Status." *Vaccine* 41, no. 29 (June 29): 4239–48. doi:10.1016/j.vaccine.2023.04.069.

Emanuel, Ezekiel J., Govind Persad, Adam Kern, Allen Buchanan, Cécile Fabre, Daniel Halliday, Joseph Heath, et al. 2020. "An Ethical Framework for Global Vaccine Allocation." *Science* 369, no. 6509 (September 11): 1309–12. doi:10.1126/science.abe2803.

Gu, Yuanyuan, Emily Lancsar, Peter Ghijben, James R. G. Butler, and Cam Donaldson. 2015. "Attributes and Weights in Health Care Priority Setting:

A Systematic Review of What Counts and to What Extent." *Social Science & Medicine* 146 (December): 41–52. doi:10.1016/j.socscimed.2015.10.005.

Jones, Gary E. 1985. "Preferential Treatment and the Allocation of Scarce Medical Resources." *Philosophical Quarterly* 35, no. 141 (October): 382–93. doi:10.2307/2219473.

Jonsen, Albert R. 1986. "Bentham in a Box: Technology Assessment and Health Care Allocation." *Law, Medicine & Health Care* 14, nos. 3–4 (September): 172–74. doi:10.1111/j.1748-720x.1986.tb00974.x.

Kant, Immanuel. 1996. *Groundwork of the Metaphysics of Morals*. In *Practical Philosophy*, translated and edited by Mary J. Gregor, 41–108. Cambridge: Cambridge University Press.

Locke, John. 1980. *Second Treatise of Government*. Edited by C. B. Macpherson. Indianapolis: Hackett.

"McMorris Rodgers Leads Legislation to Ban QALYs, Protect Individuals with Disabilities from Discrimination." 2023. https://mcmorris.house.gov/posts/mcmorris-rodgers-leads-legislation-to-ban-qalys-protect-individuals-with-disabilities-from-discrimination.

Moss, Alvin H., and Mark Siegler. 1991. "Should Alcoholics Compete Equally for Liver Transplantation?" *JAMA: Journal of the American Medical Association* 265, no. 10 (March 13): 1295–98. doi:10.1001/jama.1991.03460100097032.

National Academies of Sciences, Engineering, and Medicine. 2020. *Framework for Equitable Allocation of COVID-19 Vaccine*. Washington, DC: National Academies Press. https://www.ncbi.nlm.nih.gov/books/NBK562672/pdf/Bookshelf_NBK562672.pdf.

National Council on Disability. 2019. *Quality-Adjusted Life Years and the Devaluation of Life with Disability*. Washington, DC: National Council on Disability. https://www.ncd.gov/report/quality-adjusted-life-years-and-the-devaluation-of-life-with-a-disability/.

New York State Department of Health, Task Force on Life and the Law. 2015. "Ventilator Allocation Guidelines." November. https://nysba.org/app/uploads/2020/05/2015-ventilator_guidelines-NYS-Task-Force-Life-and-Law.pdf.

Organ Procurement and Transplantation Network. 2015. "Ethical Principles in the Allocation of Human Organs." June. https://optn.transplant.hrsa.gov/professionals/by-topic/ethical-considerations/ethical-principles-in-the-allocation-of-human-organs/.

———. n.d. "National Data: Removal Reasons by Year." Accessed January 15, 2025. https://optn.transplant.hrsa.gov/data/view-data-reports/national-data/#.

Persad, Govind, Alan Wertheimer, and Ezekiel Emanuel. 2009. "Principles for Allocation of Scarce Medical Interventions." *Lancet* 373, no. 9661 (January 31): 423–31. doi:10.1016/S0140-6736(09)60137-9.

Rawls, John. 1999. *A Theory of Justice*. Rev. ed. Cambridge, MA: Belknap.
Rockwood, Kenneth, and Olga Theou. 2020. "Using the Clinical Frailty Scale in Allocating Scarce Health Care Resources." *Canadian Geriatrics Journal* 23, no. 3 (September 1): 210–15. doi:10.5770/cgj.23.463.
Rosenthal, Brian M., Mark Hansen, and Jeremy White. 2025. "Organ Transplant System 'in Chaos' as Waiting Lists Are Ignored." *New York Times*. February 26. https://www.nytimes.com/interactive/2025/02/26/us/organ-transplants-waiting-list-skipped-patients.html.
Ross, W. D. 2002. *The Right and the Good*. Edited by Philip Stratton-Lake. Oxford: Clarendon.
Sarkar, Supriya, Phaedra Corso, Shideh Ebrahim-Zadeh, Patricia Kim, Sana Charania, and Kristin Wall. 2019. "Cost-Effectiveness of HIV Prevention Interventions in Sub-Saharan Africa: A Systematic Review." *eClinicalMedicine* 10 (April): P10–31. doi:10.1016/j.eclinm.2019.04.006.
Statista. 2023. "Number of Deceased Organ Donors in the United States in 2021, by Age Group." November 3. https://www.statista.com/statistics/398442/total-number-of-us-organ-donors-by-age-group/.
Taurek, John M. 1977. "Should the Numbers Count?" *Philosophy & Public Affairs* 6, no. 4 (Summer): 293–316. https://www.jstor.org/stable/2264945.
United Network for Organ Sharing. 2023. "Policy: Lung: Continuous Distribution." March 9. https://unos.org/news/new-lung-allocation-policy-in-effect/.
University of Pittsburgh, Department of Critical Care Medicine. 2020a. "Allocation of Scarce Critical Care Resources during a Public Health Emergency." March 23. https://bioethics.pitt.edu/sites/default/files/Univ%20Pittsburgh%20-%20Allocation%20of%20Scarce%20Critical%20Care%20Resources%20During%20a%20Public%20Health%20Emergency.pdf.
——— . 2020b. "Allocation of Scarce Critical Care Resources during a Public Health Emergency." April 15. https://pair.upenn.edu/uploads/attachments/ckevsfhlc45vbszu09p4z0r9o-allocation-of-scarce-critical-care-resources-during-a-public-health-emergency.pdf.
Vergano, Marco, Guido Bertolini, Alberto Giannini, Giuseppe R. Gristina, Sergio Livigni, Giovanni Mistraletti, Luigi Riccioni, and Flavia Petrini. 2020. "Clinical Ethics Recommendations for the Allocation of Intensive Care Treatments in Exceptional, Resource-Limited Circumstances: The Italian Perspective during the COVID-19 Epidemic." *Critical Care* 24: article no. 165. doi:10.1186/s13054-020-02891-w.
Washington State Department of Health and the Northwest Healthcare Response Network. 2020a. "Scarce Resource Management & Crisis Standards of Care." March 16.
——— . 2020b. "Scarce Resource Management & Crisis Standards of Care." December.

———. 2021. "Washington State Crisis Standards of Care Triage Team Operational Guidebook." October. https://doh.wa.gov/sites/default/files/2022-02/821-151-CSC-TT-guidebook.PDF.

World Health Organization. 2022. "Global Covid-19 Vaccination Strategy in a Changing World." July. https://www.who.int/publications/m/item/global-covid-19-vaccination-strategy-in-a-changing-world--july-2022-update.

Zeckhauser, Richard, and Donald Shepard. 1976. "Where Now for Saving Lives?" *Law and Contemporary Problems* 40, no. 4 (Autumn): 5–45. doi:10.2307/1191310.

Zhou, Fei, Ting Yu, Ronghui Du, Guohui Fan, Ying Liu, Zhibo Liu, Jie Xiang, et al. 2020. "Clinical Course and Risk Factors for Mortality of Adult Inpatients with COVID-19 in Wuhan, China: A Retrospective Cohort Study." *Lancet* 395, no. 10229 (March 28): P1054–62. doi:10.1016/S0140-6736(20)30566-3.

## Further Reading

Arras, John D. 2005. "Rationing Vaccine during an Avian Influenza Pandemic: Why It Won't Be Easy." *Yale Journal of Biology and Medicine* 78, no. 5 (October): 287–300. https://pmc.ncbi.nlm.nih.gov/articles/PMC2259161/.
    Proposes that, during interpandemic vaccine shortages, we should target those most at risk for mortality and hospitalization—that is, those most in need. During a pandemic, however, we should think more broadly about maintaining the function of social institutions. We should balance protection of the most vulnerable against other priorities, such as protecting healthcare workers and others who are crucial to crisis response; protecting key social functions, such as police departments and food producers; maximizing economic benefits by vaccinating the working population; and giving younger people an equal opportunity to live a full life (fair innings).

Childress, James F. 1970. "Who Shall Live When Not All Can Live?" *Soundings* 53, no. 4 (Winter): 339–55. https://www.jstor.org/stable/41178062.
    Rejects allocation schemes that prioritize people based on social benefit. Childress argues that, first, we should exclude those who will not benefit from the treatment. Among those who remain—the "medically acceptable"—we should choose randomly, with either a lottery or first-come, first-served. Random selection respects everyone's equal right to be saved, establishes equality of opportunity, and preserves a relationship of trust between candidates and decision-makers.

Emanuel, Ezekiel, Andrew Steinmetz, and Harald Schmidt, eds. 2018. *Rationing and Resource Allocation in Healthcare: Essential Readings*. Oxford: Oxford University Press.

    Extensive collection of readings on the allocation of scarce medical resources. The book is divided into three parts: the first defines key terms and excerpts classic works in ethics; the second sets out principles of rationing and examines policies regarding organ transplants and vaccine allocations in emergencies; and the last focuses on different aspects of healthcare policy, bedside rationing, personal responsibility for health, and global health priorities.

Emanuel, Ezekiel J., Govind Persad, Ross Upshur, Beatriz Thome, Michael Parker, Aaron Glickman, Cathy Zhang, Connor Boyle, Maxwell Smith, and James P. Phillips. 2020. "Fair Allocation of Scarce Medical Resources in the Time of Covid-19." *New England Journal of Medicine* 382 (May 21): 2049–55. doi:10.1056/NEJMsb2005114.

    Written shortly after the COVID-19 outbreak was declared a pandemic by the WHO, this article adopts four fundamental values for allocating scarce resources: "maximizing the benefits produced by scarce resources, treating people equally, promoting and rewarding instrumental value, and giving priority to the worst off." The authors then apply those values to make specific recommendations in the context of the COVID-19 pandemic.

Engelhardt, H. Tristram Jr., and Michael A. Rie. 1986. "Intensive Care Units, Scarce Resources, and Conflicting Principles of Justice." *JAMA: Journal of the American Medical Association* 255, no. 9 (March 7): 1159–64. doi:10.1001/jama.1986.03370090081025.

    Proposes an allocation system for beds in the ICU. How should we weigh possibility of survival, quality of life after discharge, and length of survival, all while under conditions of uncertainty in prognosis, when making allocation decisions? The authors have us consider social policy around ICU bed allocation like an insurance policy against losses at the natural lottery (natural abilities and disabilities) and social lottery (social circumstances that lead to privileges or disadvantages). We would invest little public resources for great benefit (good chance of survival, good quality of life for many years) and avoid incurring additional communal costs for marginal benefits.

Harris, John. 1987. "QALYfying the Value of Life." *Journal of Medical Ethics* 13, no. 3 (September): 117–23. doi:10.1136/jme.13.3.117.

    Raises several objections to the use of QALYs in resource allocation. Appealing to QALYs assumes that an individual preference can be generalized to group decisions; it pays no attention to their distribution, only their total amount; it devalues persons; it is ageist, racist, and sexist; it subjects people with poor quality of life to further victimization; and it makes no distinction between life-saving and life-enhancing treatment.

Krütli, Pius, Thomas Rosemann, Kjell Y. Törnblom, and Timo Smieszek. 2016. "How to Fairly Allocate Scarce Medical Resources: Ethical Argumentation under Scrutiny by Health Professionals and Lay People." *PLoS One* 11, no. 7 (July 27): e0159086. doi:10.1371/journal.pone.0159086.

    Empirical survey of how laypeople, general practitioners, medical students, and other healthcare professionals evaluate ten potential allocation principles. The results varied depending on people's medical backgrounds. While laypeople rated sickest first as most fair, general practitioners rated prognosis as most fair. Both groups rated lottery, reciprocity, and instrumental value as very unfair.

Sönmez, Tayfun, Parag A. Pathak, M. Utku Ünver, Govind Persad, Robert D. Truog, and Douglas B. White. 2021. "Categorized Priority Systems: A New Tool for Fairly Allocating Scarce Medical Resources in the Face of Profound Social Inequities." *CHEST* 159, no. 3 (March): P1294–99. doi:10.1016/j.chest.2020.12.019.

    Claims that most allocation guidelines adopted during the COVID-19 pandemic reinforced healthcare disparities. The authors propose a categorized priority system (or reserved system) instead. An equitable allocation system would establish different categories, including separate categories for disadvantaged groups such as disabled people and those who are socially vulnerable, and then assign resources to and distribute them within each category.

Strech, Daniel, Matthis Synofzik, and Georg Marckmann. 2008. "How Physicians Allocate Scarce Resources at the Bedside: A Systematic Review of Qualitative Studies." *Journal of Medicine and Philosophy* 33, no. 1 (February): 80–99. doi:10.1093/jmp/jhm007.

    Surveys many empirical studies on how physicians decide what to do for patients when resources are stretched thin. The authors found that physicians' decisions depend on context-related factors such as time of day, the number of hospital beds, and the hospital's operating budget; doctor-related factors such as whether they consider the patient "good" or "bad"; and patient-related factors such as patients' ability to articulate their wishes. The authors conclude that there are no existing standards for bedside rationing and insist that explicit rationing strategies should be developed.

White, Douglas B., Mitchell H. Katz, John M. Luce, and Bernard Lo. 2009. "Who Should Receive Life Support during a Public Health Emergency? Using Ethical Principles to Improve Allocation Decisions." *Annals of Internal Medicine* 150, no. 2 (January 20): 132–38. doi:10.7326/0003-4819-150-2-200901200-00011.

> Surveys and critiques existing allocation strategies, claiming that they are overly concerned with the utilitarian goal of maximizing the number of people who survive to hospital discharge. The authors reject appeals to social value and instrumental value; first-come, first-served; sickest first; and QALYs and DALYs (which, they claim, could not realistically be calculated during a public health crisis). They instead adopt a pluralistic approach: saving the most lives, saving the most life years, and giving individuals equal opportunity to live through life's stages (youngest first).

# CHAPTER 11
# Racial Disparities in Healthcare

**Key topics in this chapter:**

- How racialized hierarchies affect respect for autonomy and beneficence
- Racial disparities in health outcomes and their causes
- The history of racialized medical experimentation in the U.S. and its contemporary legacy
- Racial prejudice in public health campaigns
- How the history of medical racism impacts contemporary clinical interactions
- Weathering as a social determinant of health

## Introduction

Cornel West describes racism as the battleground where what it means to be human and who counts as human are contested (2002, 90). If, fundamentally, medicine as a practice attempts to reduce human suffering, then it should not be surprising that those who have been excluded from full personhood—in the United States, particularly Indigenous people and people of African ancestry—have also been excluded from the moral attention that motivates medical prevention and treatment. The first American study of racial health disparities was W. E. B. Du Bois's *The Philadelphia Negro* (1899), which examines the lives of people in Philadelphia's Seventh Ward. As part of a systematic sociological analysis, Du Bois documents the contagious diseases and other threats to the health of Black people who lived in this community and emphasizes the economic and environmental conditions that allowed them to proliferate. He attributes these disparities to a basic neglect of Black people's welfare: "The most difficult social problem in the matter of Negro health is the peculiar attitude of the nation toward the well-being of the race. There have . . . been few other cases in the history of civilized peoples where human suffering has been viewed with such peculiar indifference" (Du Bois 1899, 116). In 1903, Du Bois would come to experience that indifference sharply when, in segregated Atlanta, his two-year-old son Burghardt fell ill from diphtheria and died ten days later due to lack of access to adequate medical services—a common problem for Black Americans (Du Bois 1903, ch. 11). In reviewing statistics of medical disparities, we need to remember that differential treatment impacts particular people and the families and communities around them.

As a social practice, medicine reflects and reinforces the norms of its surrounding culture. For much of the last several centuries, people of color have been vulnerable to explicit and systemic medical racism: excluded from medical training, targeted for unsafe and unnecessary medical experimentation, subject to intensified medical surveillance, and denied access to quality healthcare. In more recent decades, since the end of legalized discrimination, medical racism has continued in more covert but still significant forms, often as the result of physician-patient relationships diminished by mistrust or implicit bias. In these ways, contemporary inequalities in medical care reveal the long legacy of racial oppression and discrimination.

## Health Outcomes

Racial disparities in health outcomes are longstanding and well-documented. The single most glaring disparity is in overall life expectancy. In 1900, Black Americans had a life expectancy of thirty-three years, while whites lived on average for forty-eight years. The racial longevity gap decreased through the course of the twentieth century as Black Americans made economic gains and secured greater access to healthcare ("Over the Past Century" 2021). As of 2019, overall life expectancy was 85.6 years for Asian Americans, 81.9 years for Latino/as, 78.8 years for non-Hispanic whites, 74.8 years for Black Americans, and 71.8 years for American Indians/Alaskan Natives (Arias and Xu 2022, 3). During the COVID-19 pandemic, however, Black and brown people were disproportionately impacted. In the United States, age-adjusted death rates from COVID-19 were 605 people per 100,000 for Indigenous people, 507 for Latino/as, 486 for Black Americans, 308 for non-Hispanic whites, and 223 for Asian Americans (Gawthrop 2023). Between 2019 and 2021, non-Hispanic whites had on average lost 2.4 years of longevity, dropping to 76.7, but Black Americans had lost 4 years, dropping to 71.2 (Hill, Ndugga, and Artiga 2024). Apart from broader issues such as access to adequate healthcare, one specific cause of this disparity was that pulse oximeters overestimated the oxygen saturation levels of people of color, because they are less accurate in people with dark skin pigmentation, thus delaying their eligibility for COVID-19 therapies (Fawzy et al. 2022). This kind of error is emblematic of how white bodies have been prioritized in medical research.

A range of health disparities contribute to differential longevity. Infant mortality rates as of 2022 were 4.5 per 1,000 live births for non-Hispanic whites, 4.9 for Hispanics, 9.1 for Native Americans, and 10.9 for Black Americans (Centers for Disease Control and Prevention 2024). The overall maternal mortality rate in 2021 was 32.9 deaths per 100,000 live births (an increase from 17.4 in 2018), but the rate for non-Hispanic whites was 26.6, 28.0 for Latino/as, and 69.9 for Black Americans (Hoyert 2023).

Black Americans are significantly more likely to die of preventable heart disease (Ferdinand et al. 2017); have higher mortality rates for the most common kinds of cancer (Tong, Hill, and Artiga 2024); are more likely to suffer from asthma, along with Native Americans (American Lung Association 2024); are more likely to suffer from diabetes, along with Latino/as (Rodríguez and Campbell 2017); and have a mortality rate from HIV/AIDS seven times higher than whites (Centers for Disease Control and Prevention 2022). With regard to mental health, Black Americans are 2.4 times more likely to be diagnosed with schizophrenia than whites are, and they are much more likely to be diagnosed with other forms of psychosis (Cohen and Marino 2013; see also Faber et al. 2023). These persistent disparities may be caused by misdiagnosis stemming from implicit bias (people of color are more likely to be interpreted as aggressive by healthcare professionals and police officers), the psychological effects of enduring racism, difficulty accessing mental health services, or some combination of these.

Lack of consistent access to quality healthcare is a major driver of all these disparate outcomes. Black Americans enrolled in managed care organizations are significantly more likely to be denied insurance authorization for emergency department visits than white patients (Lowe et al. 2001). They are less likely to receive screenings or other forms of preventive medicine (Matthew 2015, 57–58). They are less likely to be offered kidney transplants or coronary bypass operations, and they are more likely to be diagnosed at later stages of cancer (58–60). They are on average discharged earlier from hospital stays, adjusted for the diagnoses and treatments they receive. Black Americans with diabetes are more likely to have a limb amputated, and Black Americans with prostate cancer are more likely to have both testicles amputated (Gornick et al. 1996). There are also racial disparities in post-surgical cancer care. Black women are less likely to receive rehabilitation support services following mastectomy (Diehr et al. 1989), and Black colorectal cancer patients are less likely to receive post-treatment surveillance care (Lafata et al. 2001). A study of heart patients "found Black and Latino patients were more likely to be admitted to general care, while white patients were admitted to cardiology service. After 30 days, the minority patients were more likely to be readmitted, a proxy for quality of care" (Blanding 2022). Overall, children from minoritized racial and ethnic groups receive worse healthcare than white children, from preventive care to diagnostic tests to surgical outcomes (Slopen et al. 2024). This is only a sample of racial disparities in medical treatment.

It may be intuitive to attribute these differences to socioeconomic class or to individual choices as a way of avoiding how the legacy of racism persists in contemporary medicine. However, Dayna Bowen Matthew argues against this reduction:

> Although it is popular to blame the poor for their poor health by pointing to risky health behaviors, careful studies of nationally representative populations conclude that the significantly higher prevalence of cigarette smoking, alcohol consumption, obesity, and physical inactivity are only one aspect of the relationship between lower socioeconomic status and poor health. Moreover, behavioral disparities must not be taken out of their societal context where unequal exposure to the stress of discrimination, inequitable access to healthy food and built environments, and inferior access to resources generally are integrally associated with many racial and ethnic differences in health behavior. (2015, 1)

Even when controlling for insurance status and socioeconomic class, racial disparities persist. A study of two million California births found that, for families in the highest income bracket, Black mothers and their babies are twice as likely to die as white mothers and their babies (Kennedy-Moulton et al. 2023). Although significant racial disparities exist between whites and most people of color, the division between Black and white Americans remains the widest (Villarosa 2022b, 62).

## Medical Experimentation

To begin with an issue at the center of medical research, prevention, and treatment, responding to pain has been racialized historically and continues to impact medical practice in the present. In the eighteenth and nineteenth centuries, anthropologists, geneticists, and newly professionalized medical doctors attempted to justify the claim that people of color were less sensitive to pain with pseudoscientific evidence. Scientific racism was used to legitimize existing socially imposed hierarchies as biological, immutable facts by treating race as a heritable marker of identity that determined a wide range of personal characteristics, including sensitivity to pain, intelligence, and physical stamina (Hutchinson 2013). This narrative had practical implications for how people of color interacted with medical professionals, both researchers and clinicians. In the United States, people of African ancestry were particularly targeted by these claims about decreased sensitivity to pain—not surprisingly, given the nation's economic dependence on enslaved and then oppressed labor, and the forms of physical violence necessary to maintain those economic institutions.

Prior to the codification of medical ethics and governmental regulation in the twentieth century, medical experimentation was often performed on enslaved people (Washington 2006, 52–74). The paradox at the heart of these experiments is that slaves were recognized as human beings biologically, because the intended beneficiaries of these experiments were whites, but they were excluded from the normative status of persons. The same paradox plagues the notorious medical experiments in Nazi Germany on concentration camp prisoners, which in theory were intended to benefit those who understood themselves to be part of the master race, superior to (according to eugenicist claims) and yet similar enough to those whose bodies were being used to gain such medical knowledge.

In a largely agrarian society, healthy childbirth was economically profitable, so in the eighteenth- and nineteenth-century United States, gynecology and obstetrics became two of the medical specializations in which enslaved women were pervasively used as experimental subjects. In the

1840s, the so-called "father of gynecology," J. Marion Sims, developed a treatment for vesico-vaginal fistulas (a tear between the bladder and the vagina) by experimenting, without anesthesia, on enslaved women. From his records, we know three of their first names: Anarcha, Lucy, and Betsey. As a teenager, Anarcha underwent more than thirty surgeries in five years (Washington 2006, 63–66). In his memoirs, Sims describes one of his experimental surgeries: "Lucy's agony was extreme. She was much prostrated, and I thought that she was going to die. . . . After she had recovered entirely from the effects of this unfortunate experiment, I put her on a table, to examine" (quoted in Domonoske 2018). The awareness of Lucy's pain and medical exigency did not generate enough of Sims's moral attention to protect her from the infliction of further pain, much less the infringement on her autonomy to decide whether to be examined. The enslaved women involved in Sims's experiments were also made to serve as nurses in between their own surgeries and work as field hands. Sims then used the treatments that resulted from these experiments on wealthy white women in the United States and Europe, with anesthesia—although, to be fair, Sims initially did not think anesthesia would be necessary for any women.

Some of these experiments on enslaved women were called into question because they were done on Black women. A doctor in the early 1800s criticized experiments on removing ovarian tumors: "All of the women operated upon . . . were negresses, and they will bear cutting with nearly, if not quite, as much impunity as dogs and rabbits" (Owens 2017, 31). Wealthy white women, by contrast, were thought to be extremely fragile and sensitive to pain. That is, enslaved women were seen as sharing the pain tolerance of nonhuman animals that were typically and uncontroversially used in research, and this presumed biological difference from white women (the primary intended beneficiaries) invalidated the experiments' usefulness.

The juxtaposition of recognizing enslaved women as biologically human and rejecting their moral considerability placed these women and other racially marginalized experimental subjects in the category of what Charles Mills calls **subpersons**:

> The peculiar status of a subperson is that it is an entity which, because of phenotype, seems (from, of course, the perspective of the categorizer) human in some respects but not in others. It is a human (or, if this word already seems normatively loaded, a humanoid) who, though adult, is

not fully a person. And the tensions and internal contradictions in this concept capture the tensions and internal contradictions of the black experience in a white-supremacist society. (1998, 6–7)

The key characteristic of subpersons is their social exclusion from the moral community. If the pain of others typically provokes moral attention, then the moral significance of the pain of subpersons must be contained and diminished—a social imperative reflected in the beliefs that Black people were less sensitive to pain or were prone to exaggerating their pain for self-interested purposes.

The most infamous of all U.S. medical experiments is the Tuskegee syphilis study, conducted by the United States Public Health Service from 1932 to 1972 in Tuskegee, Alabama, into which six hundred low-income Black men were recruited. Of those six hundred men, 399 were identified as being already infected with advanced syphilis. In the American cultural imaginary, treating syphilis was quite different from treating heart disease or cancer: notions of sin and shame surrounded sexually transmitted infections, and Black men were typically animalized as beings incapable of controlling themselves. James Jones emphasizes this dehumanization: study administrators referred to Tuskegee as a "'sick farm' where diseased and dying men could be maintained without further treatment and herded together for inspection at the yearly roundups. The health officer who conducted the 1970 roundup even spoke of 'corraling' the men for study" (1981, 187).

The study observed the course of the (mostly) untreated disease in these men, even after penicillin was discovered to be an effective cure. Just as this medical innovation had no impact on the continuing project, the moral principles set out by the Nuremberg Code were also taken not to apply. The design and implementation of the research did not recognize the research subjects' autonomy by securing their informed consent and did not protect their well-being. The men were told that they were being treated for "bad blood" when, in fact, they were simply being observed (with regular blood tests and physical examinations) and given pink aspirin pills as a semblance of treatment. During World War II, some of them were tested by the military and received letters offering treatment; the Public Health Service got the men deferred from the draft instead. Rather than researchers attempting to protect the test subjects from injury or death, they were expected eventually to succumb to the disease. Because it was built into the study design itself, the research was literally a "forty-year death watch," as a headline later described it ("Forty Year Death Watch" 1972).

The Tuskegee study participants had the social status of "death-bound-subjects," people whose lives seem so worthless or so inherently associated with violence that their deaths are treated as natural features of reality rather than attracting any moral attention (JanMohamed 2005). Treating subjects as death-bound normalizes moral inattention, including by medical professionals, and the reduction of human persons to subpersons to be used in research without concern for their well-being or consent. It also frames that category as natural and immutable rather than the product of social forces and individual decisions, which are open to moral critique and institutional reform.

The U.S. Public Health Service published many journal articles about the Tuskegee study without controversy. It was not until 1972, when a young public health service physician laid out the whole history of the study for a journalist, that it was called to the public's attention. After a wave of scandals involving medical research on vulnerable or marginalized populations (principally the Willowbrook hepatitis study and the Jewish Chronic Disease Hospital cancer study), the Belmont Report established legally enforceable principles of human experimentation and mechanisms to regulate medical research.

It is worth mentioning that the live cancer cells injected into elderly patients at the Jewish Chronic Disease Hospital—some of whom were Shoah survivors, spoke little or no English, and were cognitively incompetent—were cultured from the line of cancer cells taken from Henrietta Lacks, a Black woman in Baltimore who went to the segregated wards of Johns Hopkins University Hospital for treatment of her cervical cancer, from which she quickly died. Her cancer cells were kept and used for research without her informed consent. In the last sixty years, approximately twenty tons of those cells—called the HeLa cell line—have been replicated for research into the polio vaccine, cancer, HIV, Parkinson's, and gene mapping (Skloot 2011).

Finally, racialized mass incarceration intersects with medical experimentation in prisons. Many researchers have conducted studies on prisoners—most notoriously, at Holmesburg Prison, where between 1951 and 1974, a dermatologist working at the University of Pennsylvania conducted a series of experiments on what he characterized as "acres of skin" (Hornblum 1998). Without informed consent, prisoners were exposed to a variety of pathogens (including radioactive and chemical warfare agents) and then subjected to dermatological testing. We discuss these cases in more detail in Chapter 14 (on human experimentation).

As these experiments show, medical researchers have historically treated people of color as subpersons. In this sense, medicine has reflected broader cultural judgments, including racial prejudices. At the same time, racist practices have frequently been justified using medical metaphors. For instance, intersections between racism and xenophobia contribute to continuing representations of people of color as "pathogenic," sources of disease within an otherwise healthy (white) population that therefore need to be excluded or controlled (Holt, Kjærvik, and Bushman 2022). In fact, medical authorities have actively collaborated in efforts to present racial prejudice as empirical fact. To the extent that medical researchers repeat and reinforce popular prejudices about racial hierarchies, they use the authority of science to cover over the social origins of such prejudices, including the construction of the modern conception of race itself.

Medicine is immersed in social conditions that shape which problems attract attention, how those problems are resolved, who has access to those solutions, and whose voices are treated as authoritative. The people who practice medicine, both researchers and clinicians, do so having grown up in a culture that has given them a moral education, which has trained them what to be sensitive to and what not to be sensitive to: "The experimental abuse of African Americans was not a cultural anomaly; it simply mirrored in the medical arena the economic, social, and health abuses that the larger society perpetrated against people of color, especially in slaveholding states" (Washington 2006, 56). Racialized medical experimentation has the overt purpose of acquiring medical knowledge and skills; however, it also reinforces white researchers' lack of moral accountability for failing to respect the autonomy and promote the well-being of people of color.

Outside of medical research itself, there were quasi-scientific projects such as zoos and lectures that expressed and contributed to scientific racism. The case of Ota Benga is particularly extreme. He was kidnapped in 1903 in what is now the Democratic Republic of the Congo and displayed for three years at the Bronx Zoo in the same cage as a gorilla and an orangutan, with a placard describing his height and weight and that he had "been brought from the Kasai River . . . by Dr. Samuel P. Verner" (Washington 2006, 76–77). He was regularly referred to as a "specimen" in newspapers and public lectures (77–78). He was displayed as part of a larger racist argument that Africans were closer, evolutionarily, to nonhuman apes than whites were—a straightforwardly dehumanizing description that various doctors and anthropologists tried to justify empirically. The Black ministers who protested his captivity and display as a zoo animal were accused of being anti-scientific, of denying basic facts of reality. Their protest primarily made a moral claim, but that dimension of the protest was dismissed by white scientists and physicians who claimed that Benga was a specimen that should be studied to understand evolution, as part of the triumphant progress of science.

By contrast, whites were protected as full persons in several ways. As people not enslaved, they could physically leave hospitals and other experimental contexts. As citizens, they could sue doctors, hospitals, and medical journals. And public opinion worked against the exhibition of whites (at least whites without disabilities) for medical purposes. Harriet Washington notes that there was a strong cultural prohibition against displaying white people's organs, which, apart from skin, are identical to the organs of people of color (2006, 110). When white patients' cases were published, their names and faces were not included as a way of respecting their privacy.

The juxtaposition between the experiences of white and Black research subjects contributed to different levels of trust in mainstream medicine. By the beginning of the twentieth century, many Black Americans experienced hospitals not as places of healing but as places where they were often treated as "clinical material," if they were treated at all (Washington 2006, 113). They were subject to being displayed to medical students and endured unnecessary and unanesthetized surgery for the purpose of medical education. After death, their bodies were also disproportionately stolen from cemeteries for autopsies at medical schools (119–22). That is, not only in life but in death, people of African ancestry were treated as morally inconsiderable: objects of medical or public curiosity rather than people deserving respect and care, embedded in families whose grief should be treated as socially significant.

Jones argues that, in the late twentieth century, allegations that HIV was an artificial virus deliberately spread in Black communities gained credence due to the history of Tuskegee and other medical experiments

(1981, 732–33; see also Gamble 1997). That distrust of medical authority impacts not only public health campaigns but also relationships with individual healthcare professionals. Compounded with contemporary forms of medical racism—such as limited access to quality healthcare, pharmacy deserts, and implicit biases of clinicians—this historical legacy continues to produce disparate health outcomes (Halbert et al. 2006).

## Public Health Campaigns

The history of public health campaigns similarly reflects the division between persons and subpersons, with immigrants and people of color treated as bearers of disease that threaten white populations. These prejudices are often entangled with colonialist ideas about people of color lacking rationality or being less civilized than whites and with racist stereotypes around sexuality and purity. Anxieties about the bubonic plague in 1900 led the San Francisco Board of Health to require all Chinese residents to be vaccinated or quarantined, although the resolution was later found to be unconstitutional (Matthew 2015, 18). In 1916, the "unclean habits" of Mexican railroad workers were blamed for a typhus outbreak near Los Angeles, so they were subjected to invasive health inspections, including the use of cyanide gas to kill lice (Molina 2011). The conditions under which these workers were forced to live, as an incubator of disease, were ignored. Public health measures were thus used as racialized and nativist methods of social control, normalized through scientific authority.

At an abstract level, racial hierarchies deployed the conceptual frameworks of pathology to describe racial differences so that diversity would be interpreted as deviance that needed to be managed. Eugenicist theories of the late nineteenth and early twentieth centuries gave rise to state laws allowing for **forced sterilization** (primarily of women) in the name of protecting the overall health of the nation. Sterilization laws were first directed at women who were thought to have cognitive disabilities or who flouted feminine norms, as in the *Buck v. Bell* (274 U.S. 200 [1924]) case, where the U.S. Supreme Court ruled that the state interest in protecting public health justified involuntary sterilization based on mental capacity. That precedent was then used against Indigenous women, Latinas, and Black women, especially in California, Puerto Rico, and southern states. Between the 1930s and the 1970s, almost two-fifths of Puerto Rican women of childbearing age were sterilized, and in the 1970s alone, almost a third of Indigenous American women were sterilized (Lawrence 2000, 400; Villarosa 2022b, 38). Not only were women and girls (or their families) not asked for consent, but they were often not even informed that the procedure had been done. More recently, women incarcerated in California prisons (between 2006 and 2010) and women incarcerated in an immigration detention facility in Georgia (revealed in 2020)—most of them Black and/or Latina—were forced to undergo tubal ligations (Villarosa 2022b, 41–42). Such public health campaigns highlight how medicine has been weaponized against communities of color, further eroding trust in healthcare professionals. Rather than supporting the individual, medicine has been used in racialized ways to subordinate their goals and welfare to the supposed good of the whole society.

## Clinician-Patient Relationships

In the U.S., human experimentation is now strictly regulated by federal law, which has attempted to address racial discrimination. However, diminishing the autonomy and well-being of people of color, particularly Black Americans, persists into the present. The most egregious contemporary issues arise in patient care, where bias is harder to identify and regulate, even if its impact is striking in terms of longevity, maternal and infant mortality, and quality of life (Wenneker and Epstein 1989; Lantz et al. 1998). Until recently, patients have typically been seen as individuals with certain characteristics, risk factors, and medical histories, without regard for the social determinants of health: the wide-scale socioeconomic patterns that affect a person's health, such as income and income distribution, social status, employment and working conditions, education, and housing. Rather than tracing differential health outcomes to social forces, for which the culture as a whole is responsible and which arise out of the history of racism, these disparities have been attributed to either individual decisions or innate differences.

Patients impacted by poverty, discrimination, and other forms of oppression have often been treated by clinicians as if their health conditions were the result of bad choices, thereby creating an atmosphere of blame rather than cooperation (Bervell 2023). Patients may be held responsible by clinicians for their levels of stress, for example, without taking into account how forces outside of their control contribute to the stress they experience in ways that strategies of self-care cannot mitigate. The individualistic paradigm fosters an environment that inhibits communication and trust between physician and patient. Language barriers, classism, and cultural incompetence may exacerbate those issues. In 1985, a U.S. Department of Health and Human Services report (known as the Heckler Report) documented racial health disparities, including almost 59,000 "excess deaths" among Black Americans annually, but attributed those disparities to behavioral decisions that could be improved through further public health education (Heckler 1985, 5; Villarosa 2022b, 4–5).

Unequal treatment also results from false assumptions about innate biological differences. Despite decades of consensus that race is not a useful biological category, the essentialist stereotype that Black people are less sensitive to pain, for example, persists even among contemporary medical professionals. In a 2016 study, 40 percent of first- and second-year medical students agreed with the statement that "Blacks' skin is thicker than whites'"; agreement decreased to 25 percent among medical residents (doctors in post-graduate training). Laypersons endorsed that claim at a rate of 58 percent (Hoffman et al. 2016; see also Trawalter, Hoffman, and Waytz 2012). In general, whites tend to rate the observed pain of Black people with "more stringent thresholds" (that is, taking the pain to be less serious) than the observed pain of whites, and thus—in a hypothetical scenario—recommend lower doses of analgesics (Mende-Siedlecki et al. 2019).

In actual clinical practice, Black patients are prescribed fewer painkillers than white patients. Vickie Shavers, Alexis Bakos, and Vanessa Sheppard summarize the consistent results of many empirical studies:

> Racial/ethnic minority patients are less likely than White patients to receive any pain medication, more likely to receive lower doses of pain medications, more likely to have longer wait times to receipt of pain medication in the emergency department, and less likely to receive opiates as treatment for pain despite higher pain scores, and to be treated in [a] manner consistent with the World Health Organization recommendations. They also are treated in pain clinics, under hospice care, and have pain needs adequately met while in hospice care less frequently than Whites. (2010, 179)

As a specific example, sickle cell anemia predominantly affects people of African ancestry, and it causes acute and chronic pain. But sickle cell patients are often confronted with the stigma that they are illegitimately seeking pain medication (Bulgin, Tanabe, and Jenerette 2018). A literature review by Peter Mende-Siedlecki et al. concludes that "the pain of Black patients is systematically underdiagnosed and undertreated" (2019, 864), and a review by Carmen Green et al. (2003) finds that Black patients experience lower rates of pain assessment and higher rates of undertreatment in all clinical settings and across all types of pain. The hierarchy of personhood and subpersonhood casts a long shadow in this most basic function of medical care: to reduce patients' suffering.

Racial biases may be difficult to identify and address internally by clinicians because prejudices shape how we perceive the world rather than calling critical attention to themselves. General attitudes in the culture reinforce the racial expectations of individual practitioners. Black patients are 2.54 times more likely than white patients to have negative descriptors entered into their electronic health records, which transmits stigmatizing language to multiple clinicians (Sun et al. 2022). As medical students progress through their education, they become less likely to recognize how biases operate concretely in clinician-patient interactions:

> Medical students and physicians may become less willing to ascribe the disparities reported in current medical research to unfair treatment practiced by their peers and the health care system within which they work. Acculturation into the medical profession may make students and physicians less accepting of the possibility that physicians harbor prejudice and bias and less open to acknowledging explanations for these disparities that imply discriminatory practices. (Wilson et al. 2004, 718)

In other words, the generalized acknowledgment of racial prejudice in the wider society does not entail that it is recognized in one's own behavior or that of one's colleagues, or that its impact on patients is understood. Even if such biases are not apparent to clinicians, they impact the experiences of patients, including through behavioral or verbal microaggressions (Freeman and Stewart 2024). In a 2017 study, 32 percent of Black Americans reported personally experiencing discrimination from a doctor or other healthcare professional, and 22 percent have refrained from medical care as a way to avoid discrimination (*Discrimination in America* 2017, 6, 12; see also Artiga et al. 2023). The perception of discrimination and its real effects is called "stereotype threat," and it can

> impair patient adherence [following treatment decisions and instructions]; impair patient communication skills (including fluency and ability to respond to questions); lead patients to discount feedback from providers, avoid and disengage from the health care system (including delaying or missing appointments), and disidentify with health promotion behaviors; and reinforce stereotypes held by providers, if the minority patient behaves in the way that was stereotyped. (Burgess et al. 2010, 169)

Patients' mistrust of medical authority thus contributes to poorer health outcomes and perpetuates racialized biases, such as the idea that people of color are less likely to comply with medical advice, that shape clinicians' future interactions.

The disparate treatment of people of color by doctors is one of the legacies of structural racism in the medical profession. The Flexner Report, titled *Medical Education in the United States and Canada* (1910), established stricter guidelines for medical education—increasing the prerequisites for medical training, partnering with hospitals for clinical instruction, and introducing a more stringent state licensure process. It also led to the reduction of medical schools until only two Black medical schools remained. Since Black students were not admitted to white medical schools until decades later—and they were also excluded from both local medical societies and the American Medical Association—this had a tremendous impact on racial diversity in the profession that continues to reverberate (Baker et al. 2008; Sullivan and Suez Mittman 2010). As of 2023, 5.2 percent of physicians in the U.S. are Black, 6.5 percent are Latino/a, and 0.3 percent are Native American (Association of American Medical Colleges, n.d.).

This lack of representation in the medical profession impacts how clinicians and patients interact. Black patients treated by Black clinicians receive more attentive care: those patients do more of the talking, on average, than those who meet with white clinicians; there is more shared decision-making; and practitioners take more detailed clinical notes. These differences significantly affect medical outcomes: patients are more likely to take medicines as prescribed, understand the risks of various behaviors, and consent to services such as vaccinations (Huerto and Lindo 2020). A study at Stanford University suggests that matching Black patients with Black doctors could close as much as 19 percent of the racial mortality gap related to heart disease (Alsan, Garrick, and Graziani 2019). In 2020, researchers found that Black infants are more likely to survive if they are treated by Black doctors; when treated by white doctors, they are three times more likely to die than white infants (Greenwood et al. 2020). A recent study of county-level health data concluded that every 10 percent increase in the representation of Black primary care physicians was associated, on average, with 30.6 days of greater life expectancy for Black people in that county (Snyder et al. 2023).

**Epistemic injustice** is the illegitimate refusal to see a person as a knower: dismissing their claims about what is true, misrepresenting their positions, or simply ignoring them. When someone is repeatedly silenced in this way, they can come to see themselves as lacking epistemic authority (Fricker 2007). Patients not being listened to carefully and responsively about their own health undermines the clinician-patient relationship. One possible explanation for the fact that Black women have three times the number of maternal deaths as white women is that their symptoms of preeclampsia or other life-threatening conditions are not taken as seriously when they are reported to clinicians—again, an indication of how granular dynamics of trust and communication impact health outcomes. Black women are more susceptible to uterine fibroids, and the pain and infertility that fibroids can cause are frequently ignored or undertreated by physicians (Eltoukhi et al. 2014). As Matthew notes, "Physicians' assumptions about the experience of black women as a group—their threshold for pain, their goals for family planning, or even the ordinariness of the problem they suffer—can prevent them from treating a specific black woman as a distinct individual" (2015, 100). Those patterns of differences in listening and responding may also explain the differences in treatment discussed earlier, in which people of color (especially Black people) receive more conservative, less effective, and generally inferior medical interventions.

For all these reasons, who is recruited into medical/nursing schools and the curricula they encounter both matter. Does the population of healthcare practitioners in a given community reflect the patient population in terms of race, ethnicity, and language? Have they been taught to reflect critically on their own implicit biases and to resist the practical effects of those biases? Have they learned to attend to the social determinants of health?

## Weathering

Beyond immediate medical impacts, experiencing persistent racism itself takes a physical toll on people's health, a phenomenon that has been called **weathering**. Arline Geronimus (1992, 2023b) coined the term to describe how the stress of living under conditions of racial discrimination accelerates the aging process by causing disruptions of immune, endocrine, and cardiovascular functions. She describes weathering in terms of one's level of social acceptance and support:

> Where you don't share the same assumptions or background, where the people you're working with don't appreciate all you've been through, where you're having to always be on your guard and manage how you portray yourself or present yourself to try and not fulfill stereotypes that you think people you're working with or going to school with might have about you. And that means you're at a certain level of vigilance and looking for cues everywhere of whether you belong, whether you're welcome, whether you're going to be subject to what many people call microaggressions. . . . Those experiences themselves can cause weathering. (Geronimus 2023a)

Racism causes increased levels of stress for people of color, who directly experience discrimination, harassment, or violence; indirectly observe or hear about such incidents; or feel anxious about future incidents. Experiencing elevated stress on a regular basis can lead to a wide range of conditions: "Chronically elevated blood pressure can damage arteries and veins, which can lead to hypertension, for example. A constant stream of cortisol—known as the stress hormone—can create insulin resistance, leading to diabetes. Research has suggested that chronic stress can damage DNA and even alter brain structure" (Gupta 2023). One factor in racially disparate maternal mortality rates may be that Black Americans live with chronic inflammation, the effects of which are exacerbated during pregnancy. Black women across socioeconomic groups who reported experiencing racial discrimination were twice as likely to have low-birthweight babies—under three pounds at birth (Collins et al. 2004). Chronic stress may be caused by a whole series of related issues, such as poverty, discrimination, and living with violence; however, weathering seems to affect people of color across socioeconomic classes, which explains why even high-income Black mothers are at an increased risk of mortality.

The concept of weathering resists explanations of health disparities in terms of individually chosen behaviors and lifestyles, poverty, and genetics, all of which would exonerate the culture as a whole from the socially contingent but powerful effects of racism. First, rather than attributing disparate healthcare outcomes to individual choices, the concept of weathering recognizes that racism itself is a public health issue—and that encouraging people of color to exercise more, eat nutritious foods, decrease tobacco or alcohol use, or practice emotional self-care to reduce stress are inadequate methods to address the broader interplay of economic, social, psychological, and medical issues that living in a racist society generates. Second, the patterns of accelerated aging and increased susceptibility to disease emerge independently of socioeconomic class. Linda Villarosa (2022a) recounts the work of Harold Freeman, who found that Black men in Harlem had shorter lives and lower quality of life than men in Bangladesh, thereby demonstrating that the problem was not poverty. And finally, health disparities result from social interactions and institutions in addition to inherited risk factors.

Given the contingent causes of weathering, Geronimus emphasizes a shared cultural responsibility for reducing the stress levels of people of color. In the case of maternal health, one response could be to provide doulas and midwives to coach pregnant people of color through the process and to listen for warning signs of preeclampsia and diabetes (Geronimus 2023a). By recognizing the medical impact of racism, clinicians will build trust with patients, and their interactions will be less likely to contribute further to weathering.

## Conclusion: Addressing Medical Racism

Studying this history should not leave us paralyzed by despair, but we should also not assume that we have progressed beyond it. That would be the moral equivalent of American doctors who ignored the Nuremberg Code by distancing themselves from the practices of Nazi-affiliated physicians, and then replicated some of those practices in post-war medical experimentation. As this chapter makes clear, racial disparities in healthcare stem from a variety of sources: institutional policies and practices, structural inequities in the wider society, interpersonal dynamics, and internalized prejudice, which manifests itself in stereotyping and other expectations that shape the behavior of those who are racially privileged and those who are not (Bervell 2023). We are grappling then with a systemic and complex issue that is not isolated to healthcare but is expressed significantly within it.

Many recent concrete proposals to address medical racism focus on medical education—both within medical schools and in ongoing professional development. In recent years, there has been more emphasis on ethics and anti-racism training for healthcare professionals, including educating people to recognize implicit bias. Another major strategy is to recruit a more diverse set of clinicians, with the idea that people of color are more likely to trust and receive quality healthcare from people with whom they identify. Since currently so few clinicians are people of color, this is a significant obstacle to reducing minoritized patients' disproportionately negative health outcomes. Some proposals focus more on clinical practice by educating patients to advocate for themselves, providing translation services, and adding "nudges" into electronic health records that alert clinicians to increased risks related to weathering (McFarling 2022). These reminders call attention to the health disparities that people of color objectively experience without attributing bias to individual physicians.

To ensure that minorities are represented adequately in medical studies and receive preventive care, many researchers and public health officials have recruited community leaders to encourage people of color to participate in medical research and preventive clinics. Those leaders often address the history of medical racism and the distrust that it has sown in communities of color. A similar strategy involves training community health workers, a practice developed in China and several Latin American and African countries. These people function as medical advocates, peer health educators, and community outreach workers in their own neighborhoods, often sharing ties of language, religion, and ethnic background with those who might otherwise be isolated from formal healthcare institutions.

These various solutions may work best in concert by wrestling with medical racism at the level of institutions, practitioners, patients, and communities. Both the subjective force of trust in medical professionals and more objective factors, such as access to quality healthcare, are generational influences on health outcomes. Overcoming the history of medical racism will therefore require persistent, manifold efforts to treat each patient and research subject, regardless of race, as a person in the full moral sense of that term.

# REFERENCES

Alsan, Marcella, Owen Garrick, and Grant Graziani. 2019. "Does Diversity Matter for Health? Experimental Evidence from Oakland." *American Economic Review* 109, no. 12 (December): 4071–111. doi:10.1257/aer.20181446.

American Lung Association. 2024. "Current Asthma Demographics." Last modified June 13, 2024. https://www.lung.org/research/trends-in-lung-disease/asthma-trends-brief/current-demographics.

Arias, Elizabeth, and Jiaquan Xu. 2022. "United States Life Tables, 2019." *National Vital Statistics Reports* 70, no. 19 (March 22): 1–59. https://www.cdc.gov/nchs/data/nvsr/nvsr70/nvsr70-19.pdf.

Artiga, Samantha, Liz Hamel, Ana Gonzalez-Barrera, Alex Montero, Latoya Hill, Marley Presiado, Ashley Kirzinger, and Lunna Lopes. 2023. "Survey on Racism, Discrimination and Health: Experiences and Impacts across Racial and Ethnic Groups." Kaiser Family Foundation. December 5. https://www.kff.org/racial-equity-and-health-policy/poll-finding/survey-on-racism-discrimination-and-health/.

Association of American Medical Colleges. n.d. "U.S. Physician Workforce Data Dashboard." Accessed January 15, 2025. https://www.aamc.org/data-reports/report/us-physician-workforce-data-dashboard.

Baker, Robert B., Harriet A. Washington, Ololade Olakanmi, Todd L. Savitt, Elizabeth A. Jacobs, Eddie Hoover, and Matthew K. Wynia. 2008. "African American Physicians and Organized Medicine, 1846–1968: Origins of a Racial Divide." *JAMA: Journal of the American Medical Association* 300, no. 3 (July 16): 306–13. doi:10.1001/jama.300.3.306.

Bervell, Joel. 2023. "Increasing Understanding by Listening to Overlooked Stories." Presentation at Annual Meeting of the Washington State Hospital Association, Renton, WA, October 23.

Blanding, Michael. 2022. "Revisiting the 'Unequal Treatment' Report, 20 Years Later." *Harvard Public Health*. October 3.

Bulgin, Dominique, Paula Tanabe, and Coretta Jenerette. 2018. "Stigma of Sickle Cell Disease: A Systematic Review." *Issues in Mental Health Nursing* 39, no. 8 (August): 675–86. doi:10.1080/01612840.2018.1443530.

Burgess, Diana J., Jennifer Warren, Sean Phelan, John Dovidio, and Michelle van Ryn. 2010. "Stereotype Threat and Health Disparities: What Medical Educators and Future Physicians Need to Know." In "Health Disparities Education," edited by Monica L. Lypson, Jada Bussey-Jones, Susan Glick, Arleen F. Brown, and Elizabeth A. Jacobs. Supplement, *Journal of General Internal Medicine* 25, no. S2 (May): 169–77. doi:10.1007/s11606-009-1221-4.

Centers for Disease Control and Prevention. 2022. *HIV Surveillance Report*. Vol. 23, *Diagnoses of HIV Infection in the United States and Dependent Areas, 2020*. May. https://stacks.cdc.gov/view/cdc/121127.

———. 2024. "Infant Mortality." Last modified September 16, 2024. https://www.cdc.gov/maternal-infant-health/infant-mortality/index.html.

Cohen, Carl I., and Leslie Marino. 2013. "Racial and Ethnic Differences in the Prevalence of Psychotic Symptoms in the General Population." *Psychiatric Services* 64, no. 11 (November): 1103–9. doi:10.1176/appi.ps.201200348.

Collins, James W. Jr., Richard J. David, Arden Handler, Stephen Wall, and Steven Andes. 2004. "Very Low Birthweight in African American Infants: The Role of Maternal Exposure to Interpersonal Racial Discrimination." *American Journal of Public Health* 94, no. 12 (December): 2132–38. doi:10.2105/ajph.94.12.2132.

Diehr, Paula, John Yergan, Joseph Chu, Polly Feigl, Gwen Glaefke, Roger Moe, Marilyn Bergner, and Jeff Rodenbaugh. 1989. "Treatment Modality and Quality Differences for Black and White Breast-Cancer Patients Treated in Community Hospitals." *Medical Care* 27, no. 10 (October): 942–58. doi:10.1097/00005650-198910000-00005.

*Discrimination in America: Experiences and Views of African Americans*. 2017. NPR, Robert Wood Johnson Foundation, and Harvard T. H. Chan School of Public Health. October. https://www.rwjf.org/content/dam/farm/reports/reports/2017/rwjf441128.

Domonoske, Camila. 2018. "'Father of Gynecology,' Who Experimented on Slaves, No Longer on Pedestal in NYC." *NPR*. April 17. https://www.npr.org/sections/thetwo-way/2018/04/17/603163394/-father-of-gynecology-who-experimented-on-slaves-no-longer-on-pedestal-in-nyc.

Du Bois, W. E. B. 1899. *The Philadelphia Negro: A Social Study*. Philadelphia: University of Pennsylvania Press.

———. 1903. *The Souls of Black Folk*. Chicago: McClurg.

Eltoukhi, Heba M., Monica N. Modi, Meredith Weston, Alicia Y. Armstrong, and Elizabeth A. Stewart. 2014. "The Health Disparities of Uterine Fibroid Tumors for African American Women: A Public Health Issue." *American Journal of Obstetrics & Gynecology* 210, no. 3 (March): 194–99. doi:10.1016/j.ajog.2013.08.008.

Faber, Sonya C., Anjalika Khanna Roy, Timothy I. Michaels, and Monnica T. Williams. 2023. "The Weaponization of Medicine: Early Psychosis in the Black Community and the Need for Racially Informed Mental Healthcare." *Frontiers in Psychiatry* 14 (September 9): 1098292. doi:10.3389/fpsyt.2023.1098292.

Fawzy, Ashraf, Tianshi David Wu, Kunbo Wang, Matthew L. Robinson, Jad Farha, Amanda Bradke, Sherita H. Golden, Yanxun Xu, and Brian T.

Garibaldi. 2022. "Racial and Ethnic Discrepancy in Pulse Oximetry and Delayed Identification of Treatment Eligibility among Patients with COVID-19." *JAMA Internal Medicine* 182, no. 7 (July 1): 730–38. doi:10.1001/jamainternmed.2022.1906.

Ferdinand, Keith C., Kapil Yadav, Samar A. Nasser, Helene D. Clayton-Jeter, John Lewin, Dennis R. Cryer, and Fortunato Fred Senatore. 2017. "Disparities in Hypertension and Cardiovascular Disease in Blacks: The Critical Role of Medication Adherence." *Journal of Clinical Hypertension* 19, no. 10 (October): 1015–24. doi:10.1111/jch.13089.

Flexner, Abraham. 1910. *Medical Education in the United States and Canada: A Report to the Carnegie Foundation for the Advancement of Teaching*. New York: Carnegie Foundation for the Advancement of Teaching. http://archive.carnegiefoundation.org/publications/pdfs/elibrary/Carnegie_Flexner_Report.pdf.

"The Forty Year Death Watch." 1972. *Medical World News*. August 18: 15–17.

Freeman, Lauren, and Heather Stewart. 2024. *Microaggressions in Medicine*. New York: Oxford University Press. doi:10.1093/oso/9780197652480.001.0001.

Fricker, Miranda. 2007. *Epistemic Injustice: Power and the Ethics of Knowing*. New York: Oxford University Press. doi:10.1093/acprof:oso/9780198237907.001.0001.

Gamble, Vanessa Northington. 1997. "Under the Shadow of Tuskegee: African Americans and Health Care." *American Journal of Public Health* 87, no. 11 (November): 1773–78. doi:10.2105/ajph.87.11.1773.

Gawthrop, Elizabeth. 2023. "The Color of Coronavirus: COVID-19 Deaths by Race and Ethnicity in the U.S." APM Research Lab. October 19. https://www.apmresearchlab.org/covid/deaths-by-race.

Geronimus, Arline T. 1992. "The Weathering Hypothesis and the Health of African-American Women and Infants: Evidence and Speculations." *Ethnicity & Disease* 2, no. 3 (Summer): 207–21. https://www.jstor.org/stable/45403051.

———. 2023a. "How Poverty and Racism 'Weather' the Body, Accelerating Aging and Disease." Interview by Dave Davies. *Fresh Air*. March 28. https://www.npr.org/sections/health-shots/2023/03/28/1166404485/weathering-arline-geronimus-poverty-racism-stress-health.

———. 2023b. *Weathering: The Extraordinary Stress of Ordinary Life in an Unjust Society*. New York: Little, Brown.

Gornick, Marian E., Paul W. Eggers, Thomas W. Reilly, Renee M. Mentnech, Leslye K. Fitterman, Lawrence E. Kucken, and Bruce C. Vladeck. 1996. "Effects of Race and Income on Mortality and Use of Services among Medicare Beneficiaries." *New England Journal of Medicine* 335, no. 11 (September 12): 791–99. doi:10.1056/NEJM199609123351106.

Green, Carmen R., Karen O. Anderson, Tamara A. Baker, Lisa C. Campbell, Sheila Decker, Roger B. Fillingim, et al. 2003. "The Unequal Burden of Pain: Confronting Racial and Ethnic Disparities in Pain." *Pain Medicine* 4, no. 3 (September): 277–94. doi:10.1046/j.1526-4637.2003.03034.x.

Greenwood, Brad N., Rachel R. Hardeman, Laura Huang, and Aaron Sojourner. 2020. "Physician-Patient Racial Concordance and Disparities in Birthing Mortality for Newborns." *Proceedings of the National Academy of Sciences of the United States of America* 117, no. 35 (April 17): 21194–200. doi:10.1073/pnas.1913405117.

Gupta, Alisha Haridasani. 2023. "How 'Weathering' Contributes to Racial Health Disparities." *New York Times*. April 12. https://www.nytimes.com/2023/04/12/well/live/weathering-health-racism-discrimination.html.

Halbert, Chanita Hughes, Katrina Armstrong, Oscar H. Gandy Jr., and Lee Shaker. 2006. "Racial Differences in Trust in Health Care Providers." *Archives of Internal Medicine* 166, no. 8 (April 24): 896–901. doi:10.1001/archinte.166.8.896.

Heckler, Margaret M. 1985. *Report of the Secretary's Task Force on Black & Minority Health*. Washington, DC: U.S. Department of Health and Human Services.

Hill, Latoya, Nambi Ndugga, and Samantha Artiga. 2024. "Key Data on Health and Health Care by Race and Ethnicity." Kaiser Family Foundation. Last modified June 11, 2024. https://www.kff.org/racial-equity-and-health-policy/report/key-data-on-health-and-health-care-by-race-and-ethnicity/.

Hoffman, Kelly M., Sophie Trawalter, Jordan R. Axt, and M. Norman Oliver. 2016. "Racial Bias in Pain Assessment and Treatment Recommendations, and False Beliefs about Biological Differences between Blacks and Whites." *Proceedings of the National Academy of the Sciences* 113, no. 16 (April 4): 4296–301. doi:10.1073/pnas.1516047113.

Holt, Lanier Frush, Sophie L. Kjærvik, and Brad J. Bushman. 2022. "Harming and Shaming through Naming: Examining Why Calling the Coronavirus the 'COVID-19 Virus,' Not the 'Chinese Virus,' Matters." *Media Psychology* 25, no. 5: 639–52. doi:10.1080/15213269.2022.2034021.

Hornblum, Allen M. 1998. *Acres of Skin: Human Experiments at Holmesburg Prison*. New York: Routledge.

Hoyert, Donna L. 2023. "Maternal Mortality Rates in the United States, 2021." Centers for Disease Control and Prevention. Last modified March 16, 2023. https://www.cdc.gov/nchs/data/hestat/maternal-mortality/2021/maternal-mortality-rates-2021.htm#Table.

Huerto, Ryan, and Edwin Lindo. 2020. "Minority Patients Benefit from Having Minority Doctors, but That's a Hard Match to Make." *The Conversation*.

February 13. https://theconversation.com/minority-patients-benefit-from-having-minority-doctors-but-thats-a-hard-match-to-make-130504.

Hutchinson, Janis Faye. 2013. "Racism: Medical." In *Encyclopedia of Race and Racism*, edited by Patrick L. Mason, 440–45. New York: Macmillan.

JanMohamed, Abdul R. 2005. *The Death-Bound-Subject: Richard Wright's Archeology of Death*. Durham, NC: Duke University Press. doi:10.1215/9780822386629.

Jones, James H. 1981. *Bad Blood: The Tuskegee Syphilis Experiment*. New York: Free Press.

Kennedy-Moulton, Kate, Sarah Miller, Petra Persson, Maya Rossin-Slater, Laura Wherry, and Gloria Aldana. 2023. "Maternal and Infant Health Inequality: New Evidence from Linked Administrative Data." NBER Working Paper 30693. September. https://www.nber.org/system/files/working_papers/w30693/w30693.pdf.

Lafata, Jennifer Elston, Christine Cole Johnson, Tamir Ben-Menachem, and Robert J. Morlock. 2001. "Sociodemographic Differences in the Receipt of Colorectal Cancer Surveillance Care Following Treatment with Curative Intent." *Medical Care* 39, no. 4 (April): 361–72. doi:10.1097/00005650-200104000-00007.

Lantz, Paula M., James S. House, James M. Lepkowski, David R. Williams, Richard P. Mero, and Jieming Chen. 1998. "Socioeconomic Factors, Health Behaviors, and Mortality: Results from a Nationally Representative Prospective Study of US Adults." *JAMA: Journal of the American Medical Association* 279, no. 21 (June 3): 1703–8. doi:10.1001/jama.279.21.1703.

Lawrence, Jane. 2000. "The Indian Health Service and the Sterilization of Native American Women." *American Indian Quarterly* 24, no. 3 (Summer): 400–419. doi:10.1353/aiq.2000.0008.

Lowe, Robert A., Sheetal Chhaya, Kathleen Nasci, Laurence J. Gavin, Kathy Shaw, Mark L. Zwanger, et al. 2001. "Effect of Ethnicity on Denial of Authorization for Emergency Department Care by Managed Care Gatekeepers." *Academic Emergency Medicine* 8, no. 3 (March): 259–66. doi:10.1111/j.1553-2712.2001.tb01302.x.

Matthew, Dayna Bowen. 2015. *Just Medicine: A Cure for Racial Inequality in American Health Care*. New York: New York University Press.

McFarling, Usha Lee. 2022. "The Nation Hasn't Made Much Progress on Health Equity. These Leaders Forged Ahead Anyway." *STAT News*. February 24. https://www.statnews.com/2022/02/24/little-progress-health-equity-these-leaders-forged-ahead-anyway/.

Mende-Siedlecki, Peter, Jennie Qu-Lee, Robert Backer, and Jay J. Van Bavel. 2019. "Perceptual Contributions to Racial Bias in Pain Recognition." *Journal of Experimental Psychology: General* 148, no. 5 (May): 863–89. doi:10.1037/xge0000600.

Mills, Charles W. 1998. *Blackness Visible: Essays on Philosophy and Race.* Ithaca, NY: Cornell University Press.

Molina, Natalia. 2011. "Borders, Laborers, and Racialized Medicalization: Mexican Immigration and US Public Health Practices in the 20th Century." *American Journal of Public Health* 101, no. 6 (June): 1024–31. doi:10.2105/AJPH.2010.300056.

"Over the Past Century, African American Life Expectancy and Education Levels Have Soared." 2021. *Economist.* May 20. https://www.economist.com/graphic-detail/2021/05/20/over-the-past-century-african-american-life-expectancy-and-education-levels-have-soared.

Owens, Dierdre Cooper. 2017. *Medical Bondage: Race, Gender, and the Origins of American Gynecology.* Athens: University of Georgia Press.

Rodríguez, José E., and Kendall M. Campbell. 2017. "Racial and Ethnic Disparities in Prevalence and Care of Patients with Type 2 Diabetes." *Clinical Diabetes* 35, no. 1 (January): 66–70. doi:10.2337/cd15-0048.

Shavers, Vickie L., Alexis Bakos, and Vanessa B. Sheppard. 2010. "Race, Ethnicity, and Pain among the U.S. Adult Population." *Journal of Health Care for the Poor and Underserved* 21, no. 1 (February): 177–220. doi:10.1353/hpu.0.0255.

Skloot, Rebecca. 2011. *The Immortal Life of Henrietta Lacks.* New York: Doubleday.

Slopen, Natalie, Andrew R. Chang, Tiffani J. Johnson, Ashaunta T. Anderson, Aleha M. Bate, Shawnese Clark, Alyssa Cohen, et al. 2024. "Racial and Ethnic Inequities in the Quality of Paediatric Care in the USA: A Review of Quantitative Evidence." *Lancet: Child & Adolescent Health* 8, no. 2 (February): 147–58. doi:10.1016/S2352-4642(23)00251-1.

Snyder, John E., Rachel D. Upton, Thomas C. Hassett, Hyunjung Lee, Zakia Nouri, and Michael Dill. 2023. "Black Representation in the Primary Care Physician Workforce and Its Association with Population Life Expectancy and Mortality Rates in the US." *JAMA Network Open* 6, no. 4 (April 14): e236687. doi:10.1001/jamanetworkopen.2023.6687.

Sullivan, Louis W., and Ilana Suez Mittman. 2010. "The State of Diversity in the Health Professions a Century after Flexner." *Academic Medicine* 85, no. 2 (February): 246–53. doi:10.1097/ACM.0b013e3181c88145.

Sun, Michael, Tomasz Oliwa, Monica E. Peek, and Elizabeth L. Tung. 2022. "Negative Patient Descriptors: Documenting Racial Bias in the Electronic Health Record." *Health Affairs* 41, no. 2 (February): 203–11. doi:10.1377/hlthaff.2021.01423.

Tong, Michelle, Latoya Hill, and Samantha Artiga. 2024. "Racial Disparities in Cancer Outcomes, Screening, and Treatment." Kaiser Family Foundation.

Last modified June 11, 2024. https://www.kff.org/racial-equity-and-health-policy/issue-brief/racial-disparities-in-cancer-outcomes-screening-and-treatment/.

Trawalter, Sophie, Kelly M. Hoffman, and Adam Waytz. 2012. "Racial Bias in Perceptions of Others' Pain." *PLoS ONE* 7, no. 11: e48546. doi:10.1371/journal.pone.0048546.

Villarosa, Linda. 2022a. "'1619 Project' Journalist Lays Bare Why Black Americans 'Live Sicker and Die Quicker.'" Interview by Dave Davies. *Fresh Air*. June 14. https://www.npr.org/transcripts/1103935147.

———. 2022b. *Under the Skin: The Hidden Toll of Racism on Health in America*. New York: Penguin.

Washington, Harriet A. 2006. *Medical Apartheid: The Dark History of Medical Experimentation on Black Americans from Colonial Times to the Present*. New York: Doubleday.

Wenneker, Mark B., and Arnold M. Epstein. 1989. "Racial Inequalities in the Use of Procedures for Patients with Ischemic Heart Disease in Massachusetts." *JAMA: Journal of the American Medical Association* 261, no. 2 (January 13): 253–57. doi:10.1001/jama.1989.03420020107039.

West, Cornel. 2002. "A Genealogy of Modern Racism." In *Race: Critical Theories, Text and Context*, edited by Philomena Essed and David Theo Goldberg, 90–112. Malden, MA: Blackwell.

Wilson, Elisabeth, Kevin J. Grumbach, Jeffrey Huebner, Jaya Agrawal, and Andrew B. Bindman. 2004. "Medical Student, Physician, and Public Perceptions of Health Care Disparities." *Family Medicine* 36, no. 10 (November–December): 715–21. https://www.stfm.org/familymedicine/vol36issue10/Wilson715.

## FURTHER READING

Anderson, Warwick. 2006. *Colonial Pathologies: American Tropical Medicine, Race, and Hygiene in the Philippines*. Durham, NC: Duke University Press. doi:10.1215/9780822388081.

> A historical account of American medical practice in the Philippines between the late nineteenth century and the 1930s, and the intersections of public health concerns, racial and colonial ideology, and conceptions of science as a tool of civilization. Anderson discusses attempts to "Americanize" Filipino bodies, and also anxieties about the parallel effects of living in the Philippines on American colonial masculinity.

*Birthing while Black: Examining America's Black Maternal Health Crisis*. 2021. Hearing before the Committee on Oversight and Reform, House of

Representatives, 117th Cong., First Session, May 6. Washington, DC: U.S. Government Publishing Office.

    Testimony of physicians, public health officials, politicians, advocates, and ordinary citizens on racial disparities in maternal health. The witnesses provide evidence for the disparities, attempt to explain them, and suggest solutions.

Blackstock, Uché. 2024. *Legacy: A Black Physician Reckons with Racism in Medicine.* New York: Viking.

    A memoir of a Black physician whose mother was also a Black physician. Blackstock weaves together her family's experiences as Black women patients (her mother died young of leukemia) with her experiences as a clinician. The book focuses on how medical racism has been and continues to be normalized in the U.S. and offers recommendations for how to repair those inequities.

Carten, Alma J., Alan Siskind, and Mary Pender Greene, eds. 2016. *Strategies for Deconstructing Racism in the Health and Human Services.* New York: Oxford University Press.

    An anthology directed at healthcare and social service administrators and clinicians, by scholars and clinicians. The chapters cover some theoretical background on how racism has shaped society through personal bias, structural racism, and institutional racism. It then focuses on effective strategies to dismantle those inequities, including educating staff members and revising institutional policies.

Faissner, Mirjam, and Esther Braun. 2024. "The Ethics of Coercion in Mental Healthcare: The Role of Structural Racism." *Journal of Medical Ethics* 50, no. 7 (July): 476–81. doi:10.1136/jme-2023-108984.

    Argues that a history of representing people of color as more dangerous or irrational than whites leads to more coercive measures in response to mental health issues, thereby devaluing their autonomy. Faissner and Braun then suggest how clinicians can counteract those disparities by being more critical of discriminatory biases.

Galarneau, Charlene. 2022. "Recognizing Racism in US Bioethics as the Subject of Bioethical Concern." *Canadian Journal of Bioethics/Revue Canadienne de Bioéthique* 5, no. 1: 62–67. doi:10.7202/1087204ar.

    Evaluates forms of racial discrimination not in medicine itself but in U.S. bioethical discourse since the 1970s. Galarneau discusses the prevalence and modes of critiques of racism in medicine in different decades. She argues that understanding race in the history of bioethics will help to build an anti-racist ethical discourse in the present.

Hoberman, John. 2012. *Black and Blue: The Origins and Consequences of Medical Racism*. Berkeley: University of California Press.
   Analyzes how medical racism is perpetuated in the physician-patient relationship, primarily focusing on the attitudes and behaviors of physicians toward Black patients, but also exploring how professional organizations and editorial boards have contributed to the problem. Hoberman argues that racism in the United States is the root cause of medical disparities. The final chapter proposes an anti-racist medical school curriculum.

Powell, Wizdom, Jennifer Richmond, Dinushika Mohottige, Irene Yen, Allison Joslyn, and Giselle Corbie-Smith. 2019. "Medical Mistrust, Racism, and Delays in Preventive Health Screening among African-American Men." *Behavioral Medicine* 45, no. 2: 102–17. doi:10.1080/08964289.2019.1585327.
   Examines the levels of medical mistrust as a result of everyday racism and perceived racism among Black men, in comparison to medical mistrust among non-Hispanic white men across the United States. The authors link these attitudes to delays in preventive health and suggest that addressing medical racism will directly impact the overall health of people of color.

Roberts, Dorothy E. 2017. *Killing the Black Body: Race, Reproduction, and the Meaning of Liberty*. New York: Pantheon.
   Provides a history of the control and violence directed at Black women's bodies in the United States. Originally published in 1997 and updated twenty years later, the book focuses on forms of reproductive injustice and cultural representations of Black motherhood. Roberts discusses reproductive injustices suffered by enslaved women, the eugenicist history of birth control, the criminalization of pregnancy during the war on drugs, the image of the welfare mother, and the commodification of Black women in surrogacy and in vitro fertilization.

Smedley, Brian D., Adrienne Y. Stith, and Alen R. Nelson, eds. 2003. *Unequal Treatment: Confronting Racial and Ethnic Disparities in Health Care*. Washington, DC: National Academies Press. doi:10.17226/12875.
   A systematic discussion of racial disparities in U.S. medicine by the Institute of Medicine's Committee on Understanding and Eliminating Racial and Ethnic Disparities in Health Care. Their analysis focuses on the clinician-patient interaction and how beliefs and behaviors on each side contribute to health outcomes. The study concludes that people of color tend to receive a lower quality of care than white people. The authors offer a range of solutions, including improving clinicians' cultural understanding and supporting community-based treatment.

# CHAPTER 12
# Pediatric Ethics

**Key topics in this chapter:**

- How parents and clinicians can respect emerging autonomy and promote the well-being of pediatric patients, and how to manage conflicting judgments
- The difference between consent and assent, and when minors can make medical decisions for themselves
- How these principles apply to specific clinical decisions: vaccination, intersex treatment and genital surgeries, and transgender care
- Legal regulations and ethical concerns in research on children
- Children as a vulnerable population, and how race and other identity factors intensify this vulnerability

## Introduction

When patients are children, the framing of issues in medical ethics shifts significantly. Moral deliberation must take into account parents' wishes and role in decision-making, as well as patients' developing autonomy. The unique vulnerabilities of children complicate even those principles that are well-established in medical ethics as they pertain to competent adults, such as the right to refuse life-sustaining treatment. In some cases, clinicians and parents must also navigate state regulations that attempt to protect the well-being of a vulnerable population. This chapter grapples with overarching concerns that shape pediatric ethics—namely, the interaction between beneficence and autonomy, and the role of families and healthcare practitioners. We then consider specific ethical issues that arise in this area, including infant elective surgery, puberty blockers and gender-affirming treatment for transgender minors, and pediatric research.

## Beneficence and Emerging Autonomy

In the case of cognitively capable adults, medical ethics in the last half-century has emphasized the principle of respect for autonomy. In general, patients have the right to make medical decisions concerning their own health and well-being, even if those decisions are medically unjustified or otherwise unreasonable. In the case of adults who have at some point been capable, decisions can be made based on previously expressed wishes or by a medical proxy. In the case of people who have never been capable and for whom there is no expectation of future capacity, protecting the patient's well-being becomes the priority—although ideally one also takes into account the patient's wishes, desires, and values (to the extent that they can be ascertained). Children do not fit straightforwardly into this model. When parents act as proxies for children, it is different from family members acting as proxies for once-capable patients. Among other things, there is likely to be little information about pediatric patients' values, priorities, and prior medical decisions. And what information is available about children's preferences may be difficult to disentangle from what their parents want (Miller 2003, 52).

In the case of children, families and clinicians are caring for patients who are expected to become capable of making medical decisions and to become legally recognized as competent: the "pre-competent" or "proto-competent," in Richard Miller's terms (2003, 52–53). As children cognitively develop, the weight placed on autonomy and confidentiality will strengthen as they are able to understand their medical situations and the options available to them, ask questions of their clinicians, and come to decisions based on their fundamental values (Miller 2003). They have **emerging autonomy**. But infants and young children are typically seen as incapable of informed consent and autonomous decision-making. Their parents or guardians make everyday decisions for them, such as what they eat, how they dress, and with what and with whom they play. It seems like a natural extension of such authority to allow parents to make medical decisions on their behalf. That is, paternalism by parents seems appropriate in the case of not-yet-capable patients.

The needs of children thus speak to the limits of the assumption that patients are individual, self-determining agents. To varying degrees, healthcare practitioners must consider the pediatric patient's embeddedness within a family, which can cause tensions and conflicts that are less likely to arise with adult patients. From the perspective of pediatric clinicians, "the patient is a member of a social unit rather than a freestanding agent" (Miller 2003, 2). This is true of all patients, but it is more clearly manifested with children, in part because clinicians may be primarily or exclusively communicating with parents and trying to build a "therapeutic alliance" with them (2). In complicating the principle of respect for autonomy, the issues raised by pediatric ethics open up broader questions about how to address the medical needs of vulnerable populations such as people with cognitive disabilities, people with limited literacy, and people with mental health disorders.

## The Roles of Parents and Clinicians

Although colloquially and sometimes legally parents are described as "consenting" on behalf of their children to medical treatment or participation in research, some bioethicists have recommended calling it **informed permission** instead because it raises different ethical issues than informed consent (Committee on Bioethics 1995; Committee on Clinical Research Involving Children 2004; Katz et al. 2016). Two related reasons justify this distinction. First, one (or one's proxy) can only consent for oneself. Second, there are constraints on what parents can agree to on behalf of their child—they have parental responsibilities, not only parental rights—since they have a legally defined goal: to promote the child's interests (Dworkin 1982). For example, a patient or proxy can refuse life-sustaining treatment, but parents generally cannot do so for their children. Therefore, we use the language of parental permission rather than parental consent to recognize the special obligations raised by the emerging autonomy of pediatric patients.

Ideally, healthcare professionals or researchers will communicate clearly and thoroughly with parents about a pediatric patient's current situation, options for treatment or participation in research, and the risks and benefits of each option. Those discussions should involve the child or adolescent in age-appropriate ways. And (again, ideally) a decision regarding treatment or research participation would emerge from those discussions based on a shared understanding of the child's present and future well-being. Informed permission on the part of parents will be supplemented by **assent** from the child. Assent involves the child in medical decisions "to the extent that they are able" (Miller and Nelson 2006, S25). It does not place final decision-making authority with minors, who in legal terms are assumed to be incompetent—with the notable exception of mature minors, which we discuss later in the chapter. Children do not have the power to decline treatment that the parents and physicians have decided is medically necessary. But soliciting a child's assent demonstrates respect for their emerging autonomy and builds trusting relationships with family and clinicians (Spriggs 2023). In sum, the ideal scenario involves clinicians receiving informed permission from parents and assent from the child for treatment that meets the clinicians' judgment of what serves the patient's best interests.

The paternalism that dominated the clinician-patient dynamic until recent decades meant that sometimes parents themselves were not given full information about their child's medical situation, or they were presented with one recommendation without other alternatives. To take a prominent example, in the middle of the twentieth century, once "gender-correcting" surgery was possible for infants with disorders of sex development (intersex infants), parents were typically told that such interventions would protect the psychosocial well-being of the child, without full disclosure of the risks, such as scar tissue from multiple surgeries or the psychological impact of repeatedly being examined by clinicians and researchers. That is, the paternalistic tendency to dispense information as medicine, in only those doses that would benefit patients, extended to parents. With the recent emphasis on patient autonomy, that tendency has been roundly criticized, and parental permission—when parents are informed enough to make decisions for their children—is usually respected.

Even beyond the issues caused by clinician paternalism, each element of the ideal sketched above may be derailed. Parents accustomed to making decisions not only about what their children do but also what they know may seek to limit children's access to information about their medical situations, most commonly out of a desire to protect them from psychological harm. Along the same lines, parents may actively lie to their children and attempt to recruit healthcare professionals into such deceptions. Children and parents may disagree about treatment and the basic values that inform medical decisions. Clinicians and parents may disagree about the treatments that will best serve the well-being of the children. Children may have trouble questioning the authority of parents or clinicians, or detaching their own judgments from the desire to meet the real or projected expectations of those adults. With each of these concerns, there is a balance to be struck between the tendency to infantilize all minors (that is, for parents or clinicians to revert to medical paternalism) and to treat minors as small autonomous adults (Miller 2003, 180).

Miller (2003) warns that parents and healthcare practitioners, especially when confronted with children who are sick, are primed to underestimate the extent to which children can participate in decision-making. This is a form of epistemic injustice, which devalues children as knowers (Carel and Györffy 2014). One element of emerging autonomy is children's ability to understand the medical options and their implications. Even very young children have some awareness of their own symptoms, are attuned to their parents' emotional reactions, and are affected by disruptions to their usual routines—including the very mundane facts of being in a doctor's office, research lab, or hospital; interacting with unfamiliar adults clad in white coats; and being treated differently than siblings or peers. Older children can understand simplified diagnoses, treatment options, and risks. Ignoring this spectrum of comprehension dismisses the developing authority that children possess.

Children need help making sense of their experiences to reduce the isolation and confusion caused by illness rather than having adults shield them from such understanding. Discussing their medical situations in age-appropriate ways is beneficial in building their sense of autonomy: "Children who have not been given the opportunity to understand their illness exhibit significantly greater distress, more internalization of problems, and increased symptoms of depression" (Fleischman 2016, 128). Clinicians should not lie to children, even if parents want them to. Trusting physicians and nurses is in children's long-term best interests. This does not entail, however, that children should be treated as if they were already adult, fully autonomous patients. They must be included in decision-making in ways that match their cognitive and emotional development.

For pediatric patients even more than adults, the principles of beneficence and respect for autonomy are not easily separable. Protecting a child's health is a way of supporting their future autonomy, which may mean overriding impulsive or short-sighted preferences in some situations. In Joel Feinberg's terms, children have "an open future": "[An adult's] present autonomy takes precedence even over his probable future good, and he may use it as he will, even at the expense of the future self he will one day become. Children are different. Respect for the child's future autonomy, as an adult, often requires preventing his free choice now" (1980, 127). But protecting children's well-being also means treating them as people with developing autonomy rather than valuable objects without agency.

In most cases, parents or guardians can be assumed to prioritize the child's well-being and emerging autonomy. Empowering the decisions of caregivers is generally in the child's best interests; usually, family members dispense medication or provide basic healthcare at home, make decisions about preventive and follow-up care, and decide when a child urgently needs to be seen by a professional. Clinicians thus need to take seriously the goal of reaching consensus with parents or other caregivers rather than adopting an adversarial approach by which parents may be legally compelled to enact clinicians' judgments. This may be effective in the short term but typically does not serve the child's long-term health needs.

Bryanna Moore and Rosalind McDougall (2022) suggest that medical personnel should seek to reconcile disparate judgments by understanding the different roles that parents and clinicians play in the child's life. This approach focuses on resolving conflicts between parents and medical staff, in the recognition that the child's health will be best supported if professional and nonprofessional caregivers function as a team, which requires trust and communication. Parents are unlikely to have the medical knowledge that professionals use to understand a child's situation and treatment options, so they need to be respectfully educated about those matters. Parents also are likely to come into medical decisions with motivations that do not apply to most physicians: they are particularly committed to the well-being of their child, they are attuned to the psychological and emotional state of their child, and their ideas about what a "good parent" would do may be deeply wrapped up in their religious tradition, family history, or other core aspects of their identity. On the other hand, physicians and nurses may be motivated by a sense of obligation to multiple patients and a duty to temper unrealistic expectations. Recognizing these differing roles and articulating the values behind them can help resolve conflicts by engaging rather than overriding the parents' perspective. Parents' sense of their roles and responsibilities can evolve, especially when their child has a long-term illness (Moore and McDougall 2022, 42). And clinicians' sense of the child's well-being may also shift to take into account the family's ethical commitments. This kind of conversation may help to avert a breakdown in trust, which would lead to an antagonistic decision-making process:

Working to reframe the case in this way has the potential to shift the dynamics between parents and the team out of battle mode, where the team's goal is to get the parents to do what the team thinks is in this child's best interests, and into a more flexible approach in which the team asks, how can we care for this patient in a way that helps these parents to feel that they are fulfilling their responsibilities to their child? (Moore and McDougall 2022, 39)

Again, for the long-term best interests of the child, ideally parents and clinicians would reach consensus about the goals and methods of treatment.

In other instances, however, healthcare professionals need to act as pediatric patients' advocates to guard against the excesses of parental authority. Parents may demand overtreatment—medically futile, experimental, or otherwise unjustified interventions—or undertreatment, such as a religiously based refusal of life-sustaining blood transfusions. What complicates the decision to override a parent's judgment is what Ezekiel Emanuel (1987) calls "pluralism" regarding best interests: reasonable and competent decision-makers can disagree about what the principle of beneficence requires. However, uncontroversial primary goods include physical health, avoidance of pain, and the means to develop future autonomy.

## Resolving Ethical Conflicts

In recent decades, bioethicists have attempted to balance beneficence toward the child and respect for parental autonomy, and also to specify what the principle of beneficence entails. Three of the most prominent standards are

1. the best interests standard, in which clinicians are obligated to promote the child's medical and nonmedical interests (Malek 2009);

2. the harm principle, in which medical personnel protect a minimum standard of care (to do no harm) but respect parental decisions outside of that domain (Diekema 2004); and

3. the standard of respecting parental autonomy, as long as those judgments are autonomous in the Kantian sense of that term—that is, parents are accountable for making rational decisions (Ross 2007).

Grounded in consequentialist and deontological ethics, these standards function as ways to navigate conflicts between clinicians' and parents' judgments.

Applying these standards in concrete situations can be difficult. For example, should parents be able to implement a Do Not Resuscitate (DNR) order for newborns with severe congenital abnormalities? On the other hand, should parents be able to demand all possible treatments for a seriously ill child? These issues of undertreatment or overtreatment raise the need for clinicians' judgment about a child's best interests, perhaps in consultation with a hospital ethics committee.

Decisions to withdraw or withhold life-sustaining treatment are particularly fraught, and ones in which conflicts between the judgments of parents and clinicians are most likely. The legal history relevant to such decisions illuminates the ethical issues involved. One key case is that of Baby Doe in 1982—an infant born with Down syndrome and a tracheoesophageal fistula (an opening between the trachea and the esophagus). Without repair of the fistula, the infant would have difficulty swallowing food and would be at risk of serious lung infections. With repair, the child would be expected to live without significant after-effects. The obstetrician advised the parents against the surgery, and the parents agreed with that decision. The infant's pediatrician objected on the grounds that the surgery would likely be successful and that therefore the infant was being discriminated against because of his disability. As the legal process to override the parents' decision was initiated through local and state courts, Baby Doe died of dehydration and pneumonia.

In response to this and similar cases, a report of the President's Commission for the Study of Ethical Problems in Medicine and Biomedical and Behavioral Research made the following judgment, prioritizing beneficence over parental autonomy:

> When treatment is clearly beneficial, it should be provided regardless of whether or not parents agree, but for cases in which the benefits of treatment are ambiguous or uncertain, parents should have the authority to determine whether treatment is provided or foregone. When treatment is considered futile, cannot provide benefit, and may only prolong or increase suffering, life-extending treatment should not be provided, even if parents insist on it. (Fleischman 2016, 66; see President's Commission 1983, 214–23)

In 1984, the U.S. government instituted the more specific rule that medical treatment can only be withheld from an infant if

> (A) the infant is chronically and irreversibly comatose; (B) the provision of such treatment would (i) merely prolong dying, (ii) not be effective in ameliorating or correcting all of the infant's life-threatening conditions; or (iii) otherwise be futile in terms of survival of the infant; or (C) the provision of such treatment would be virtually futile in terms of the survival of the infant and the treatment itself under such circumstances would be inhumane. (Pub. L. 98-457)

The terms "virtually futile" and "inhumane" still require interpretation in each case. In line with these principles, parents may choose treatments for infants and young children within certain parameters—namely, within the domain of what is medically justified, or meeting the legal standard of care. They should alleviate unnecessary suffering and avoid treatments that would inflict or prolong such suffering.

There will still be situations when legal redress is required: if parents are endangering the child's life by refusing medical care that would be effective (undertreatment) or are demanding ineffective interventions (overtreatment). For instance, Jehovah's Witnesses generally do not consent to blood transfusions due to their interpretation of a biblical injunction against consuming blood. For capable adults, even if blood transfusions are necessary to sustain their health, that refusal is morally and legally binding, assuming their decision is informed by an understanding of the risks of nontreatment. For children, however, such refusals are problematic because they endanger children's present well-being and future autonomy. Sometimes alternatives can be found: certain "minor" blood products (not whole blood or plasma, but albumin or clotting factors) and reinfusion of a patient's own blood under certain circumstances are religiously acceptable. But if these alternatives will not be effective in protecting the child's health, the overriding priority is the patient's physical well-being, even if parents are convinced that medically necessary blood transfusions will endanger their child in a spiritual sense (Woolley 2005). Clinicians usually respect parents' religious beliefs as long as the child's health is not in danger; at that point, a court order is sought. In this sense, parental control over the health of pediatric patients is conditional and limited by the harm principle.

In cases where the child's well-being is not being protected due to social determinants of health, clinicians must also act as advocates for the family as a whole, including referring them to social services that may address unsafe housing or housing insecurity, food insecurity, domestic violence, and child abuse. Legally, clinicians are mandated reporters of suspected abuse or neglect of children or vulnerable adults because they are uniquely positioned to encounter evidence of abuse or neglect and to intervene against it. Pediatric healthcare practitioners also play a significant role in securing psychosocial support for patients who may be suffering from eating disorders, anxiety and depression, or other mental health problems, and in assisting families to promote healthy behaviors around eating, physical activity, sexuality, and substance use.

## Mature Minors

When do children become capable of making decisions for themselves? As with many ethical and legal questions, the gradual development of autonomy that characterizes childhood complicates attempts to draw a clear line. Children are not simply autonomous or heteronomous but somewhere on a spectrum of developing the cognitive processes that support autonomy. Recent studies have demonstrated that children as young as seven are cognitively capable of assenting to medical decisions and that around the age of fourteen, adolescents' cognitive capacities relevant to decision-making match those of capable adults (Grisso and Vierling 1978; Weithorn and Campbell 1982; Committee on Bioethics 1995; Schachter, Kleinman, and Harvey 2005). But each child is different, and the specific circumstances in which those decisions are made may impact a minor's ability to assent or consent. Are they given information in an age-appropriate way? Are they given time to deliberate and ask questions? Are they given the psychological space to deliberate, apart from the entrenched desire to please parents or other caregivers? These variables make it more difficult to determine whether they have decision-making capacity. Problems often emerge when adolescents (who are almost adults) and their parents or guardians disagree about medical decisions.

Legally, people do not have the right to make medical decisions for themselves until the age of majority—in the United States, on the day they turn eighteen—unless a court grants them an exception. However, thirty-five states currently consider some adolescents to be **mature minors** who can make decisions concerning contraception and pregnancy (including abortion), sexually transmitted infections, and substance use without requiring parents to be informed about or permit treatment. These provisions recognize that allowing adolescents this limited autonomy ultimately protects their well-being because they may be hesitant to discuss these issues with parents. Mature minor laws developed out of the *Smith v. Seibly* (72 Wn. 2d 16 [1967]) court case in Washington state, in which a physician performed a vasectomy on an eighteen-year-old at their request (the legal age of competence in the state was twenty-one at the time). The patient later claimed not to have been capable of consenting and had not understood that the procedure had permanent consequences. The court found that the patient was competent:

> A married minor, 18 years of age, who has successfully completed high school and is the head of his own family, who earns his own living and maintains his own home, is emancipated for the purpose of giving a valid consent to surgery if a full disclosure of the ramifications, implications and probable consequences of the surgery has been made by the doctor in terms which are fully comprehensible to the minor. Thus, age, intelligence, maturity, training, experience, economic independence or lack thereof, general conduct as an adult and freedom from the control of parents are all factors to be considered in such a case. (21)

Mature minor laws vary from state to state. Some states designate that anyone over a particular age (typically fourteen or sixteen) can request contraceptive services without parental notification or permission, and some states say that minors can demonstrate their legal competence to make medical decisions, either to clinicians or to a court. Fourteen states allow people of any age to get abortions without parental permission or notification. Some states articulate a precise age at which mature minor exceptions apply, while others refer to life circumstances, such as having graduated from high school or being "unaccompanied" (experiencing homelessness). Such laws attempt to recognize the emerging capacity for autonomy and the particular areas in which respecting it in adolescents will significantly impact their present and future well-being. Finally, if a minor between fourteen and seventeen is legally emancipated from their parents' custody, they are able to make medical decisions for themselves.

## Childhood Vaccination and Screening

How to apply the principles of respect for autonomy and beneficence can be further illuminated by analyzing particular issues in pediatric ethics. Some of these issues arise in every childhood, such as vaccination, and some of them arise in particular populations, such as intersex and transgender children.

Since the advent of inoculation in the fifteenth century, when people deliberately exposed themselves to smallpox, the medical community has promoted the value of childhood vaccination, mainly because children are more vulnerable to diseases that are not life-threatening to adults. In 1796, Edward Jenner developed a smallpox vaccine derived from cowpox. It was first tested on his gardener's eight-year-old son and then repeated on other children, including his own eleven-month-old child and forty-eight children living in an almshouse (Moreno and Kravitt 2010). At the time, smallpox was globally endemic, with approximately 75 percent of adults having survived exposure to it. Smallpox disproportionately killed infants and children, and in medieval and early modern Europe, the disease was responsible for approximately 10 percent of all deaths (Razzell 1977). Polio, measles, and diphtheria are also typically diseases of childhood, and prior to the development of vaccines in the nineteenth and twentieth centuries, they would permanently disable or kill millions of children. Because of the health risks, childhood vaccinations are now often required by school districts and childcare facilities.

The protection offered to each child is one major justification for vaccination, but a second strand of reasoning involves herd immunity. Some children and adults will not be able to be vaccinated against some infectious diseases due to conditions that compromise their immune systems or inadequate access to preventive healthcare. **Herd immunity** (or collective immunity) occurs when enough of the population is inoculated against a disease that an infected individual is unlikely to encounter an uninoculated individual and pass the infection onward. For instance, for measles, one of the most contagious diseases in humans, approximately 94–95 percent of a population must be immunized to shut down transmission (Pandey and Galvani 2023). This is an issue where parental autonomy or liberty (the authority to make medical decisions on behalf of one's children) may conflict with the wider obligation of justice: their medical decisions impact the level of risk that others face.

**Vaccine hesitancy and refusal** on the part of parents impairs herd immunity and the eventual eradication of infectious diseases. Measles was declared eradicated (no disease transmission for the past twelve months) in the United States in 2000, but since then, there have been periodic outbreaks of measles due to decreasing proportions of young children being vaccinated against it. Vaccine hesitancy and refusal can be generated by spurious scientific reports and the "truth decay" associated with social media—in the case of measles (typically bundled with vaccinations against mumps and rubella as the MMR vaccine), a much-criticized and since-retracted paper suggesting a link between the MMR vaccine and increased risk of autism (see DeStefano and Shimabukuro 2019; Kavanaugh 2021). Suspicion about vaccines may also thrive when medical authority becomes politicized, such as during the COVID-19 pandemic in the United States and in South Africa.

Vaccine debates are typically framed as a conflict between parental liberty and the public good, weighing the immediate well-being of the individual child against increased risk for other children. Johan Bester (2018) argues that this focus deflects attention from what a just society owes children and whether vaccinations fall within those obligations. Children are a vulnerable group in the sense that they depend on others to make decisions about their well-being. As we have discussed, their physical health in early childhood affects their ability to thrive throughout their lives in terms of cognitive and physical development. Preventing them from contracting lethal diseases supports their future capacity (Bester 2018, 613–14). In addition, parents have obligations to prevent not only their own children but also children in the wider society from contracting those diseases. According to Bester, this generates strong individual and collective obligations:

> Vaccination is something that is owed to children, and is not a matter of individual choice or liberty. Those who are in positions of care and positions of authority over children are obligated to provide children with timely and safe vaccination. Failure to do so is unjust, is immoral, and necessitates a societal response. This means that there are obligations resting on parents, health care professionals, and governments to ensure vaccination happens. (2018, 618)

The principle of beneficence obligates us to protect children's health and future prospects, and the principle of justice obligates us to mandate vaccinations for children who attend daycare and school with other children. These duties limit the scope of parental autonomy.

As with the conflicts described in the previous section, in addressing parents' vaccine hesitancy, clinicians should acknowledge that parents are generally motivated by the desire to protect their children. Clinicians must share the real risks and side effects of vaccination, as well as the risks of non-vaccination. Many who describe themselves as vaccine-hesitant may delay vaccinations or partially vaccinate their children and therefore may be open to conversations with trusted clinicians about how best to safeguard their children's health (Shen and Dubey 2019).

A closely related issue is that of **mandatory newborn screening**. Every U.S. state requires that newborns be tested for serious but treatable conditions for which there is a reliable test, though the specific conditions vary by state. These disorders usually do not show symptoms at birth, but early detection and treatment can prevent severe disability or death. In the case of phenylketonuria (PKU), beginning a special diet at birth prevents progressive brain damage. A blood test for PKU was developed in the 1960s, and this became a paradigm for other mandated newborn screening tests. States also screen for congenital adrenal hyperplasia, sickle cell anemia, and cystic fibrosis, among other conditions. These screenings typically do not require parental permission, although parents may refuse on religious grounds. States may keep blood spot cards (with the infant's identifying information) for several decades for public health purposes. Requests to use such samples for genetic research, however, raise further ethical concerns about sharing private medical information (Pelias, n.d; see also Fleischman 2016, 95).

## Medical Responses to Intersex

If treatments are medically necessary for pediatric patients, ethical problems are unlikely to arise as long as the parents, clinicians, and children (to the extent that they can assent) agree on those treatments. But determining what is medically justified and what is merely socially expected introduces complications, particularly when treatments—such as surgeries—have long-term effects. The treatment of disorders of sex development is a prime example.

**Disorders of sex development (DSDs)** are "a group of congenital conditions associated with atypical development of internal and external genital structures" (Witchel 2018, 90). These conditions are also known as differences in sex development, variations in sex characteristics, and **intersex**. If all genetic and physiological atypicalities related to sex are included, DSDs happen in approximately 0.1–0.5 percent of births (García-Acero et al. 2020). Some of those conditions cause ambiguous genital anatomy, which tends to be diagnosed at birth; some of them emerge later, at puberty, when people experience delayed puberty or infertility. Atypicalities can happen at the level of chromosomes, gonads, and/or anatomy. Some DSDs can have life-threatening effects—in the case of congenital adrenal hyperplasia, the inability to regulate the amount of salt in the bloodstream. Some have medically significant effects, such as an increased risk of cancer in undescended testicles. And some have no medically significant effects but generate bodies that are sex-ambiguous.

Historically, ambiguous sex itself has been treated as a medical problem, given the social stigma that is generated by any identities, desires, and behaviors that challenge the assumption of binary, heteronormative sex. "Corrective" surgeries were developed primarily at Johns Hopkins University starting in 1930 and became more sophisticated through the middle of the twentieth century. Parents of intersex newborns were strongly encouraged to authorize such interventions based on the belief that unambiguous genitalia would promote the child's psychosocial well-being.

In many ways, surgeries on infants to address disorders of sex development illuminate the issues at the core of pediatric ethics. Parents must promote the present well-being of the child and the anticipated well-being of that child as an adult, based on the medical knowledge provided to them. The child, especially if they are still an infant, cannot participate in the decision-making, and waiting until they can participate may impact their well-being: "Postponing [a medical] decision to the age of consent . . . means closing an important window of opportunity for the child. The future adult's consent . . . will be meaningless, because no decision will undo the consequences of a waiver of treatment [or authorization of treatment] in the past" (Wiesemann et al. 2010, 673). Again, a great deal depends on how the principle of beneficence is interpreted. Does avoiding entrenched social stigma justify medical intervention? What constitutes well-being around sexuality—visible normalcy, erotic sensation, fertility, felt gender identity in alignment with one's body, or something else? Do such interventions address a medical problem, or by medicalizing a biological difference, do they illegitimately impose social norms?

Many adults who experienced "corrective" surgeries and hormone treatments as children attest to the psychological and physical consequences of these interventions: shame and confusion at repeated medical examinations of their genitalia, scar tissue from multiple surgeries, and a sense of having lost an important part of their embodied identity. To raise a relatively marginal concern, the long-term risks associated with general anesthesia for children under the age of three present an ethical objection to infant surgeries that are not medically necessary (Gardner and Sandberg 2018). Alice Dreger and David Sandberg argue that there is no evidence that "normalizing" pediatric genital surgery supports the well-being of children, in part because there is no way to collect reliable data about long-term outcomes (2010, 156). In line with critical disability theory, clinicians should help parents understand the difference between medically necessary treatments, treatments to reduce medical risk, and elective treatments (157). Many parents and clinicians may anticipate a psychosocial risk, given the intensity with which the gender binary is culturally enforced and the attendant stigmatization of intersex. But these anticipations need to be weighed against the risks of surgery or other treatments, the harm children may suffer as a result of repeated genital examinations and surgeries, and their future autonomy. Cosmetic normalizing treatments serve to reinforce social stigma, particularly if such treatments signal that intersex children are "shameful, abnormal, and unlovable" (158). Dreger argues that caring for DSDs means considering that medicine is being asked to fix what social norms have framed as a problem, but that "the child is not the wound that needs healing" (2006, 78).

In recent decades, most bioethicists have concluded that pediatric infant surgery for DSDs is unjustified based on the principles of beneficence and respect for autonomy—that, beyond urgent medical treatments, long-term interventions such as surgery and hormone treatments should be delayed until children are old enough to participate substantively in decisions about their own bodies (Kipnis and Diamond 1998). On the other hand, there is continuing debate about what constitutes a disorder of sex development and what sorts of legislation would be appropriate to limit parental autonomy around infant surgery related to such disorders (Gardner and Sandberg 2018). Beyond these debates, there is consensus that neither parents nor clinicians should deceive children or avoid telling them about any procedures that take place: "For success in deception entails that the adult patient not understand his or her medical condition. Just to the extent that these adults are misled, they cannot act rationally out of a realistic appraisal of their situation" (Kipnis and Diamond 1998, 407). Such deceptions also damage trust in the family and medical professionals.

## Other Elective Genital Surgeries

Debates about infant surgery regarding disorders of sex development raise questions about other pediatric surgeries demanded by social norms rather than medical necessity—most prominently, **male circumcision** and **female genital cutting**. Both procedures involve altering external genitalia (excising erogenous tissue) to make them visibly normal to others within the cultures in which the procedures are common. Both procedures tend to be justified within those traditions with regard to sexual purity and religious identity.

Female genital cutting (also called female genital mutilation) is traditionally practiced in parts of sub-Saharan Africa and the Middle East, and in migrant populations originating from those areas. It has been roundly condemned by international human rights organizations and Western medicine because it violates the principles of beneficence and respect for autonomy: heightening risks of infection at the time of surgery, interfering with girls' and women's sexual freedom, and reinforcing women's social subordination.

Male circumcision, by contrast, has typically been judged to be acceptable even though it is medically unnecessary. Its prevalence in Europe and migrant populations originating from there stems from a Judaic practice. In modern societies, the procedure has been justified by appealing to a slight decrease in the risk of urinary tract infections (as children) and sexually transmitted diseases (as adults). But the procedure, like female genital cutting, is clearly culturally motivated (Dustin 2010).

In both cases, genital-altering surgery that happens in a medical setting carries fewer risks of short-term infection than procedures carried out elsewhere, but the ethical question extends beyond those consequences. These procedures involve a primarily nontherapeutic surgical intervention in infants and children, with a part of their bodies that is often central to someone's identity, without any possibility of consent (Earp 2015). The relatively prominent moral criticism and legal prohibitions of female genital cutting and the relatively marginal debate around male circumcision challenge us to consider how cultural norms influence medical definitions of well-being in the minds of both clinicians and parents. They also exemplify the recent bioethical emphasis on bodily autonomy: To what extent is it justified for parents to authorize irreversible alterations, in nontherapeutic but socially accepted forms, of the bodies of their children?

## Healthcare for Transgender Minors

We now turn to treatments that children may request themselves, some of which are irreversible: surgical and hormonal treatments that affirm a child's felt gender identity, which is not reflected in the child's sex as assigned at birth. In recent decades, starting in the 1990s, there has been wider recognition that gender identity emerges early in childhood (as early as age two or three), so a sense of distress at not having that identity recognized often begins well before the traditional age of consent (Giordano 2023, 2). The bioethical implications of these treatments pose the same conundrum around time and autonomy as treatments for DSDs: if treatment is postponed until the patient has reached the traditional age of consent (eighteen years old in the United States), the window of opportunity for such treatment to be fully effective will have closed. Puberty brings about sexual differentiation that can be distressing for anyone, but especially for someone who is **transgender**, whose body (or whose anticipated future body) does not match their gender identity. To have experienced adolescence in that state of alienation and to have been continually misgendered by others can create serious psychosocial harms, including higher rates of depression, anxiety, self-harm, and suicidality in transgender youth (Clark and Virani 2021; Austin et al. 2022; Hajek et al. 2023).

Transgender identity itself has a history of being pathologized, starting with the earliest decades of psychiatry, when it was understood as a form of homosexuality. Gender identity disorder was first included in the third edition of the *Diagnostic and Statistical Manual of Mental Disorders* (*DSM-III*), which defines the symptoms and thresholds for diagnosing psychiatric disorders, in 1980. In order to depathologize and destigmatize transgender identity, the fifth edition (*DSM-5*), published in 2013, recognized the diagnosis of **gender dysphoria**, defined as psychological distress that results from "a marked incongruence between one's experienced/expressed gender and assigned gender" (American Psychiatric Association 2013, 452). Under this definition, a patient's gender expression may be "incongruent" or "nonconforming" with social gender norms and expectations without their suffering from dysphoria. That is, the distress arising from transgender identity is a psychiatric problem to be treated, but the identity itself is not: "The expression of gender characteristics, including identities, that are not stereotypically associated with one's assigned sex at birth is a common and culturally diverse human phenomenon that should not be seen as inherently negative or pathological" (Coleman et al. 2022, S6). Gender dysphoria in the United States remains categorized as a mental health condition to facilitate treatment, whereas the World Health Organization's *International Statistical Classification of Diseases* (*ICD-11*) uses the term "gender incongruence," which it classifies as a "condition related to sexual health" rather than a mental disorder (2019, § 17). It is generally recognized that the diagnosis of gender dysphoria does not undermine a patient's capacity to consent to treatment.

The World Professional Association for Transgender Health recommends treating gender dysphoria with hormonal and surgical treatments, as well as individual and family counseling, so that the patient's felt gender identity aligns with their embodied experience and social identity (Coleman et al. 2022; see also Giordano 2023). It is important to distinguish between two kinds of interventions: puberty blockers, which delay the onset of puberty by suppressing increases in estrogen or testosterone, and gender-affirming surgery or hormone treatments, which actively feminize or masculinize a patient's body. The former treatment is reversible in the sense that when puberty blockers are no longer taken, the patient's natural levels of hormones will return. The latter is not. Puberty blockers tend to be prescribed for transgender patients around the age of twelve to fourteen, whereas ideally gender-affirming care is initiated around the age of fourteen to sixteen. As we noted earlier in this chapter, research suggests that fourteen-year-olds, on average, have the cognitive capacity of adults when it comes to medical decision-making.

The proportion of young children and adolescents who experience gender dysphoria or identify as transgender has increased in recent years. In the United States, 1.4 percent of adolescents now identify as transgender, although only a small proportion (2–4 percent) seeks medical intervention (Hughes 2024). Transgender identity has also become politicized in various parts of the world, but especially in the U.S., where in 2023 alone, the following states enacted legislation restricting or prohibiting gender-affirming treatment for minors, with legal consequences for clinicians and/or parents: Arkansas, Florida, Idaho, Indiana, Iowa, Louisiana, Mississippi, Missouri, Montana, Nebraska, North Carolina, North Dakota, Ohio, Oklahoma, South Dakota, Tennessee, Texas, Utah, and West Virginia. Anti-trans legislation is often framed as protecting children (e.g., the Ohio Saving Adolescents from Experimentation [SAFE] Act [HB 68] [2024]). Such laws impact the ability of doctors, clinics, and hospitals to offer gender-affirming care to minors, even when parents support their children's decisions. Sometimes this is explicitly defined in law as medical malpractice (e.g., Arkansas SB 199 [2023]), and sometimes states have extended the statute of limitations for medical malpractice lawsuits so adults can sue clinicians well into adulthood for giving them gender-affirming care that they and their parents wanted when they were minors (e.g., Missouri SB 843 [2022]). Transgender healthcare is also sometimes legally equated with child abuse, as in the recent Texas law (SB 14 [2023]), which stipulates that parents supporting puberty blockers or gender-affirming treatments for their children will be investigated by the Department of Family Protective Services, with the possible outcome of the child being placed in foster care and (presumably) prevented from receiving such treatments. In *United States v. Skrmetti* (No. 23-477), the U.S. Supreme Court seems poised to uphold the Tennessee ban on gender-affirming care for minors, rejecting the claim that it discriminates on the basis of sex. Apart from this constitutional issue, gender transition for minors raises the question of how to apply the principles of beneficence and respect for autonomy, including parental authority: surgical and hormonal interventions carry some medical risks but also psychosocial benefits, and those interventions will be most effective prior to the traditional age of consent.

One concern that can arise on the part of parents and clinicians is that minors who transition will experience regret, especially around fertility, but also that, following irreversible gender-affirming treatments, the minor's felt gender identity will not persist—hence the designation of transgender "persisters" and "desisters." There is a range of trajectories for gender-diverse children, but if minors meet all the *DSM* criteria for gender dysphoria and the symptoms of gender dysphoria intensify around puberty, this is a strong predictor of persistence (Giordano 2023, 31). Beth Clark and Alice Virani argue that trans youth have typically had to reflect carefully on their gender identity and expression (2021, 155). Simona Giordano points out that "whereas the debate has revolved around whether or not transgender adolescents are able to consent to puberty blockers, not much attention has been paid to the fact that adolescents do not consent to puberty progression either" (2023, 154).

A second concern is the safety of hormone therapy for minors. Due to their relatively recent widespread use for transgender children and adolescents, little long-term research exists. For this reason, government commissions in the United Kingdom, France, and Sweden have discussed these treatments as "experimental" and regulated their use in national health services. The 2024 *Independent Review of Gender Identity Services for Children and Young People* (known as the Cass Review) from the United Kingdom notes the need for more research into the medical and psychological outcomes of gender transitioning. It recommends a more cautious approach to the use of puberty blockers and gender-affirming treatment, including screening for and treating mental health and neurodevelopmental conditions, counseling minors about the options for preserving their fertility, and supporting detransitioning treatments. However, the report recognizes that some minors will benefit from transitioning, provided that there is a "clear clinical rationale," such as longstanding gender incongruence, for prescribing gender-affirming hormones under the age of eighteen (*Independent Review* 2024, 35). Nonetheless, the British government decided in 2024 to indefinitely ban all puberty blockers for minors. No other European countries ban transgender care for minors—people can still seek treatment outside of the public health service.

The psychosocial benefits of transgender care for minors are clearer. Puberty blockers and gender-affirming therapy are associated with decreased depression and anxiety, increased self-acceptance, and improved quality of life (de Vries et al. 2014). And there are risks of not treating gender dysphoria, given the sharply increased prevalence of self-harm and suicide among transgender and gender-nonconforming adolescents. It is worth noting that gender-*conforming* hormone treatment (for example, to manage early puberty) has not caused moral or legal controversy.

Australia's recent legal shifts around pediatric transgender decision-making are emblematic of the increasing recognition of minors' bodily autonomy and the importance of gender-affirming therapy to their well-being. Until 2017, a minor needed court authorization to complete gender-affirming hormone treatment, even if their parents permitted it and physicians had diagnosed them with gender dysphoria and recommended such treatment. In 2017, however, the court found that the therapeutic effects of such treatment outweighed the risks and decided that no legal process is required when the minor, parents, and physicians agree on gender-affirming treatment. It left in place the need for court adjudication when the minor, parents, and physicians disagree (Feldman and Dreyfus 2017).

When parents are opposed to their child's or adolescent's desire for puberty blockers or gender-affirming treatment, the moral and legal issues become thornier. Samuel Dubin et al. (2020) argue that, like abortion or treatment for sexually transmitted infections, gender-affirming care carries relatively low risks compared to untreated gender dysphoria. Interactions with parents, siblings, peers, teachers, and clinicians deeply impact the psychological stress that transgender minors experience—whether they experience guilt, shame, and frustration, or acceptance and love. LGBTQIA+ children and adolescents are much more vulnerable to harassment, discrimination, abuse, violence, and homelessness (Giordano 2023). Dubin et al. (2020) claim that, when there is disagreement, clinicians should help facilitate agreement but ultimately should act as advocates for minors, in helping to educate parents and others about the experience of gender dysphoria and medically justified treatments for it. The question of how to address gender dysphoria should apply the core principles of beneficence and respect for autonomy, to the extent that the child is capable of participating in the medical decision: a treatment that "overall serves the child's interests, . . . minimizes current distress, . . . promotes long-term self-acceptance, . . . encourages trust in significant others, [and] . . . promotes a sense of being accepted and validated by health care professionals and the family" (Giordano 2023, 108). As in other issues in pediatric ethics, a key factor in these decisions is the person's developing autonomy—that is, determining the cognitive capacities of this particular patient at this particular age and giving commensurate weight to their desires, preferences, and values.

## Pediatric Research

As noted above, historically, medical research has involved children, such as Jenner's testing of the smallpox vaccine. Given the dominant paternalistic dynamic of medical therapy and research until the last decades of the twentieth century, questions around obtaining parental permission for children's participation in research arose as little as questions of informed consent did in the case of adults. In the nineteenth century, anti-vivisection societies argued against research on nonhuman animals and children (Fleischman 2016, 199). As paternalism began to be challenged in the latter half of the twentieth century, increasingly nuanced questions were raised about the use of research subjects who are incapable of informed consent. The first principle of the Nuremberg Code states that informed consent is necessary for any research subject. Under a strict reading of this principle, no pediatric research would be justified, since children are legally presumed to be incompetent. Children are a vulnerable population for various reasons: they have emerging but not full-fledged autonomy, and they are often psychologically primed to please caregivers and adults in authority. Institutionalized children have historically been treated as captive research subjects. Prominent examples in the U.S. include the hepatitis experiments at Willowbrook State School and the testing of the live-virus polio vaccine at Letchworth Village—both facilities for children with cognitive and physical disabilities. In general, children's vulnerability is also physical: their immune systems are immature, particularly in infancy and young childhood, and treatments may have long-term consequences on developing bodies that are unpredictable or insufficiently studied.

That last vulnerability provides a justification for experimenting on children. Children's experience of illness and injury does not mimic how those conditions show up in adults, and the treatments (including medications) that address those conditions in adults do not always have the same effects in children. Therefore, significant elements of pediatric healthcare cannot be extrapolated from research conducted with adults (Fleischman 2016, 197). For these reasons, pediatric research has been authorized by institutional review boards, but with heightened regulation in comparison to research on adults.

Following the principles in the Belmont Report, the Department of Health and Human Services (HHS) adopted the policy for the Protection of Human Subjects (45 CFR 46). Subpart D governs research involving children. It distinguishes **therapeutic research** (in which there is some likelihood that participating will benefit the child's health) from **nontherapeutic research** (in which there is little or no likely contribution to their well-being) (§ 46.405). According to these regulations, pediatric research in the U.S. must conform to the following four standards:

1. Nontherapeutic research is justifiable if it carries no more than minimal risk for children. Institutional review boards must consider both psychological and physical risks. **Minimal risk** means that study participants will encounter no more "probability and magnitude of harm or discomfort" than healthy children encounter in everyday activities, assuming they live in safe environments (§ 46.102). Examples include vision screening, classroom observation, or asking children to make minor changes to their activity levels and recording the effects on their mood.

2. More than minimal risk is justified if there is a reasonable likelihood of direct health benefits to the child. The risk must be balanced against the anticipated benefit: a risk of permanent injury cannot be justified by a minor health benefit (§ 46.405). An example of such research would be a child participating in a clinical trial for a new medication that has already proven effective in adults when existing medications are ineffective. Most clinical trials belong in this category.

3. More than minimal risk may be justified if it does not significantly increase the medical risks the child already faces, as long as there is generalizable knowledge to be gained (§ 46.406). For example, a child whose therapeutic treatment already requires repeated blood draws or tissue samples may have additional blood draws or tissue samples used purely for research—assuming that these additional samples do not pose much additional risk.

4. Research that poses more than a minor increase over minimal risk (that is, beyond what is covered by categories one to three) may be approved if it "presents [the] opportunity to understand, prevent, or alleviate a serious problem affecting the health or welfare of children." Research proposals in this category are reviewed not only by institutional review boards but also by a panel of experts from HHS (§ 46.407). Such research is rarely approved.

The key terms "minimal" and "minor" are open to interpretation and judgment by institutional review boards. In all four categories, the child's assent and the parent or guardian's permission are required. If a parent agrees but a child capable of assent does not, the minor's dissent is respected unless there is evidence of direct benefit that can only be obtained through participating in the study. Minors are defined as anyone under eighteen, with one exception: if the research concerns only treatments for which minors can give consent in their particular jurisdiction (according to the state's mature minor laws), they can consent for themselves (§ 46.402). Children who are wards—that is, institutionalized—can only serve as research subjects if the research is related to their status as wards, if they are studied alongside a majority of children who are not wards, and if permission has been given by an advocate appointed to consider the children's best interests (§ 46.409).

With the third and fourth categories, the idea is that future children will benefit from risks to the present children participating in research. On the one hand, this seems legitimate, given that today's children benefit from risks encountered by previous generations (e.g., polio vaccines). On the other hand, the Nuremberg Code and the Belmont Report forbid sacrificing anyone for the well-being of others. Some bioethicists, such as Paul Ramsey (2002), have argued that children should only be enrolled in therapeutic research. If there is no benefit for them as patients, parental permission for children is insufficient: "No parent is morally competent to consent that his child shall be submitted to hazardous or other experiments having no diagnostic or therapeutic significance for this child himself" (Ramsey 2002, 13). Parents may be enticed to have their children participate in research with financial incentives, which may include not only compensation for out-of-pocket expenses (such as transportation) but also "appreciation" for the parents' inconvenience. Under these circumstances, parental permission—especially when minors will be exposed to more than minimal risk, and especially when minors cannot themselves participate meaningfully in assenting—raises more complex issues than first-person consent:

> The history of research in the US should invest all who perform research involving children with a strong sense of humility, serving to remind us how easily the frail balance between the social value of involving children in research and the protection of children from unnecessary harms can be tipped by utilitarian thinking. Although the future health of children is dependent on the performance of clinical research in which children participate, research must be carefully designed to assure that the participants are not placed at excessive risk or denied potential benefits unfairly. (Diekema 2006, S11)

Ethical questions concerning pediatric research often have us weigh the well-being and autonomy of an individual child against the well-being of children in general, including future children. In Kantian terms, should we, or when should we, treat children as a means to promote the health of other children?

## Race and Pediatric Ethics

Bioethicists should note that patients and research subjects are not generic persons. They have identities relating to gender, race, class, religion, citizenship status, sexual orientation, disability, and so on. And those identities impact their social interactions, including in the healthcare system. So too pediatric patients and research subjects are not generic children. Childhood is a medically and socially vulnerable stage of development, but some populations of children encounter intensified vulnerability because of socially contingent hierarchies. For instance, in the middle of the twentieth century, institutionalized children with cognitive disabilities were convenient research subjects in experiments that have since been condemned as unethical. Their institutionalization, the social stigma attached to cognitive disabilities, and the paternalistic assumption that medical authorities were best positioned to make decisions about their well-being sheltered these experiments from critical judgment for many decades. Only recently have bioethical and legal discussions paid more attention to how the principles of respect for autonomy and beneficence apply to children as an overall population and to people with disabilities. In this section, we focus primarily on the impact of race in pediatric ethics, but there is philosophical work to do in analyzing how a range of identity factors affect the experience of children in the healthcare system and how those factors intersect with each other.

As we discussed in the previous chapter, in comparison to whites, people of color in the U.S. experience significant differences in treatment and disparities in health outcomes. These differences also apply to children, especially Black and Native American children. These differences span ordinary forms of care, such as preventive services, and extraordinary ones, such as organ transplants. Glenn Flores's review of the relevant literature between 1950 and March 2007 found:

Racial/ethnic disparities in children's health and health care are quite extensive, pervasive, and persistent. Disparities were noted across the spectrum of health and health care, including in mortality rates, access to care and use of services, prevention and population health, health status, adolescent health, chronic diseases, special health care needs, quality of care, and organ transplantation. (2010, e979).

These differences begin before birth: while 82.8 percent of non-Hispanic white mothers and 82.4 percent of Asian mothers receive prenatal care in the first trimester, only 72.3 percent of Hispanic mothers, 68.4 percent of Black mothers, 64 percent of American Indian or Alaska Native mothers, and 51.9 percent of Native Hawaiian or other Pacific Islander mothers do (Osterman et al. 2022). Preterm births, which are associated with a whole spectrum of poorer health outcomes throughout a person's life, are also higher for Black and Indigenous infants. Infant mortality rates align with this pattern as well: in 2021, per 1,000 live births, fewer than 5 infants die before their first birthday for whites, Asians, and Hispanics, but 7.5 for American Indians or Alaska Natives, 7.8 for Native Hawaiians or other Pacific Islanders, and 10.6 for Black Americans (Xu et al. 2022). As key indicators of race-based healthcare injustice,

> mortality-rate disparities were noted for children in all 4 major US racial/ethnic minority groups, including substantially greater risks than white children of all-cause mortality; death from drowning, from acute lymphoblastic leukemia, and after congenital heart defect surgery; and an earlier median age at death for those with Down syndrome and congenital heart defects. (Flores 2010, e979)

Between 2014 and 2020, the death rate among Black children rose by 37 percent and among Native American children by 22 percent, compared to a 5 percent increase for white children, mostly due to injuries from car accidents, homicides, and suicides (Wolf et al. 2024). Outside of the stark differences in mortality, Black children are prescribed significantly less effective pain medication (Goyal et al. 2015) and fewer antibiotics (Gerber et al. 2013), and they receive less counseling during well-child visits (Hambidge et al. 2007).

These racial disparities are likely to result from systemic injustices that curtail access to quality healthcare as well as implicit biases on the part of clinicians (Lang et al. 2016). For instance, families of racial/ethnic minorities with children in pediatric intensive care units are more likely to report "feeling unheard" and to experience feelings of discrimination than white families (DeLemos et al. 2010). Racially disparate health outcomes thus should be understood in the context of families' lack of trust in the healthcare system and their clinicians. Whether it is experienced within healthcare institutions or outside of them, racism functions as a health stressor: weathering affects children of color as well (Pachter and Coll 2009; Sabin and Greenwald 2012, 992). Resolving these issues means considering carefully how pediatric ethics intersects with medical racism more generally, how children who are part of marginalized families inherit those vulnerabilities, and how to mitigate those harms both individually and collectively.

## End-of-Life Care

As with adults, questions around end-of-life care in pediatric settings are among the most charged. When is it in the patient's best interests to pursue treatment, and when is it better to focus instead on the reduction of suffering? In pediatric ethics, an additional dimension of this question is that parents or other family members may be in denial that the child is at the end of their life and hence may demand treatments that are medically futile and/or cause unnecessary suffering. They may also attempt to hide the seriousness of the medical condition from the child themselves. Both reactions have their origin in reasonable parental impulses: to protect children from harm and not to abandon them, and to protect them from psychological distress. But those reactions may also interfere with the child's well-being and in fact be at odds with their own understanding of the situation and sense of their needs. Even well-intentioned dishonesty is likely to be harmful: "Deception does not succeed in keeping out the fears of sickness and death. It only succeeds in keeping out the loved ones, who could have helped them deal with the fears" (Cassidy 1996, 76). Not disclosing details about their diagnosis, treatment, and prognosis does not protect children from distress (Claflin and Barbarin 1991).

Like other forms of palliative treatment, pediatric end-of-life care should focus on what is valuable to the minor patient. Pediatric palliative care tends to focus on symptom management, as opposed to merely pain relief, because it often deals with terminal genetic conditions that have a prognosis of years rather than months. Decisions should not exclusively focus on the child's present or future well-being (as interpreted by parents or clinicians) but on their emerging autonomy. Even young children can understand their medical situation and express their preferences, which should be taken seriously in the decision-making process.

The family also needs to be supported in their process of grieving, which may begin with the realization that the child is dying. A purely medical focus itself can cause distress during a family's crisis: "Continued focus solely on treatment can deflect the child and the family from integrating the reality of the impending death, and can increase the child's suffering" (Fleischman 2016, 115). Clinicians must leave room for and support psychosocial engagements that promote both the pediatric patient's and the family's well-being. The family may be experiencing fear for their child's health or mental state, stress about how to care for other children, or financial anxiety, all of which may impair their ability to engage in autonomous decision-making. Trusting relationships with clinicians may alleviate some of these emotional challenges.

## Conclusion: Respect for Emerging Autonomy

With the contemporary emphasis on respect for autonomy, healthcare professionals and caregivers have to do the complex work of applying that principle to patients and research subjects who are in the process of becoming adults. The principles of nonmaleficence and beneficence carry more weight than they do with adult patients, but consideration must also be paid to the future or emerging autonomy of the infant, young child, or adolescent. Justice too enters into these discussions insofar as children's health outcomes largely reflect the social hierarchies in which their families are embedded. With pediatric patients, clinicians need to pay greater attention to their role as advocates, which sometimes means challenging and negotiating with families, and sometimes means addressing the wider social environment in which such patients live.

Some of the complexities around pediatric ethics also help to attune caregivers to issues that may be significant with any patient, including people experiencing new or chronic illness or disability, people negatively impacted by the social determinants of health, and other people with diminished autonomy. These factors include how a patient is positioned within a family and community, how a patient's autonomous capacities shift over the course of an illness, how to communicate with patients with limited language or cognitive abilities, how to earn a patient's trust, and how to destigmatize or otherwise reduce shame for behaviors or conditions that are socially proscribed. In many ways, the issues that arise in pediatric ethics are amplifications and extensions of the core issues of medical ethics more generally.

## REFERENCES

American Psychiatric Association. 1980. *Diagnostic and Statistical Manual of Mental Disorders: DSM-III*. Arlington, VA: American Psychiatric Association.
———. 2013. *Diagnostic and Statistical Manual of Mental Disorders: DSM-5*. Arlington, VA: American Psychiatric Association.
Austin, Ashley, Shelley L. Craig, Sandra D'Souza, and Lauren B. McInroy. 2022. "Suicidality among Transgender Youth: Elucidating the Role of Interpersonal Risk Factors." *Journal of Interpersonal Violence* 37, nos. 5–6 (March): NP2696–718. doi:10.1177/0886260520915554.
Bester, Johan C. 2018. "Not a Matter of Parental Choice but of Social Justice Obligation: Children Are Owed Measles Vaccination." *Bioethics* 32, no. 9 (November): 611–19. doi:10.1111/bioe.12511.
Carel, Havi, and Gita Györffy. 2014. "Seen but Not Heard: Children and Epistemic Injustice." *Lancet* 384, no. 9950 (October 4): 1256–57. doi:10.1016/s0140-6736(14)61759-1.
Cassidy, Robert C. 1996. "Tell All the Truth? Shepherds, Liberators, or Educators." In *Pediatric Ethics: From Principles to Practice*, edited by Robert C. Cassidy and Alan R. Fleischman, 67–82. Amsterdam: Harwood Academic.
Claflin, Carol J., and Oscar A. Barbarin. 1991. "Does 'Telling' Less Protect More? Relationships among Age, Information Disclosure, and What Children with Cancer See and Feel." *Journal of Pediatric Psychology* 16, no. 2 (April): 169–91. doi:10.1093/jpepsy/16.2.169.
Clark, Beth A., and Alice Virani. 2021. "'This Wasn't a Split-Second Decision': An Empirical Ethical Analysis of Transgender Youth Capacity, Rights, and Authority to Consent to Hormone Therapy." *Journal of Bioethical Inquiry* 18, no. 1 (March): 151–64. doi:10.1007/s11673-020-10086-9.
Coleman, E., A. E. Radix, W. P. Bouman, G. R. Brown, A. L. C. de Vries, M. B. Deutsch, et al. 2022. "Standards of Care for the Health of Transgender and Gender Diverse People, Version 8." *International Journal of Transgender Health* 23, no. S1: S1–259. doi:10.1080/26895269.2022.2100644.

Committee on Bioethics, American Academy of Pediatrics. 1995. "Informed Consent, Parental Permission, and Assent in Pediatric Practice." *Pediatrics* 95, no. 2 (February): 314–17. doi:10.1542/peds.95.2.314.

Committee on Clinical Research Involving Children. 2004. "Understanding and Agreeing to Children's Participation in Clinical Research." In *The Ethical Conduct of Clinical Research Involving Children*, edited by Marilyn J. Field and Richard E. Berman, 146–210. Washington, DC: National Academies Press. https://www.ncbi.nlm.nih.gov/books/NBK25560/.

De Vries, Annelou L. C., Jenifer K. McGuire, Thomas D. Steensma, Eva C. F. Wagenaar, Theo A. H. Doreleijers, and Peggy T. Cohen-Kettenis. 2014. "Young Adult Psychological Outcome after Puberty Suppression and Gender Reassignment." *Pediatrics* 134, no. 4 (October): 696–704. doi:10.1542/peds.2013-2958.

DeLemos, Destinee, Minna Chen, Amy Romer, Kyla Brydon, Kathleen Kastner, Benjamin Anthony, and K. Sarah Hoehn. 2010. "Building Trust through Communication in the Intensive Care Unit." *Pediatric Critical Care Medicine* 11, no. 3 (May): 378–84. doi:10.1097/PCC.0b013e3181b8088b.

DeStefano, Frank, and Tom T. Shimabukuro. 2019. "The MMR Vaccine and Autism." *Annual Review of Virology* 6: 585–600. doi:10.1146/annurev-virology-092818-015515.

Diekema, Douglas S. 2004. "Parental Refusals of Medical Treatment: The Harm Principle as Threshold for State Intervention." *Theoretical Medicine and Bioethics* 25, no. 4 (July): 243–64. doi:10.1007/s11017-004-3146-6.

———. 2006. "Conducting Ethical Research in Pediatrics: A Brief Historical Overview and Review of Pediatric Regulations." In "Current Controversies in Pediatric Research Ethics," edited by Douglas S. Diekema. Supplement, *Journal of Pediatrics* 149, no. S1 (July): S3–11. doi:10.1016/j.jpeds.2006.04.043.

Dreger, Alice Domurat. 2006. "Intersex and Human Rights: The Long View." In *Ethics and Intersex*, edited by Sharon Sytsma, 73–86. Dordrecht: Springer. doi:10.1007/1-4220-4314-7_4.

Dreger, Alice D., and David Sandberg. 2010. "Disorders of Sex Development." In *Pediatric Bioethics*, edited by Geoffrey Miller, 149–62. Cambridge: Cambridge University Press. doi:10.1017/CBO9780511642388.012.

Dubin, Samuel, Megan Lane, Shane Morrison, Asa Radix, Uri Belkind, Christian Vercler, and David Inwards-Breland. 2020. "Medically Assisted Gender Affirmation: When Children and Parents Disagree." *Journal of Medical Ethics* 46, no. 5 (May): 295–99. doi:10.1136/medethics-2019-105567.

Dustin, Moira. 2010. "Female Genital Mutilation/Cutting in the UK: Challenging the Inconsistencies." *European Journal of Women's Studies* 17, no. 1 (February): 7–23. doi:10.1177/1350506809350857.

Dworkin, Gerald. 1982. "Consent, Representation, and Proxy Consent." In *Who Speaks for the Child: The Problems of Proxy Consent*, edited by Willard Gaylin and Ruth Macklin, 191–208. New York: Plenum.

Earp, Brian D. 2015. "Female Genital Mutilation and Male Circumcision: Toward an Autonomy-Based Ethical Framework." *Medicolegal and Bioethics* 5: 89–104. doi:10.2147/MB.S63709.

Emanuel, Ezekiel J. 1987. "A Communal Vision of Care for Incompetent Patients." *Hastings Center Report* 17, no. 5 (October–November): 15–20. doi:10.2307/3562665.

Feinberg, Joel. 1980. "The Child's Right to an Open Future." In *Whose Child? Children's Rights, Parental Authority, and State Power*, edited by William Aiken and Hugh LaFollette, 124–53. Totowa, NJ: Rowman and Littlefield.

Feldman, Sharon, and Thomas Dreyfus. 2017. "Whose Consent Is It Anyway? A Transgender Child's Right to Transition." *Voices in Bioethics* 3. https://journals.library.columbia.edu/index.php/bioethics/article/view/6025.

Fleischman, Alan R. 2016. *Pediatric Ethics: Protecting the Interests of Children*. New York: Oxford University Press. doi:10.1093/med/9780199354474.001.0001.

Flores, Glenn. 2010. "Racial and Ethnic Disparities in the Health and Health Care of Children." *Pediatrics* 125, no. 4 (April): e979–1020. doi:10.1542/peds.2010-0188.

García-Acero, Mary, Olga Moreno, Fernando Suárez, and Adriana Rojas. 2020. "Disorders of Sexual Development: Current Status and Progress in the Diagnostic Approach." *Current Urology* 13, no. 4 (January): 169–78. doi:10.1159/000499274.

Gardner, Melissa, and David E. Sandberg. 2018. "Navigating Surgical Decision Making in Disorders of Sex Development (DSD)." *Frontiers in Pediatrics* 6 (November): article no. 339. doi:10.3389/fped.2018.00339.

Gerber, Jeffrey S., Priya A. Prasad, A. Russell Localio, Alexander G. Fiks, Robert W. Grundmeier, Louis M. Bell, Richard C. Wasserman, David M. Rubin, Ron Keren, and Theoklis E. Zaoutis. 2013. "Racial Differences in Antibiotic Prescribing by Primary Care Pediatricians." *Pediatrics* 131, no. 4 (April): 677–84. doi:10.1542/peds.2012-2500.

Giordano, Simona. 2023. *Children and Gender: Ethical Issues in Clinical Management of Transgender and Gender Diverse Youth, from Early Years to Late Adolescence*. New York: Oxford University Press. doi:10.1093/oso/9780192895400.001.0001.

Goyal, Monika K., Nathan Kuppermann, Sean D. Cleary, Stephen J. Teach, and James M. Chamberlain. 2015. "Racial Disparities in Pain Management of Children with Appendicitis in Emergency Departments." *JAMA Pediatrics* 169, no. 11 (November): 996–1002. doi:10.1001/jamapediatrics.2015.1915.

Grisso, Thomas, and Linda Vierling. 1978. "Minors' Consent to Treatment: A Developmental Perspective." *Professional Psychology* 9, no. 3 (August): 412–27. doi:10.1037/0735-7028.9.3.412.

Hajek, André, Hans-Helmut König, Elzbieta Buczak-Stec, Marco Blessmann, and Katharina Grupp. 2023. "Prevalence and Determinants of Depressive and Anxiety Symptoms among Transgender People: Results of a Survey." *Health Care* 11, no. 5 (February): article no. 705. doi:10.3390/healthcare11050705.

Hambidge, Simon J., Caroline Bublitz Emsermann, Steven Federico, and John F. Steiner. 2007. "Disparities in Pediatric Preventive Care in the United States, 1993–2002." *Archives of Pediatric and Adolescent Medicine* 161, no. 1 (January 1): 30–36. doi:10.1001/archpedi.161.1.30.

Hughes, Landon D., Brittany M. Charlton, Isa Berzansky, and Jae D. Corman. 2025. "Gender-Affirming Medications among Transgender Adolescents in the US, 2018–2022." *JAMA Pediatrics* 179, no. 3 (January 6): 342–44. doi:10.1001/jamapediatrics.2024.6081.

*Independent Review of Gender Identity Services for Children and Young People: Final Report (The Cass Review)*. 2024. NHS England. April. https://cass.independent-review.uk/wp-content/uploads/2024/04/CassReview_Final.pdf.

Katz, Aviva L., Sally A. Webb, Robert C. Macauley, Mark R. Mercurio, Margaret R. Moon, Alexander L. Okun, Douglas J. Opel, and Mindy B. Statter. 2016. "Informed Consent in Decision-Making in Pediatric Practice." *Pediatrics* 138, no. 2 (August): e20161485. doi:10.1542/peds.2016-1485.

Kavanaugh, Jennifer. 2021. "How Truth Decay Is Fueling Vaccine Hesitancy." *Rand Blog*. May 14. https://www.rand.org/pubs/commentary/2021/05/how-truth-decay-is-fueling-vaccine-hesitancy.html.

Kipnis, Kenneth, and Milton Diamond. 1998. "Pediatric Ethics and the Surgical Assignment of Sex." *Journal of Clinical Ethics* 9, no. 4 (Winter): 398–410. doi:10.1086/JCE199809409.

Lang, Kellie R., Claretta Y. Dupree, Alexander A. Kon, and Denise M. Dudzinski. 2016. "Calling Out Implicit Racial Bias as a Harm in Pediatric Care." *Cambridge Quarterly of Health Care Ethics* 25, no. 3 (July): 540–52. doi:10.1017/S0963180116000190.

Malek, Janet. 2009. "What Really Is in a Child's Best Interest? Toward a More Precise Picture of the Interests of Children." *Journal of Clinical Ethics* 20, no. 2 (Summer): 175–82. doi:10.1086/JCE200920212.

Miller, Richard B. 2003. *Children, Ethics, and Modern Medicine*. Bloomington: Indiana University Press.

Miller, Victoria A., and Robert M. Nelson. 2006. "A Developmental Approach to Child Assent for Nontherapeutic Research." In "Current Controversies in Pediatric Research Ethics," edited by Douglas S. Diekema. Supplement, *Journal of Pediatrics* 149, no. S1 (July): S25–30. doi:10.1016/j.jpeds.2006.04.047.

Moore, Bryanna, and Rosalind McDougall. 2022. "Exploring the Ethics of the Parental Role in Parent-Clinician Conflict." *Hastings Center Report* 52, no. 6 (November–December): 33–43. doi:10.1002/hast.1445.

Moreno, Jonathan D., and Alexandra Kravitt. 2010. "The Ethics of Pediatric Research." In *Pediatric Bioethics*, edited by Geoffrey Miller, 54–72. Cambridge: Cambridge University Press. doi:10.1017/CBO9780511642388.006.

Osterman, Michelle J. K., Brady E. Hamilton, Joyce A. Martin, Anne K. Driscoll, and Claudia P. Valenzuela. 2022. "Births: Final Data for 2020." *National Vital Statistics Reports* 70, no. 17 (February 7). https://stacks.cdc.gov/view/cdc/112078.

Pachter, Lee M., and Cynthia García Coll. 2009. "Racism and Child Health: A Review of the Literature and Future Directions." *Journal of Developmental and Behavioral Pediatrics* 30, no. 3 (June): 255–63. doi:10.1097/DBP.0b013e3181a7ed5a.

Pandey, Abhishek, and Alison P. Galvani. 2023. "Exacerbation of Measles Mortality by Vaccine Hesitancy Worldwide." *Lancet Global Health* 11, no. 4 (April): E478–79. doi:10.1016/S2214-109X(23)00063-3.

Pelias, Mary Kay Z. n.d. "Informed Consent for Newborn Screening & Future Uses of Tissue Samples." Eunice Kennedy Shriver National Institute of Child Health and Human Development. Accessed January 15, 2025. https://www.nichd.nih.gov/publications/pubs/pku/sub13.

President's Commission for the Study of Ethical Problems in Medicine and Biomedical and Behavioral Research. 1983. *Deciding to Forego Life-Sustaining Treatment*. Washington, DC: U.S. Government Printing Office. https://repository.library.georgetown.edu/bitstream/handle/10822/559344/deciding_to_forego_tx.pdf.

Ramsey, Paul. 2002. *The Patient as Person: Explorations in Medical Ethics*. 2nd ed. New Haven, CT: Yale University Press.

Razzell, Peter E. 1977. *The Conquest of Smallpox*. Sussex: Caliban.

Ross, Lainie Friedman. 2007. "The Moral Status of the Newborn and Its Implications for Medical Decision Making." *Theoretical Medicine and Bioethics* 28, no. 5 (October): 349–55. doi:10.1007/s11017-007-9045-x.

Sabin, Janice A., and Anthony G. Greenwald. 2012. "The Influence of Implicit Bias on Treatment Recommendations for 4 Common Pediatric Conditions: Pain, Urinary Tract Infection, Attention Deficit Hyperactivity Disorder, and Asthma." *American Journal of Public Health* 102, no. 5 (May): 988–95. doi:10.2105/AJPH.2011.300621.

Schachter, Debbie, Irwin Kleinman, and William Harvey. 2005. "Informed Consent and Adolescents." *Canadian Journal of Psychiatry* 50, no. 9 (August): 534–40. doi:10.1177/070674370505000906.

Shen, Shixin Cindy, and Vinita Dubey. 2019. "Addressing Vaccine Hesitancy: Clinical Guidance for Primary Care Physicians Working with Parents." *Canadian Family Physician/Médecin de Famille Canadien* 65, no. 3 (March): 175–81. https://www.cfp.ca/content/65/3/175.

Spriggs, Merle. 2023. "Children and Bioethics: Clarifying Consent and Assent in Medical and Research Settings." *British Medical Bulletin* 145, no. 1 (March): 110–19. doi:10.1093/bmb/ldac038.

Weithorn, Lois A., and Susan B. Campbell. 1982. "The Competency of Children and Adolescents to Make Informed Treatment Decisions." *Child Development* 53, no. 6 (December): 1589–98. doi:10.2307/1130087.

Wiesemann, Claudia, Susanne Ude-Koeller, Gernot H. G. Sinnecker, and Ute Thyen. 2010. "Ethical Principles and Recommendations for the Medical Management of Differences of Sex Development (DSD)/Intersex in Children and Adolescents." *European Journal of Pediatrics* 169, no. 6 (June): 671–79. doi:10.1007/s00431-009-1086-x.

Witchel, Selma Feldman. 2018. "Disorders of Sex Development." *Best Practice & Research Clinical Obstetrics & Gynaecology* 48 (April): 90–102. doi:10.1016/j.bpobgyn.2017.11.005.

Wolf, Elizabeth R., Frederick P. Rivara, Colin J. Orr, Anabeel Sen, Derek A. Chapman, and Steven H. Woolf. 2024. "Racial and Ethnic Disparities in All-Cause and Cause-Specific Mortality among US Youth." *JAMA: Journal of the American Medical Association* 331, no. 20 (May 28): 1732–40. doi:10.1001/jama.2024.3908.

Woolley, S. 2005. "Children of Jehovah's Witnesses and Adolescent Jehovah's Witnesses: What Are Their Rights?" *Archives of Disease in Childhood* 90, no. 7 (July): 715–19. doi:10.1136/adc.2004.067843.

World Health Organization. 2019. *International Statistical Classification of Diseases and Related Health Problems*. 11th ed. https://icd.who.int/en.

Xu, Jiaquan, Sherry L. Murphy, Kenneth D. Kochanek, and Elizabeth Arias. 2022. "Mortality in the United States, 2021." NCHS Data Brief, No. 456. December. https://www.cdc.gov/nchs/data/databriefs/db456.pdf.

## Further Reading

Bavdekar, Sandeep B. 2013. "Pediatric Clinical Trials." *Perspectives in Clinical Research* 4, no. 1 (January–March): 89–99. doi:10.4103/2229-3485.106403.

Discusses the historical context for regulating medical research with pediatric subjects and the contemporary need for further clinical trials of pharmaceuticals for children. Bavdekar argues that certain kinds of medications should be prioritized for clinical trials and outlines the safeguards that will minimize risk to research subjects. The article also covers a range of issues related to pediatric research: parental permission and pediatric assent, financial incentives for research participants, effective and just recruitment strategies, and emergency and neonatal research.

Brierley, Joe, Jim Linthicum, and Andy Petros. 2013. "Should Religious Beliefs Be Allowed to Stonewall a Secular Approach to Withdrawing and Withholding Treatment in Children?" *Journal of Medical Ethics* 39, no. 9 (September): 573–77. doi:10.1136/medethics-2011-100104.

Reviews cases in the United Kingdom over a three-year period in which physicians recommended ceasing "aggressive" or "invasive" treatments for children on the grounds that they were medically futile. The authors specifically focus on cases in which parents opposed the withdrawal of such treatments because of religious beliefs in divine intervention—that children should be kept alive to allow time for a miraculous cure, for instance. The article describes the resolution of these cases through reconciliation among clinicians, parents, and ethics committees; in discussions with religious leaders; or through legal proceedings.

Etchegary, Holly, Stuart G. Nicholls, Laure Tessier, Charlene Simmonds, Beth K. Potter, Jamie C. Brehaut, and Daryl Pullman. 2016. "Consent for Newborn Screening: Parents' and Health-Care Professionals' Experiences of Consent in Practice." *European Journal of Human Genetics* 24, no. 11 (November): 1530–34. doi:10.1038/ejhg.2016.55.

Reports on a qualitative study done in two Canadian provinces with parents of newborns offered newborn screenings (a bloodspot taken by a heel prick) and healthcare professionals involved in those screenings. Such screenings are often presented as routine treatment of newborns rather than requiring an explicit informed consent process. The authors recommend that more substantive information be provided to parents at a time when they can absorb it, and that the consent process be taken seriously.

Feder, Ellen. 2014. *Making Sense of Intersex: Changing Ethical Perspectives in Biomedicine*. Bloomington: Indiana University Press.

Provides historical context of how intersex has been understood and addressed. Feder enriches the standard ethical debates around autonomy and beneficence by using a wider range of philosophical lenses—including feminist, virtue ethicist, and Foucauldian approaches—to understand the experiences of intersex children and their parents.

Griffith, Richard. 2016. "What Is Gillick Competence?" *Human Vaccines & Immunotherapies* 12, no. 1 (January): 244–47. doi:10.1080/21645515.2015.1091548.

> In 1986, a court in the United Kingdom found that children under sixteen could consent to medical treatment if they met minimum requirements for competence. This has come to be known as the Gillick competence standard, which assesses the child's ability to understand medical information, considers long-term risks and benefits of medical treatments, and separates their judgment from external sources of pressure. Griffith illustrates this concept by applying it to decisions around immunization.

Horowicz, Edmund. 2019. "Transgender Adolescents and Genital-Alignment Surgery: Is Age Restriction Justified?" *Clinical Ethics* 14, no. 2 (June): 94–103. doi:10.1177/1477750919844508.

> Argues that the current recommendation to delay genital-alignment surgery until the age of majority (eighteen)—which is the standard medical recommendation and, in some jurisdictions, a legal requirement—is unjustified. The surgical risks and risks around regret or evolving gender identity are outweighed by the need to respect the autonomy and protect the well-being of capable adolescents.

Kittay, Eva Feder. 2011. "Forever Small: The Strange Case of Ashley X." *Hypatia* 26, no. 3 (Summer): 610–31. doi:10.1111/j.1527-2001.2011.01205.x.

> In 2002, the parents of a prepubescent girl with severe cognitive and physical disabilities had doctors remove her uterus and breast buds, and administered high doses of estrogen to stunt her growth so that she could be more easily cared for. Kittay discusses this case in relation to her own experience as the parent of an adult child with disabilities. She draws on care ethics to argue against the core assumptions justifying the Ashley Treatment—for instance, that the body and its growth are irrelevant to a person's identity.

Nortjé, Nico, and Johan C. Bester, eds. 2022. *Pediatric Ethics: Theory and Practice*. Cham: Springer. doi:10.1007/978-3-030-86182-7.

> Discusses the theoretical principles behind pediatric ethics and applies those principles to case studies on a range of issues, including immunizations, access to healthcare, and end-of-life care. Written primarily for clinicians, contributors propose guidelines for how clinicians, children, and family members can engage in moral deliberation, and they emphasize how pediatric ethics involves complex relations among those roles as well as the state.

Weaver, Meaghann S., Shiven Sharma, and Jennifer K. Walter. 2023. "Pediatric Ethics Consultation Services, Scope, and Staffing." *Pediatrics* 151, no. 3 (March): e2022058999. doi:10.1542/peds.2022-058999.
> Study of pediatric ethics consultations at U.S. children's hospitals that surveyed how such consultations are supported and for what sorts of issues such consultations are requested. Many children's hospitals have minimal support for ethics programs. Consultations were most frequently requested for moral distress among clinicians, end-of-life issues, when the risks or burdens outweighed the benefits, conflicts between parents and clinicians, and questions around autonomy.

Wendler, David. 2010. *The Ethics of Pediatric Research*. New York: Oxford University Press. doi:10.1093/acprof:oso/9780199730087.001.0001.
> Explores the core dilemma of pediatric research: that biomedical research depends on nontherapeutic experimentation, but also that children incapable of consent should not be exploited for the benefit of others. Wendler evaluates various arguments addressing this dilemma and offers an original approach by emphasizing what children may gain (within the bounds of minimized risk and a compelling justification for each specific study) by knowing that they are contributing to the well-being of others.

# CHAPTER 13
# Nursing Ethics

**Key topics in this chapter:**
- Why a distinct focus on nursing ethics is necessary
- Gender norms, physician authority, and the historical subordination of nurses
- The concept of care and how it informs nurses' obligations
- The significance of nurses' perspectives for applying the four principles
- Nurses' experience of moral distress and how to address it

## Introduction

The very phrase "nursing ethics" may raise the question of why a separate discussion of ethics in the nursing profession is necessary. Nurses face the same moral issues as other healthcare practitioners. Their actions are also governed by the same overarching principles. The International Council of Nurses (ICN) Code of Ethics (2021) clearly expresses adherence to the principles of respect for autonomy, nonmaleficence, beneficence, and justice. However, studying ethical practice for nurses affords us insight into the institutional context in which medicine is lived out. Nurses have traditionally been expected to focus on the immediate *care* of patients—attending to basic needs such as food and hygiene, managing symptoms, and administering medication—whereas physicians have focused on *cure*—diagnosing the cause of symptoms, presenting treatment options, and then providing specialized treatment. In contemporary practice, these functions of care and cure cannot be cleanly delineated, but the history of the two professions remains influential. That history also continues to shape clinical decision-making and patient interactions. Although nurses spend more time with patients and have a wider view of the social and interpersonal dynamics that impact patients' health, nurses tend to have less epistemic authority than physicians, even regarding moral (as opposed to technical) issues. In sum, the distinctive perspective of nursing work has the potential to shift how the basic principles of medical ethics are interpreted and applied. The issues germane to nursing ethics provoke us to reflect on the purposes of medicine and how different clinicians should collaborate to fulfill those purposes.

## The Gendered History of Nursing

The term "nurse" derives from the Latin word for nourishment, and specifically a feminine form (*nutricia*) of *nutricius*, "a person who nourishes." This explains the additional denotation of breastfeeding (or nursing) infants. It also emphasizes the deeply gendered history of nursing in Western cultures. Women have been seen as uniquely capable, at a biological level, of caring for children and, by extension, others who are physically vulnerable—the disabled, the injured, the elderly, and those who are pregnant and bear children. Women have also been seen as uniquely capable of such care at both a psychological and emotional level. This means that nursing care has often been culturally interpreted as instinctive or intuitive rather than requiring the cultivation of any particular skill. At least the core traits of nursing were understood to belong to the nature of femininity itself, although specific skills such as wound dressing must be taught (Kuhse 1997, 16). Even breastfeeding in contemporary culture is frequently described as natural and instinctive, although new parents know it takes practice, patience, and support to develop successful breastfeeding routines. So too nursing as a profession has historically been described as an extension of femininity, exhibiting the virtues of gentleness, emotional care, concern for each patient as a singular person, provision of physical comfort, and self-sacrifice.

Florence Nightingale and other leaders in the establishment of the modern nursing profession tended to use these associations to legitimate the participation of (largely single) women in education and then employment in the public sphere, primarily in military and civilian hospitals. The reasoning was that these activities did not radically overturn the "angel of the hearth" image of femininity but extended it in ways that supported traditionally masculine pursuits. The nurse-patient relationship would thus be understood through the frame of the mother-child relationship: in their vulnerability, the patient has returned to a state of childlike dependence, which may be psychological as well as physical. And that relationship is governed by the judgments of paternal figures.

In medieval Europe, the earliest hospitals were founded by religious orders. The word "hospital" derives from charitable institutions that would provide medical care for the sick and basic needs (shelter and food) for the poor (*hospes*, Latin for "host"). Monks and nuns offered these services as spiritual, ascetic practices that renounced self-interested activity to care for others, including those suffering from leprosy or bubonic plague (Kuhse 1997, 13–33; Wall, n.d.). Modern nursing also was deeply influenced by its usefulness in military settings—for example, Florence Nightingale's work in the Crimean War or Clara Barton's work in the American Civil War, the Franco-Prussian War, and the Spanish-American War. This historical trajectory illuminates how nursing continues to be understood and practiced: nurses follow the orders of physicians in a shared battle waged against infection, injury, and death (Kuhse 1997, 22–23).

The militaristic model of nursing seems to be at odds with the maternal and religious models, but all three emphasize the virtues of obedience to authority, discipline, and self-sacrifice. As Helga Kuhse argues, they share

> the notion that the nurse is not autonomous or self-determining, but in one way or another subservient—to God, if her role is seen as that of a nun or religious ascetic; to a military authority, if her role is regarded as that of a soldier fighting disease; to a husband or father if her role is seen as that of a wife and mother in a patriarchal family; to a master if her role is seen as that of a domestic servant; and to the physician if her role is equated with that of doctor's handmaiden. (1997, 17)

The content of nursing ethics has thus been often reduced to the image of the "good nurse," defined through these various roles of gendered subordination. The social and institutional hierarchies that have been historically created between physicians and nurses shape the relative epistemic authority that each group can claim.

Through the first half of the twentieth century, nurses were taught that obedience to physicians was their overarching obligation. They needed no more complex ethical commitment than deference to physicians' decisions. A 1901 article in the *Journal of the American Medical Association* describes the nurse as "a sort of useful parasite," fundamentally dependent on doctors' expertise but functioning as an intelligent extension of their will ("Unsentimental Nurse" 1901, 33). In a 1917 article in the *American Journal of Nursing*, a nurse describes obedience as

> the first law and the very cornerstone of good nursing. And here is the first stumbling block for the beginner. No matter how gifted she may be, she will never become a reliable nurse until she can obey without question. The first and most helpful criticism I ever received from a doctor was when he told me that I was supposed to be simply an intelligent machine for the purpose of carrying out his orders. (Dock 1917, 394)

The image of the "intelligent machine"—whose thought and judgment should only be used in service to the decisions of experts—is itself invoked through the authority of an unnamed male physician. A nurses' handbook published in 1950 echoes this subordination in terms of loyalty, where loyalty is not to the patient or the profession but to the doctor one is assisting:

> Loyalty is the first essential.... your training and the lectures you receive are given so that you can intelligently cooperate with the doctor in the treatment of your patient. The little knowledge you will have gained during your years in hospital in no way fits you to diagnose disease or to prescribe treatment, nor does it place you in a position to criticise the doctor or his methods. Accord to him always that deference and respect which is his due. (Burbridge 1950, 26–27)

The intricate weighing of authority that runs through this passage illuminates the ambiguous position of the nurse, which persists through most of the history of the profession. Nursing education and experience are valued, but only to make the nurse a better instrument of the physician's decisions and directives. The phrase "intelligently cooperate with the doctor" is a charged one, with the mutuality implied by the term "cooperation" sharply undermined by the sentences that follow, which place epistemic and moral authority in the physician alone. This language is repeated in the 1965 International Code of Nursing Ethics: "The nurse is under an obligation to carry out the physician's orders intelligently and loyally" (quoted in Kuhse and Singer 1998, 7). In sum, nurses historically have been warned against questioning a physician's judgment or engaging in independent reasoning.

There has instead been a focus on correctly and reliably following set procedures—administering medications prescribed by physicians and monitoring their efficacy and side effects; keeping patients clean, hydrated, and fed; preventing infection; and so on (Hunt 1994a, 3–4). In this way, traditional, paternalistic approaches to medicine respect the autonomy of neither patients nor nurses (8).

The gendering of nursing work is intensified by the fact that medicine has been historically and still is dominated by men. When medicine was professionalized in the early nineteenth century in Europe and North America, women (who had frequently served as midwives and healers) were almost entirely excluded from physician education, training, and certification. Although the formal exclusion began to erode in the late nineteenth century, its legacy persists. In 1955, only 5 percent of graduates from medical schools were women; by 1990, that number had increased to 40 percent. As of 2021, 37 percent of active physicians are women, while 47 percent of residents and fellows are women (Boyle 2021). It is worth noting that women physicians tend to specialize in pediatrics, family medicine, obstetrics and gynecology, and child/adolescent psychiatry—areas of medicine most closely associated with traditional feminine roles.

Despite the increasing gender equality among physicians, nursing has been and continues to be a predominantly female profession. Although more men are becoming nurses—composing 2.2 percent of the U.S. workforce in 1960 and 11.9 percent now—nurses and personal care professionals are overwhelmingly female, with women making up 87.4 percent of registered nurses, 89.8 percent of nurse practitioners, 90.1 percent of nursing assistants, and 87.2 percent of home health aides (Munnich and Wozniak 2020; Bureau of Labor Statistics 2024). Globally, 90 percent of nurses are women (World Health Organization 2020, xvii). The highly gendered nature of nursing as a profession shapes the challenges that nurses face in relation to patients and other clinicians:

> Female nurses, together with other women in the health workforce, face more barriers at work than their male colleagues. . . . These include biased perceptions of women's roles in caregiving, social gender norms, gender bias and stereotyping, all of which undermine nurses' ability to obtain good working conditions, receive fair pay and equal treatment, participate in decision-making, and become leaders within health care. (World Health Organization 2020, 30)

As a recent World Health Organization (2019) report summarizes, in global terms, healthcare is "delivered by women, led by men." In the United States, nurses are also paid approximately 25–30 percent of what physicians make, an economic disparity that contributes to differences in epistemic authority (Robertson 2022).

These gendered and socioeconomic hierarchies often result in the devaluation of nurses' perspectives in healthcare decision-making. It is important to distinguish between medical and moral expertise. Physicians may have more technical training and experience in diagnosis, prognosis, and treatment, but on moral issues such as whether a patient with terminal cancer should continue to pursue aggressive treatments, the physician may have no more expertise than a nurse. Nurses experience different kinds of epistemic injustice, such as testimonial injustice, which involves being dismissed as an authority on some particular knowledge area, and hermeneutical injustice, which arises from a lack of conceptual resources to make one's specific perception of moral issues understood:

> Testimonial injustice was evident in the *silencing* found by Pavlish [et al.] (2013) in their explorations of moral distress among ICU and oncology unit nurses in their attempts to discuss their ethical concerns about patients. From a literature review, researchers [Bryon, de Casterlé, and Gastmans 2008] described nurses as being sidelined in the decision-making processes involving end-of-life care despite having relevant expertise and knowledge to contribute to the deliberations. Hermeneutical injustice was particularly evident in moral distress research with reports of nurses experiencing decreased self-worth and confidence in their own knowledge and ability to interpret and articulate their experiences with patients (Wiegand & Funk, 2012). (Reed and Rishel 2015, 242; see also Fricker 2007)

Essentially, in cases of epistemic injustice, nurses' perspectives are not taken seriously. Despite their traditional position in medical hierarchies, nurses usually have intimate knowledge of patients' physical, psychological, emotional, and social needs, which is crucial to treatment: not only which options should be presented to patients or their families, but how those options should be communicated and then enacted.

Nurses' authority may also be diminished by their racial, ethnic, and immigration demographics. In the United States, registered nurses (among the most educated and highest-paid nurses) are 72.6 percent white, 15.6 percent Black, 8.9 percent Asian, and 8.9 percent Hispanic/Latino. By contrast, home health aides (among the lowest-paid nurses) are 53.3 percent white, 29.8 percent Black, 14 percent Asian, and 24.9 percent Hispanic/Latino (Bureau of Labor Statistics 2024). Immigrants are also disproportionately represented in nursing, especially in the categories of home health aides and personal care aides (39.8 percent and 28.1 percent, respectively), whereas the proportion of foreign-born registered nurses mirrors the overall healthcare employment picture, at around 16 percent (Batalova 2023). If people have experienced epistemic injustice in their personal lives as persons of color and/or immigrants, then that same diminishment of their perspective is likely to extend into their professions as nurses in interactions with patients, physicians, and administrators.

Although the language of subordination has largely disappeared from codes of nursing, in practice physicians typically carry greater epistemic authority than nurses—this despite the fact that some nurses have longer, more relevant experience than some doctors. The problem is well-illustrated by the comment of a nurse in a study on moral distress: "Some days, our moral foundation is to advocate for what is best for our patient and because we spend so much time with the patients, we feel we have good insight on that, but then we do not have a say" (McCracken et al. 2021, E40). In a wide range of studies, nurses raise concerns about not being fully informed about patients' prognosis or possible treatments so that they can communicate effectively with patients or their family members, and not being given opportunities to participate in decision-making about medical care (Kälvemark et al. 2004; Pauly et al. 2009; Huffman and Rittenmeyer 2012; Savel and Munro 2013). The historical image of nursing as an extension of instinctive femininity, defined by self-sacrifice and obedience to external authority, leaves little room for nursing ethics as a serious domain within medical ethics. But that legacy has begun to be challenged in recent decades.

## Codes of Ethics

Alongside the questioning of paternalism in the physician-patient relationship, codes of nursing in the 1960s and 1970s began to reimagine the nurse as a patient's advocate rather than a physician's subordinate. The preamble to the ICN Code of Ethics (2021) states that nurses have four fundamental responsibilities: "To promote health, to prevent illness, to restore health, and to alleviate suffering and promote a dignified death" (Preamble). This code requires nurses to act as moral agents who can make judgments about how to provide the best possible care for patients. In emergency situations, nurses (and others) may need simply to follow the orders of physicians, but many medical decisions do not demand this level of urgency, so they can involve dialogue and careful consideration within an interdisciplinary clinical team that includes nurses (see Benjamin and Curtis 1992, 99–100). Some patients may want a maternal figure for physical and psychological support, but "their needs are more likely to be met by a nurse who not only provides them with professional nursing care, but who also refuses to surrender her professional intelligence and autonomy to the doctor to protect the patient from potential harm" (Kuhse 1997, 59). As patient advocates, nurses will ideally draw their insights, questions, and concerns from more frequent, less formal interactions with the patient and their family—interactions that may provide a richer picture of the patient's changing symptoms, the wider context of their lives, their anxieties and hopes, and the support network (or lack thereof) to which the patient will have access once discharged.

David Seedhouse defines **patient advocacy** as "support[ing] people by providing or helping them obtain some of their basic human needs" (2000, 16–17). This holistic approach means that nurses need to cultivate the skill of responding to verbal and nonverbal information about what is causing distress or promoting healing. Providing for a patient's emotional needs may mean distracting one patient with conversation during an IV insertion and providing silent, competent care to another patient who finds such chatter condescending. Nurses learn to interact with patients with widely varying interpersonal capabilities: infants, teenagers unwilling to communicate with their parents about health issues, people with cognitive impairment, those who are terminally ill, those who are worried about getting referred to law enforcement or public health authorities, people who are intoxicated, people who are dealing with acute mental illnesses, those who have experienced trauma, and patients who are distrustful of medical institutions.

## Advantages and Disadvantages of the Concept of Care

The term "care" has long been associated with the principal function of nursing. In engaging with feminist approaches to ethics, theorists and practitioners have asked what care means in the professional nursing setting and whether it provides robust guidelines for ethical decision-making. As described in Chapter 1, care ethics contests the idea that an abstract set of rules determines right actions—rules that should be impartially used by and applied to all rational individuals. An ethics of care instead emphasizes the basic forms of dependence, vulnerability, and relationality that human beings share and, from that vantage point, asks how one should respond to others' needs. It recognizes the moral significance of context, particularity, and connection. To take a somewhat simplified example, a traditional ethics of justice might ask, "Do people have a right to medical aid in dying?" and apply the answer to any patient claiming such a right. Care ethics would start from the particular patient's experiences and take into account their relationships with others. Carol Gilligan describes the distinction as follows:

> Hypothetical dilemmas, in the abstraction of their presentation, divest moral actors from the history and psychology of their individual lives and separate the moral problem from the social contingencies of its possible occurrence. In so doing, these dilemmas are useful for the distillation and refinement of objective principles of justice and for measuring the formal logic of equality and reciprocity. However, the reconstruction of the dilemma in its contextual particularity allows the understanding of cause and consequence which engages the compassion and tolerance repeatedly noted to distinguish the moral judgment of women. (1982, 100)

Gilligan's description highlights aspects of care ethics that align with the practice of nursing, since nursing requires attending to the needs of patients in all their singularity, as whole social and emotional persons. She also stresses the gendered quality of these two conceptions of ethics—a gendering that most care ethicists argue is not innate or immutable but instead deeply habituated due to cultural training.

This focus on the vulnerability of patients emerges in many discussions of what care means in professional nursing: "In nursing we interact with human beings made 'more than ordinarily vulnerable' . . . by illness, disease, or other life circumstances. These human beings need our professional help and care. Good nursing practice therefore requires us to engage at a human as well as a professional level" (Sellman 2011, 67). As Gilligan (1982) and Nel Noddings (1984) describe it, caring involves a willingness to attend actively to others and respond appropriately. More specifically, nursing care frequently means interpreting technical explanations in accessible ways for patients and their families; helping them navigate institutional procedures that may seem overwhelming; planning for self-care or social support after medical supervision ends (such as connecting patients to social workers); responding to patients' concerns and communicating with physicians about those concerns; observing patients' patterns of sleep, digestion, and pain symptoms; and discerning unarticulated needs, such as mental health or addiction issues (Savel and Munro 2013; Reed and Rishel 2015; Gallagher 2017, 57). Joan Tronto describes four dimensions of caring activity: (1) attentiveness: recognizing that a person needs care; (2) responsibility: moving to address that need; (3) competence: having the skills to respond to that need; and (4) responsiveness: the attitude toward the one cared for (1993, 117). In French, "to take care of" is *s'occuper de*—literally, to be occupied with or by another person (Lavoie, De Koninck, and Blondeau 2006, 228). Care is not an activity with clear temporal boundaries but responds to ongoing, shifting, and longitudinal needs. This is reflected in the typical nursing workflow, in which there are no designated appointments or rounds but continuous engagement with patients.

Approached in this way, patients are not malfunctioning organisms needing maintenance or consumers exchanging money for technical services. The focus is not primarily on diagnosing the cause of symptoms and eliminating that cause, which "dissects, fragments and depersonalises" patients (Marles 1988, 25–26). Linda Hanford puts the distinction between curing and caring in the following terms:

> Diseases can be cured by the skilful application of technical and chemical means but the illness, regarded as an affront to one's sense of self, requires that the patient be met with sympathy as a suffering individual and helped to find meaning in his experience, in order that it be accommodated or resolved. (1994, 187)

Autonomy is recognized here not only in the relatively simple sense of respecting the patient's purposes but also in the more complex register of treating them as meaning-making agents in their own lives. Nursing informed by an ethics of care is well positioned, therefore, to respond to the subjective significance of illness, disability, and mortality.

Despite the centrality of the concept of care to nursing ethics, there are many debates about the strengths of care ethics or what it can offer to nursing, including whether justice and care are alternative or complementary approaches to ethics; whether healthcare professionals should separate caring *for* patients from caring *about* patients (Kuhse 1997, 145–46); what role self-care plays, given the continuities between the self-sacrificial feminine ideal and the ethics of care; and whether care ethics can effectively account for simultaneous obligations to multiple patients and to a wider society. Some scholars worry that the asymmetrical, nonreciprocal focus of care ethics reinstates the mother-child model that dominated the early history of nursing, with all its moral and social liabilities (see Kuhse 1997, 162–66). Among other theorists, Kuhse suggests combining the advantages of care ethics and justice-based ethics, with the idea of "dispositional" or professionally mediated care, tempered by attention to the principles of medical ethics to navigate and resolve moral problems (1997, 150–52).

## From Intelligent Machines to Moral Agents

As we discussed earlier, the traditional image of nurses as "intelligent machines" diminishes the activity of moral reasoning. As in other professions, nursing ethics is sometimes presented as a series of procedures to be followed, to align individual and team behavior with legal and institutional policies. However, the work that nurses do requires moral judgment. The ICN Code of Ethics (2021) lists a number of duties that cannot be discharged with merely technical expertise—for example, respecting the privacy and confidentiality of patients and colleagues (1.5), serving as patient advocates (2.7), challenging unethical clinical and research practices (3.5), and promoting healthcare as a human right (4.1). To fulfill such obligations, nurses must claim moral agency to apply these abstract duties to the particular situations they encounter. Developing and supporting moral agency among nurses resists the association between professional nursing care and (supposedly) instinctive feminine behaviors. The question is whether nursing education cultivates those moral capacities and whether the culture of the institutions where nurses work encourages their moral agency. Given nurses' commitment to care, they may have more practice in collaborative, dialogic decision-making than is taught and expected among physicians (Baggs et al. 1997; Vazirani et al. 2005; Hamric and Blackhall 2007; Thomson 2007).

Nurses may also intervene critically in medical experimentation when researchers' goals or methods are morally questionable. To take a historical example, the Tuskegee syphilis study enlisted a local Black nurse, Eunice Rivers. Starting in 1932 and over several decades, she worked to recruit men into the study and then functioned as the facilitator between the subjects, their families, and the U.S. Public Health Service researchers. She exemplifies the common situation that nurses are more likely to understand their patients' lives and are more likely to be deeply embedded in their patients' communities than physicians or public health officials are. By all accounts, Rivers was a talented and dedicated nurse. She attended to the wider needs of the Tuskegee subjects, including providing food and clothing, and there is "some evidence that she may have advised [people outside the study] to seek penicillin treatment to cure their potentially fatal disease" (Sanford 2021). Alongside these praiseworthy actions, however, she worked diligently to keep subjects enrolled in the study. Her caring labor enabled the continuation of unethical research. We should recognize that, as a Black woman working as a nurse in the segregated South, Rivers faced intersectional epistemic injustice. Any overt moral challenge or resistance to the study's methods she might have mustered was unlikely to shift its trajectory. And yet her story is a reminder of how important it is for nurses to be empowered to advocate for their patients. Her moral perspective, which is not part of the historical record, carried no weight in the design or implementation of the study. Rivers represents the traditional ideal of the nurse: subordinate to physicians' judgments, technically competent, and performing the caring work of an intermediary. But because she could not effectively raise moral questions about the project, all these gendered functions contributed to the objectification and harming of human subjects.

Nurses' intimate and rich knowledge may serve as a check when medical orders violate patients' interests or ethical values. Affirming nurses' moral autonomy may lead to discussions about how health and illness are defined, more careful communication with patients and families, greater focus on the social determinants of health, and critical reflection on the effects of institutional policies and how the healthcare industry as a whole is organized (Hunt 1994a, 4). In the context of medical research, nurses are also well-positioned to attend to both the rights of individual subjects and the overarching goals of the experiment (Kennedy 1994, 107).

## Moral Problems Central to Nursing Ethics

Given their positions in the clinical environment and the emphasis on care, the kinds of ethical issues that nurses confront frequently differ from the concerns of physicians. First, nurses are typically expected to care for multiple patients simultaneously. In settings such as intensive care units or emergency departments, often many patients urgently need their attention. This pressure intensifies when hospitals make staffing decisions that prioritize cost reductions over patient care. The notorious case of Mid-Staffordshire Hospital in the United Kingdom provoked a government inquiry that found that severe staffing cuts (especially of highly skilled nurses) and a culture of bullying (rather than responding to patient and staff complaints) led to substandard care and increased mortality rates between 2005 and 2008 (Francis 2013; see also Wells 2024). As we saw in Chapter 2, morally significant decisions on the part of individual nurses can be supported or hindered by organizational priorities, especially when a focus on efficiency results in shorter patient hospital stays or staffing shortages (planned or unplanned). For-profit hospitals in particular may trim nursing staff to reduce labor costs, since nursing care is not billed to insurance in the same way as physicians' services. Those conditions mean that nurses have less time to learn patients' needs and respond to them, or to have substantive conversations with physicians, other nurses, family members, and patients themselves. Nurses "floated" to another department or travel/per diem nurses have less time to develop the familiarity of working in a professional team. Within the policies of their employing institution, nurses must navigate how to care for each individual patient adequately when their time and attention is a scarce resource. Regardless of personal characteristics—such as age, demeanor, political affiliation, vaccination status, or mental state—every patient has to be treated as worthy of care (Felzmann 2017, 36). This commitment runs against the utilitarian intuitions behind triage and other attempts to rank patients when allocating resources. Nurses are also responsible for raising concerns if organizational policies are violated or if those policies interfere with nurses' duties to patients or to themselves.

The second moral challenge emerges out of the history of nursing ethics. Nurses typically function as intermediaries between physicians and patients, so they must advocate for patients while also explaining physicians' recommendations to them. Nurses must make morally significant decisions about what to communicate "downward" to patients and "upward" to physicians, and how to communicate that information effectively. This obligation may be complicated if patients express one desire to a nurse ("I don't want any more treatment and am ready to die") and a different desire to a physician ("I want to keep fighting"). In this situation, a nurse is caught in a conflict between defending what the patient says they want (to the nurse) and carrying out what the physician thinks they want.

Third, nurses have to be mindful that, even though patients are in a vulnerable position, they also deserve respect. Despite the ways that nurses have often been devalued in paternalistic hierarchies, they may also act paternalistically toward patients if the obligation to care is used to infantilize or objectify them. In the name of beneficence, nurses may be tempted to withhold negative information from patients and emphasize hopeful outcomes. As with many issues in medical ethics, the principle of respect for autonomy should mitigate how beneficence may be misapplied—that is, when clinicians listen to what patients say they want, the therapeutic decision is more likely to align with patients' best interests. Nurses need to be committed to treating patients as self-determining persons who deserve full information about their conditions and the options available to them, as well as time and support to make sense of that information. Nurses must develop the skills to communicate that information effectively, given the particular patient's situation and attitude (Tronto 1993, 143; Sellman 2017, 50–51). That same commitment to informed consent means resisting the "empty ritual" of having patients sign consent forms, which may serve the bureaucratic and legal ends of the hospital but not patient comprehension: "If patients are to make a considered and informed decision they must be asked at the best time for them, and be given time to reflect, sort out their feelings and, if possible, discuss with spouses, friends and relatives" (Taplin 1994, 33). Nurses asking patients to explain their situation and options in their own terms is a way to confirm their comprehension and give patients space to break out of the passive "sick role" that habitually defers to medical authority (Segall 1976).

Fourth, balancing respect for autonomy and beneficence takes on highly concrete forms in nursing care. Focusing on care for vulnerable people may prime nurses (and healthcare organizations more generally) to undermine patient autonomy by prioritizing safety over self-determination. Attempts to control a patient's ailment at a medical level can interfere with attempts to support them as self-determining agents (Smith 1994, 59). As Geoffrey Hunt argues, beneficence must take into account the patient's biological health as only one moral value among others: "Medical talk of the 'interest of the patient' is in the doctor's mind talk about the biological interest of the human body—which is where medical expertise lies. But there's an unsustainable dualism here. When the doctor talks of my body he talks of *me*" (1994a, 14). For instance, hospitals and long-term care facilities may be so concerned that elderly patients will fall that they institute policies that overly restrict patients' activity—which not only threatens patient autonomy but also their overall health in terms of muscle mass, coordination, flexibility, and balance. Patients with psychiatric disorders may be prescribed medications that control symptoms but have the side effect of dampening their ability to interact with others or retain a sense of themselves.

Nurses can be patient advocates in the broad sense of promoting overall well-being. Atul Gawande (2014) criticizes the tendency of nursing homes to focus exclusively on the health and safety of patients (narrowly conceived) without considering the sources of value in their lives. He describes an experiment in which a nursing home in upstate New York introduced "one hundred parakeets, four dogs, two cats, plus a colony of rabbits and a flock of laying hens. There were also hundreds of indoor plants and a thriving vegetable and flower garden. The home has on-site child care for the staff and a new after-school program" (123). Some of these innovations had to be initiated as research, since they violated state health codes. The experiment found that interactions with nonhuman animals, plants, and children significantly lowered patients' need for medications, decreased mortality rates, and raised their quality of life (123–24). Addressing loneliness and depression among elderly patients may mean supporting social interaction and purposeful activities, as opposed to primarily treating the serious physical symptoms that arise from those psychological states (Fenton 1994, 86). Attending to this wider sense of well-being may sometimes result in simple fixes—for instance, minimizing overnight interruptions to protect patients' sleep or removing tripping hazards to allow patients more mobility. But often the situation is more complicated. Many elderly and injured patients desperately want to return home rather than spend more time in medical settings. In those cases, nurses and other staff need to assess whether patients' homes will offer enough social and medical support to make that option reasonably safe (Greaney and O'Mathúna 2017, 89–90). Since legally patients cannot be held against their will, there is an inclination to allow them to leave when they want, regardless of their living situation. However, there is also a countervailing tendency to keep them in the hospital to avoid lawsuits for discharging them too early.

Given their longer and less formal interactions with patients, nurses have a special responsibility to uphold patient autonomy at a bodily level. Nurses encounter patients from a variety of cultural and religious backgrounds, and patients who are experiencing their bodies as wounded, vulnerable, or traumatized. Therefore, nurses are obligated to approach issues of privacy and bodily self-determination with particular sensitivity: as Paul Wainwright puts it, they have to "renegotiate socially the various norms, values, taboos, beliefs and learned ways of behaving with respect to the body" (1994, 44). Nurses can model how to care for the body's needs without shame or judgment, but they also need to be attentive to patients' attitudes regarding the body—for instance, giving a patient who has experienced a sexual assault some measure of control over an examination, or taking their cues from a transgender adolescent about pronouns and bodily self-relation.

Even with this emphasis on patient autonomy, some patients require more paternalistic care to support the possibility of regaining self-determination in the future. Patients who are intoxicated, delirious, experiencing acute psychiatric episodes, or attacking staff or other patients may require coercive measures, such as giving them medication or restraining them, to prevent them from harming themselves or others. Nurses are frequently targets of workplace violence, and they are also the ones who carry out physicians' orders for coercive measures. Physicians must order restraints, for example, but the type of restraint is determined by the nurses, who decide what is least invasive in a given situation. In this sense, they are the ones negotiating between respecting autonomy and promoting safety. These measures aim to stabilize patients until they can participate more substantively in their own decision-making. Any coercive intervention is likely to cause harm to patients' sense of self-determination and trust in others, but communicating with them frequently and using the least coercive interventions possible, in following the principles of nonmaleficence and beneficence, may mitigate that damage (O'Brien and Golding 2003).

Finally, nurses are particularly well-positioned to care for patients at the end of life. When patients or their families choose to stop seeking a cure and instead receive **hospice care**, focusing on comfort and quality of life, the holistic and interpersonal skills of nursing are crucial: communicating with patients and families, listening to what each patient desires and values, and working with a wider support network to meet their needs. Kuhse makes the radical suggestion that, in the realm of hospice care, nurses should have more authority than physicians in deciding how to fulfill patients' goals, since curing is no longer the medical priority. Nurses are more likely to have "particularized insights into the patient's wishes at the end of the life" (Kuhse 1997, 217). In attending to the specific needs of patients, nurses are likely to conceive of their role less in terms of doing battle—so that death or referrals to hospice care are framed as failures of medicine—and more in terms of doing what they can for this individual patient given their condition and place in their life cycle. Noddings encourages clinicians to ask, in end-of-life decisions, when a cognitively capable patient no longer wishes to live: "What should I do in the face of this reality? In particular . . . what should I do in the face of extreme suffering when there is a well-grounded judgment of hopelessness?" (1989, 130). How nurses (and others) answer that question may refer to moral principles or core values, including patient autonomy, but the key idea is that the moral question begins from responding to the particular person, in all their emotional, psychological, and social complexity.

Like physicians and other healthcare professionals, nurses should be encouraged to engage in reflection and collaborative discussions when confronting these moral problems. This process of moral reasoning might best be located in hospital ethics committees, which should have nurse representation. No one comprehensive method will resolve every moral question; Simone de Beauvoir reminds us that ethics cannot be reduced to "recipes" or algorithms (2015, 144–45). Instead, nurses and others involved in decision-making need to gather all relevant information, clarify the core values on which their moral intuitions are founded, and discuss which outcome best lives out their commitments. Sometimes even sharply differing values produce converging judgments about what action should be taken.

For this reason, clinicians and ethics committees should primarily emphasize the practical outcome of these discussions.

## Moral Distress and Compassion Fatigue

When nurses' moral agency is hindered or undermined, they are likely to experience moral distress. The concept was first defined by Andrew Jameton: "When one knows the right thing to do, but institutional constraints make it nearly impossible to pursue the right course of action" (1984, 6). Although more recent discussions have extended the definition of moral distress to include cases of moral uncertainty ("uncertainty-distress"), under the traditional definition, moral distress arises from not being able to enact what one knows to be right ("constraint-distress") (Fourie 2017). It threatens a person's sense of moral agency in their professional life. It could result from working routinely under conditions of scarce resources, not being heard when one raises concerns about patient safety, or functioning under legal or organizational constraints that seem unjustified. It is often tied to the issue of epistemic injustice—one's moral judgment not being taken seriously in medical decision-making. One major cause of moral distress among nurses is aggressive treatment that does not ultimately benefit the patient, perhaps by intensifying suffering or prolonging a patient's life without regard to the quality of that life (Elpern, Covert, and Kleinpell 2005).

Patricia Reed and Cindy Rishel (2015) distinguish between internal and external constraints that contribute to moral distress. Internal constraints involve a person's subjective sense of powerlessness, including the feeling that their perspective will not be heard or anxiety that they will face retaliation from supervisors for voicing concerns. External constraints involve institutional limitations, including poor communication, lack of decision-making power, and inadequate staffing (241). The two dimensions are clearly related: personally experiencing external constraints or witnessing others experience them contributes to an internal sense of limited moral agency. During the COVID-19 pandemic, when clinicians lacked resources to care adequately for the influx of patients and could not transfer them to other facilities, their sense of obligation came into conflict with very real limitations of space, staffing, and equipment. Colleen McCracken et al. list the following causes of moral distress, based on their qualitative work with oncology nurses: "Conflicts about goals of care, inadequate communication, false hope, and the challenge of moving from cure to comfort, . . . a lack of palliative care or ethics involvement during situations of conflict, the healthcare hierarchy, the organization's business agenda, and a culture where death is considered a failure" (2021, E37). In sum, moral distress results from inadequate support for moral reflection about what healthcare practitioners are trying to accomplish and how they should accomplish it, or from the inability to act in alignment with those judgments. Clinicians across a variety of disciplines experience moral distress, often due to institutional pressure to increase the number of patients seen or to wider social failures to provide access to the medical care that patients need— economic barriers such as lack of insurance or under-insurance, or legal barriers such as state bans on abortion or gender-affirming care for transgender minors. But nurses face an additional source of moral distress: a less powerful position within medical hierarchies, which often means a diminished voice in decision-making alongside the expectation that they will enact the decisions of others.

Reed and Rishel (2015) note that moral distress is particularly prevalent among nurses caring for patients at the end of life. They attribute this correlation to the way that nursing has been defined, both in terms of the central virtue of caring and the subordination to physicians' authority:

> The ubiquity of moral distress is not surprising, considering nurses' highly regarded moral status coupled with situations in which bedside nurses must provide expert care around the clock, sometimes without full disclosure of treatment decisions, yet expected to advocate for patients and their families—all within the highly-charged moral context of end-of-life. (241)

Jameton (2017) describes as a "common flash point" for moral distress the experience of having to participate in curative measures, such as resuscitating a patient, when such efforts seem futile and produce unnecessary suffering. Caring for patients at the end of life itself does not seem to provoke moral distress: "Nurses have been found to be able to cope with a patient's death most easily when they can tell themselves, with justice, that nothing more could have been done. . . . There was surprisingly little sense of 'failure' when a patient died" under those conditions (Dickenson 1994, 210).

But when aggressive medical interventions or under-staffing undermine the focus on caring for patients, nurses are primed for moral distress.

If moral distress comes to dominate a person's professional experience, it can lead to moral injury, the psychological harm that arises from repeated compromising of one's moral values. Either moral distress on its own or the more persistent condition of moral injury can cause burnout. As noted in Chapter 4, the term "burnout" seems to name an individual pathology, an inadequacy on the part of some particular employee, who experiences "mental or physical exhaustion, mental distance from the job, cynicism about the job, and reduced efficacy in the workplace" (American Nurses Association 2024). Yet a 2020 study found that 62 percent of nurses experience burnout, including 69 percent of nurses under the age of twenty-five (American Nurses Association 2022). We should therefore understand burnout as a predictable reaction to wider institutional and systemic inadequacies. The COVID-19 pandemic exacerbated existing problems for nurses' work environment but should not be read as an aberration that will recede without intervention, since nursing burnout rates are strongly correlated with the number of patients cared for, insufficient staffing, and inadequate pay (Galanis et al. 2021; Sullivan et al. 2022). Moral distress speaks to the deeply interpersonal nature of nursing work. Nurses who cannot support each other at an emotional level, who quit their permanent jobs to become locum tenens or travel nurses, or who leave the profession entirely may contribute to the burden on other nurses.

Over the last several decades, healthcare organizations have increasingly recognized the impact of moral distress, moral injury, and burnout, and they have begun to address it. Some of their solutions emphasize individual strategies: self-care techniques and access to social and psychological support. But these issues cannot be effectively resolved solely at this level, since they speak to pervasive challenges within the healthcare industry as it currently exists and within cultural attitudes toward health, disability, and mortality. Broader solutions involve institutional changes, such as improving communication among clinicians and fostering a culture in which all of them—physicians, advanced practice clinicians, and nurses—feel comfortable raising moral concerns. Practices such as involving the entire care team in treatment decisions and debriefing afterward can mitigate the power imbalances among clinicians and allow team members an opportunity to express their cognitive and emotional reactions. Some of those solutions involve shifts in nursing education, including giving nurses more practice in collaborative decision-making (Jameton 2017). Reed and Rishel argue that moral distress can be effectively addressed by involving nurses in discussions around medical care, including end-of-life care, as a way of improving treatment for the patient, supporting families, and respecting nurses as moral agents (2015, 243; see also McCracken et al. 2021, E38).

Another factor that can interfere with effective nursing care is **compassion fatigue**. Sometimes described as secondary trauma, compassion fatigue refers to the "cost of caring," the psychological effects of responding to the suffering of others (Figley 1995, 7). Most at risk are physicians, nurses, therapists, social workers, and others in "caring professions" who work directly with individual patients or clients (Cocker and Joss 2016). Compassion fatigue may manifest in emotional and/or physical ways, such as numbing, anxiety, feelings of helplessness or powerlessness, sleep disturbances, and headaches. The cumulative psychological effects of caring for patients who have experienced traumatic events or who are at the end of life sometimes cannot be effectively processed by clinicians. In this way, compassion fatigue resembles post-traumatic stress disorder (PTSD), in which overwhelming experiences (in this case, responding to the trauma of others) lead the mind to utilize primitive coping mechanisms, including avoidance and desensitization. Neither of these responses to psychological exhaustion is helpful for patients or ultimately constructive for the clinicians themselves. Strong social support networks tend to reduce these effects (Haik et al. 2017). Institutions can address this problem by establishing mentoring relationships (since older and more experienced healthcare workers seem to be less vulnerable to compassion fatigue), offering psychosocial support in the workplace, and providing adequate staffing.

## Conclusion: Nursing as a Moral Profession

Discussions of nursing ethics allow us to look beyond the physician-patient dyad to the larger context in which medical treatment occurs: institutional hierarchies and collaborations, interpersonal networks, and communication patterns, all of which may support or hinder patient autonomy and healing. Hunt sounds a somewhat pessimistic note in asking whether the history of subordination that nurses have experienced has yet been overcome: "Although the word 'obedience' is generally avoided with some embarrassment one has to ask whether it is still in actuality the first principle of nursing practice" (1994b, 131–32). If obedience or loyalty is a nurse's primary obligation, nursing ethics cannot develop into a particularly complex or philosophically rigorous discursive field. To validate nurses as moral agents is to recognize the particular responsibilities, perspectives, and challenges that arise within the activity of nursing, and that can enrich the moral reflection that happens in healthcare settings.

Mark Lazenby argues that nursing is defined by its deep moral and social significance: nurses have an obligation to care for each patient and for all patients, no matter who they are (2020, xv). Their work begins from the singular, vulnerable person in front of them but also broadens to treat the underlying causes of suffering: supporting public health, attempting to reform institutions, and arguing for a more just distribution of healthcare resources. Other healthcare professionals share these goals, but the particular tenor of nursing brings it into focus. Nursing interacts with embodied, mortal, distressed human beings and responds (ideally) by treating each one as a person worthy of care. In Lazenby's terms, nursing arises from a recognition of common humanity—the moral considerability of all—as its ethical foundation. All the ordinary acts of comfort and astonishingly complex medical interventions proceed from that normative ground.

## References

American Nurses Association. 2022. *Pulse on the Nation's Nurses Survey Series: COVID-19 Two-Year Impact Assessment Survey.* March 1. https://www.emergingrnleader.com/wp-content/uploads/2022/03/COVID-19-Two-Year-Impact-Assessment-Written-Report-Final.pdf.

———. 2024. "What Is Nurse Burnout? How to Prevent It." April 25. https://www.nursingworld.org/content-hub/resources/workplace/what-is-nurse-burnout-how-to-prevent-it/.

Baggs, J. G., M. H. Schmitt, A. I. Mushlin, D. H. Eldredge, D. Oakes, and A. D. Hutson. 1997. "Nurse-Physician Collaboration and Satisfaction with the Decision-Making Process in Three Critical Care Units." *American Journal of Critical Care* 6, no. 5 (September 1): 393–99. doi:10.4037/ajcc1997.6.5.393.

Batalova, Jeanne. 2023. "Immigrant Health-Care Workers in the United States." Migration Policy Institute. April 7. https://www.migrationpolicy.org/article/immigrant-health-care-workers-united-states.

Beauvoir, Simone de. 2015. *The Ethics of Ambiguity*. Translated by Bernard Frechtman. New York: Philosophical Library.

Benjamin, Martin, and Joy Curtis. 1992. *Ethics in Nursing: Cases, Principles, and Reasoning*. 3rd ed. New York: Oxford University Press.

Boyle, Patrick. 2021. "Nation's Physician Workforce Evolves: More Women, a Bit Older, and toward Different Specialties." American Association of Medical Colleges. February 2. https://www.aamc.org/news/nation-s-physician-workforce-evolves-more-women-bit-older-and-toward-different-specialties.

Bryon, E., B. Dierckx de Casterlé, and C. Gastmans. 2008. "Nurses' Attitudes towards Artificial Food or Fluid Administration in Patients with Dementia and in Terminally Ill Patients: A Review of the Literature." *Journal of Medical Ethics* 34, no. 6 (June): 431–36. doi:10.1136/jme.2007.021493.

Burbridge, G. N. 1950. *Lectures for Nurses*. 4th ed. Glebe, Australia: Australasian Medical Publishing.

Bureau of Labor Statistics. 2024. "Labor Force Statistics from the Current Population Survey, Table 11: Employed Persons by Detailed Occupation, Sex, Race, and Hispanic or Latino Ethnicity." U.S. Department of Labor. Last modified January 26, 2024. https://www.bls.gov/cps/cpsaat11.htm.

Cocker, Fiona, and Nerida Joss. 2016. "Compassion Fatigue among Healthcare, Emergency and Community Service Workers: A Systematic Review." *International Journal of Environmental Research and Public Health* 13, no. 6 (June): 618–35. doi:10.3390/ijerph13060618.

Dickenson, Donna. 1994. "Nurse Time as a Scarce Health Care Resource." In *Ethical Issues in Nursing*, edited by Geoffrey Hunt, 207–17. New York: Routledge.

Dock, Sarah E. 1917. "The Relation of the Nurse to the Doctor and the Doctor to the Nurse." *American Journal of Nursing* 17, no. 5 (February): 394–96. doi:10.2307/3405170.

Elpern, Ellen H., Barbara Covert, and Ruth Kleinpell. 2005. "Moral Distress of Staff Nurses in a Medical Intensive Care Unit." *American Journal of Critical Care* 14, no. 6 (November): 523–30. doi:10.4037/ajcc2005.14.6.523.

Felzmann, Heike. 2017. "Utilitarianism as an Approach to Ethical Decision Making in Health Care." In *Key Concepts and Issues in Nursing Ethics*, edited by P. Anne Scott, 29–41. Cham: Springer. doi:10.1007/978-3-319-49250-6_3.

Fenton, Julie. 1994. "Caring for Patients Who Cannot or Will Not Eat." In *Ethical Issues in Nursing*, edited by Geoffrey Hunt, 73–89. New York: Routledge.

Figley, Charles R. 1995. "Compassion Fatigue as Secondary Traumatic Stress Disorder: An Overview." In *Compassion Fatigue: Coping with Secondary Traumatic Stress Disorder in Those Who Treat the Traumatized*, edited by Charles R. Figley, 1–20. New York: Routledge.

Fourie, Carina. 2017. "Who Is Experiencing What Kind of Moral Distress? Distinctions for Moving from a Narrow to a Broad Definition of Moral Distress." *AMA Journal of Ethics* 19, no. 6 (June): 578–84. doi:10.1001/journalofethics.2017.19.6.nlit1-1706.

Francis, Robert. 2013. *Report of the Mid Staffordshire NHS Foundation Trust Public Inquiry: Executive Summary*. February. London: Stationery Office. https://assets.publishing.service.gov.uk/government/uploads/system/uploads/attachment_data/file/279124/0947.pdf.

Fricker, Miranda. 2007. *Epistemic Injustice: Power and the Ethics of Knowing*. New York: Oxford University Press. doi:10.1093/acprof:oso/9780198237907.001.0001.

Galanis, Petros, Irene Vraka, Despoina Fragkou, Angeliki Bilali, and Daphne Kaitelidou. 2021. "Nurses' Burnout and Associated Risk Factors during the COVID-19 Pandemic: A Systematic Review and Meta-analysis." *Journal of Advanced Nursing* 77, no. 8 (August): 3286–302. doi:10.1111/jan.14839.

Gallagher, Ann. 2017. "Care Ethics and Nursing Practice." In *Key Concepts and Issues in Nursing Ethics*, edited by P. Anne Scott, 55–68. Cham: Springer. doi:10.1007/978-3-319-49250-6_5.

Gawande, Atul. 2014. *Being Mortal: Medicine and What Matters in the End*. New York: Henry Holt.

Gilligan, Carol. 1982. *In a Different Voice: Psychological Theory and Women's Development*. Cambridge, MA: Harvard University Press.

Greaney, Anna-Marie, and Dónal P. O'Mathúna. 2017. "Patient Autonomy in Nursing and Healthcare Contexts." In *Key Concepts and Issues in Nursing Ethics*, edited by P. Anne Scott, 83–99. Cham: Springer. doi:10.1007/978-3-319-49250-6_7.

Haik, Josef, Stav Brown, Alon Liran, Denis Visentin, Amit Sokolov, Isaac Zilinsky, and Rachel Kornhaber. 2017. "Burnout and Compassion Fatigue: Prevalence and Associations among Israeli Burn Clinicians." *Neuropsychiatric Disease and Treatment* 13: 1533–40. doi:10.2147/NDT.S133181.

Hamric, Ann B., and Leslie J. Blackhall. 2007. "Nurse-Physician Perspectives on the Care of Dying Patients in Intensive Care Units: Collaboration, Moral Distress, and Ethical Climate." *Critical Care Medicine* 35, no. 2 (February): 422–29. doi:10.1097/01.CCM.0000254722.50608.2D.

Hanford, Linda. 1994. "Nursing and the Concept of Care: An Appraisal of Noddings' Theory." In *Ethical Issues in Nursing*, edited by Geoffrey Hunt, 181–97. New York: Routledge.

Huffman, Delores M., and Leslie Rittenmeyer. 2012. "How Professional Nurses Working in Hospital Environments Experience Moral Distress: A Systematic Review." *Critical Care Nursing Clinics of North America* 24, no. 1 (March): 91–100. doi:10.1016/j.ccell.2012.01.004.

Hunt, Geoffrey. 1994a. "Introduction: Ethics, Nursing and the Metaphysics of Procedure." In *Ethical Issues in Nursing*, edited by Geoffrey Hunt, 1–18. New York: Routledge.

———. 1994b. "Nursing Accountability: The Broken Circle." In *Ethical Issues in Nursing*, edited by Geoffrey Hunt, 129–47. New York: Routledge.

International Council of Nurses. 2021. *The ICN Code of Ethics for Nurses*. https://www.icn.ch/sites/default/files/2023-06/ICN_Code-of-Ethics_EN_Web.pdf.

Jameton, Andrew. 1984. *Nursing Practice: The Ethical Issues*. Englewood Cliffs, NJ: Prentice Hall.

———. 2017. "What Moral Distress in Nursing History Could Suggest about the Future of Health Care." *AMA Journal of Ethics* 19, no. 6 (June): 617–28. doi:10.1001/journalofethics.2017.19.6.mhst1-1706.

Kälvemark, Sofia, Anna T. Höglund, Mats G. Hansson, Peter Westerholm, and Bengt Arnetz. 2004. "Living with Conflicts: Ethical Dilemmas and Moral Distress in the Health Care System." *Social Science & Medicine* 58, no. 6 (March): 1075–84. doi:10.1016/s0277-9536(03)00279-x.

Kennedy, Ann. 1994. "Ethical Issues in HIV/AIDS Epidemiology: A Nurse's Perspective." In *Ethical Issues in Nursing*, edited by Geoffrey Hunt, 106–25. New York: Routledge.

Kuhse, Helga. 1997. *Caring: Nurses, Women and Ethics*. Malden, MA: Blackwell.

Kuhse, Helga, and Peter Singer. 1998. "What Is Bioethics? A Historical Introduction." In *A Companion to Bioethics*, edited by Helga Kuhse and Peter Singer, 3–11. Malden, MA: Blackwell. doi:10.1002/9781444307818.ch1.

Lavoie, Mireille, Thomas De Koninck, and Danielle Blondeau. 2006. "The Nature of Care in Light of Emmanuel Levinas." *Nursing Philosophy* 7, no. 4 (October): 225–34. doi:10.1111/j.1466-769X.2006.00279.x.

Lazenby, Mark. 2020. *Toward a Better World: The Social Significance of Nursing*. New York: Oxford University Press. doi:10.1093/med/9780190695712.001.0001.

Marles, F. 1988. *Report of the Study of Professional Issues in Nursing*. Melbourne: Health Department of Victoria.

McCracken, Colleen, Natalie McAndrew, Kathryn Schroeter, and Katie Klink. 2021. "Moral Distress: A Qualitative Study of Experiences among Oncology Team Members." *Clinical Journal of Oncology Nursing* 25, no. 4 (August): E35–43. doi:10.1188/21.CJON.E35-E43.

Munnich, Elizabeth, and Abigail Wozniak. 2020. "What Explains the Rising Share of US Men in Registered Nursing?" *Industrial & Labor Relations Review* 73, no. 1 (January): 91–123. doi:10.1177/0019793919838775.

Noddings, Nel. 1984. *Caring: A Feminine Approach to Ethics and Moral Education*. Berkeley: University of California Press.

———. 1989. *Women and Evil*. Berkeley: University of California Press.

O'Brien, A. J., and C. G. Golding. 2003. "Coercion in Mental Healthcare: The Principle of Least Coercive Care." *Journal of Psychiatric and Mental Health Nursing* 10, no. 2 (April): 167–73. doi:10.1046/j.1365-2850.2003.00571.x.

Pauly, Bernadette, Colleen Varcoe, Janet Storch, and Lorelei Newton. 2009. "Registered Nurses' Perceptions of Moral Distress and Ethical Climate." *Nursing Ethics* 16, no. 5 (September): 561–73. doi:10.1177/0969733009106649.

Pavlish, Carol L., Joan Henriksen Hellyer, Katherine Brown-Saltzman, Anne G. Miers, and Karina Squire. 2013. "Barriers to Innovation: Nurses' Risk Appraisal in Using a New Ethics Screening and Early Intervention Tool." *Advances in Nursing Science* 36, no. 4 (October–December): 304–19. doi:10.1097/ANS.0000000000000004.

Reed, Patricia G., and Cindy J. Rishel. 2015. "Epistemic Injustice and Nurse Moral Distress: Perspective for Policy Development." *Nursing Science Quarterly* 28, no. 3 (July): 241–44. doi:10.1177/0894318415585634.

Robertson, Marcus. 2022. "Nurse Pay vs. Physician Pay for Each State." *Becker's ASC Review*. May 18. https://www.beckersasc.com/asc-news/nurse-pay-vs-physician-pay-for-each-state.html.

Sanford, Ezelle III. 2021. "Remembering Nurse Eunice Rivers Laurie, the Black Face of the Tuskegee Syphilis Study, and Why She Is an Important Figure for Students to Know." *Common Reader*. November 12. https://commonreader.wustl.edu/remembering-nurse-eunice-rivers-laurie-the-black-face-of-the-tuskegee-syphilis-study-and-why-she-is-an-important-figure-for-students-to-know/.

Savel, Richard H., and Cindy L. Munro. 2013. "Conflict Management in the Intensive Care Unit." *American Journal of Critical Care* 22, no. 4 (July 1): 277–80. doi:10.4037/ajcc2013857.

Seedhouse, David. 2000. *Practical Nursing Philosophy: The Universal Ethical Code*. Chichester, UK: Wiley.

Segall, Alexander. 1976. "The Sick Role Concept: Understanding Illness Behavior." *Journal of Health and Social Behavior* 17, no. 2 (June): 162–69. doi:10.2307/2136342.

Sellman, Derek. 2011. *What Makes a Good Nurse: Why the Virtues Are Important for Nurses*. London: Kingsley.

———. 2017. "Virtue Ethics and Nursing Practice." In *Key Concepts and Issues in Nursing Ethics*, edited by P. Anne Scott, 43–54. Cham: Springer. doi:10.1007/978-3-319-49250-6_4.

Smith, Linda. 1994. "Choice and Risk in the Care of Elderly People." In *Ethical Issues in Nursing*, edited by Geoffrey Hunt, 55–72. New York: Routledge.

Sullivan, Debra, Virginia Sullivan, Deborah Weatherspoon, and Christine Frazer. 2022. "Comparison of Nurse Burnout, before and during the COVID-19

Pandemic." *Nursing Clinics of North America* 57, no. 1 (March): 79–99. doi:10.1016/j.cnur.2021.11.006.

Taplin, Deborah. 1994. "Nursing and Informed Consent: An Empirical Study." In *Ethical Issues in Nursing*, edited by Geoffrey Hunt, 21–37. New York: Routledge.

Thomson, Stacy. 2007. "Nurse-Physician Collaboration: A Comparison of the Attitudes of Nurses and Physicians in the Medical-Surgical Patient Care Setting." *Medsurg Nursing* 16, no. 2 (April): 87–91, 104.

Tronto, Joan C. 1993. *Moral Boundaries: A Political Argument for an Ethics of Care*. New York: Routledge.

"The Unsentimental Nurse." 1901. *JAMA: Journal of the American Medical Association* 37, no. 1 (July 6): 33. doi:10.1001/jama.1901.02470270039013.

Vazirani, Sondra, Ron D. Hays, Martin F. Shapiro, and Marie Cowan. 2005. "Effect of a Multidisciplinary Intervention on Communication and Collaboration among Physicians and Nurses." *American Journal of Critical Care* 14, no. 1 (January 1): 71–77. doi:10.4037/ajcc2005.14.1.71.

Wainwright, Paul. 1994. "The Observation of Intimate Aspects of Care: Privacy and Dignity." In *Ethical Issues in Nursing*, edited by Geoffrey Hunt, 38–54. New York: Routledge.

Wall, Barbra Mann. n.d. "History of Hospitals." University of Pennsylvania School of Nursing. Accessed January 15, 2025. https://www.nursing.upenn.edu/nhhc/nurses-institutions-caring/history-of-hospitals/.

Wells, Kate. 2024. "After His Wife Died, He Joined Nurses to Push for New Staffing Rules in Hospitals." *NPR*. February 22. https://www.npr.org/sections/health-shots/2024/02/22/1231926415/after-his-wife-died-he-joined-nurses-to-push-for-new-staffing-rules-in-hospitals.

Wiegand, Debra L., and Marjorie Funk. 2012. "Consequences of Clinical Situations That Cause Critical Care Nurses to Experience Moral Distress." *Nursing Ethics* 19, no. 4 (July): 479–87. doi:10.1177/0969733011429342.

World Health Organization. 2019. *Delivered by Women, Led by Men: A Gender and Equity Analysis of the Global Health and Social Workforce*. Geneva: World Health Organization. https://www.who.int/publications/i/item/9789241515467.

———. 2020. *State of the World's Nursing 2020: Investing in Education, Jobs and Leadership*. Geneva: World Health Organization. https://www.who.int/publications/i/item/9789240003279.

## Further Reading

Čartolovni, Anto, Minna Stolt, P. Anne Scott, and Riitta Suhonen. 2021. "Moral Injury in Healthcare Professionals: A Scoping Review and Discussion." *Nursing Ethics* 28, no. 5 (August): 590–602. doi:10.1177/0969733020966776.

A survey of recent empirical studies on moral injury, with specific emphasis on the COVID-19 pandemic. The authors discuss how nurses are at particular risk for moral injury because nursing ethics tends to prioritize the duty to care, and they may experience patient suffering more immediately than other clinicians. The article relates the concept of moral injury to other psychological descriptors, such as regret, ethical suffering, and moral residue.

Fowler, Marsha, ed. 2015. *Guide to the Code of Ethics for Nurses: Interpretation and Application.* 2nd ed. Silver Spring, MD: American Nurses Association.

The American Nurses Association's official guide to nursing ethics, intended for practicing nurses. The text describes the history of the code of ethics and analyzes each of its nine provisions with reference to ethical and legal restrictions, case studies, and different interpretations of each provision. In the process, the authors discuss the role of nurses in medical research, social justice, and systems of authority and accountability.

Fry, Sara T., and Robert M. Veatch. 2011. *Case Studies in Nursing Ethics.* 4th ed. Sudbury, MA: Jones & Bartlett.

Surveys basic ethical principles in medicine and applies those principles in a multitude of examples relevant to nursing care, categorized thematically. The authors emphasize the development of moral reasoning skills by exploring how to analyze these cases rather than offering a settled solution to each one.

Grace, Pamela June. 2023. *Nursing Ethics and Professional Responsibility in Advanced Practice.* 4th ed. Burlington, MA: Jones & Bartlett.

A textbook intended for nursing students, written by nursing educators. Following an introductory discussion of moral reasoning and the goals of nursing, ethical questions relating to a wide range of issues are presented, including the nurse-patient relationship, medical research, pediatric and adolescent patients, psychiatric care, and palliative care.

Heaslip, Vanessa, and Julie Ryden, eds. 2013. *Understanding Vulnerability: Nursing and Healthcare Approach.* Chichester, UK: Wiley-Blackwell.

An edited volume examining how nursing care can ethically respond to vulnerability as part of the human condition, as well as the increased vulnerability of particular groups created by social conditions. Vulnerability is considered in its physical, psychological, and psychosocial dimensions. The authors, who are mainly nursing practitioners, focus on past failures and opportunities to improve the British healthcare system.

Kohlen, Helen, and Joan McCarthy, eds. 2020. *Nursing Ethics: Feminist Perspectives.* Cham: Springer. doi:10.1007/978-3-030-49104-8.

Analyzes nursing as a profession through feminist theoretical lenses, including a consideration of workplace power dynamics, the links between family and professional care, and conceptions of autonomy and agency. Chapters focus on specific issues, such as how gender roles shape nurse-patient and nurse-physician interactions, the history and contemporary role of midwives as skilled obstetrical nurses, and the broader attention that nurses have paid to the social determinants of health and social justice.

Lipscomb, Martin, ed. 2023. *Routledge Handbook of Philosophy and Nursing*. Abingdon, UK: Taylor & Francis.

A wide-ranging edited volume considering moral distress, the role of nurses in medical research, the need for cultural literacy, and the significance of empathy and compassion. Many of the chapters focus on the theoretical elements of nursing, such as the proper role of care, epistemic injustice, and concepts of personhood at work in contemporary nursing practice.

Monteverde, Settimio, ed. 2017. "End of Life Ethics." Special issue, *Nursing Ethics* 24, no. 1 (February).

Analyzes the role of nurses in end-of-life care, including how to preserve patient dignity in emergency departments (an under-studied aspect of end-of-life care), how decisions about medical futility are handled in Iranian hospitals, the process of surrogate planning and decision-making, nursing attitudes toward euthanasia, and issues around truth-telling. The authors focus on how nurses' perspectives, life experiences, and priorities can shift debates in medical ethics and improve patient care at the end of life.

Peter, Elizabeth, and Joan Liaschenko. 2013. "Moral Distress Reexamined: A Feminist Interpretation of Nurses' Identities, Relationships, and Responsibilities." *Journal of Bioethical Inquiry* 10, no. 3 (October): 337–45. doi:10.1007/s11673-013-9456-5.

Applies the feminist epistemological work of Hilde Lindemann Nelson and Margaret Urban Walker to the problem of moral distress in nursing, and suggests possible solutions. One key recommendation is to allow nurses to develop counternarratives to their subordination as a way of articulating their own values and moral identities.

Tingle, John, and Alan Cribb, eds. 2014. *Nursing Law and Ethics*. 4th ed. Chichester, UK: Wiley.

Considers the intersection between the laws governing nursing care and ethical debates in that field. Contributors focus on the British healthcare context and discuss issues such as midwives, consent, mental health nursing, and end-of-life care. The various chapters extensively utilize case studies, and each topic is addressed from both legal and ethical perspectives.

# CHAPTER 14
# Experimentation on Human Subjects

**Key topics in this chapter:**

- The historical origins of ethical principles governing human subjects research
- Twentieth-century moral failures in medical experimentation
- How that history precipitated attempts to regulate research, including the Nuremberg Code and the Belmont Report, and the principles expressed in those documents
- What the Common Rule requires of U.S. researchers

## Introduction

The foundational ethical principles and debates around medical experimentation emerged out of a series of horrific moral failures that treated human beings as disposable resources for medical research—especially those who were enslaved, poor, disabled, institutionalized, and/or socially marginalized by their race or ethnicity. The primary purpose of medicine is healing human beings, but the history of medical experimentation serves as a powerful warning that individuals or populations may be acknowledged to belong to the human species, and thus have biological commonality with those whom medical experiments seek to benefit, without being acknowledged normatively as persons whose autonomy and well-being need to be considered. Frequently, such dehumanization has located biological inferiority in intangible qualities such as sensitivity to pain, ability to control emotion or impulse, or intelligence, while conveniently acknowledging the commonality of anatomy, thus rendering the dehumanized (or de-personalized) subjects useful for experimentation.

For much of the history of medicine, research has made use of animals and cadavers, which generate their own debates. Which species of animals are morally considerable and on what basis? What are our obligations to the dead? How medical research is conducted reminds us of how living human beings have sometimes been instrumentalized. Medical experiments implicitly appeal to a utilitarian calculation that the expenditure of resources, sometimes including human suffering or injury, will produce generalizable knowledge that will improve the health of many others. Medical experimentation tests techniques, pharmaceuticals, and equipment in order to improve the powers of medicine to treat or prevent pathology. Such research tries to discover new knowledge, so inherently it carries the risk of no positive benefits. Especially over the last eight decades, codes of research ethics have insisted that the well-being and autonomy of human subjects should not be sacrificed for the "greater good." Such codes demand that we confront the ethical costs of research. What makes it worthwhile or gratuitous? If the risks and outcomes have yet to be discovered, can research subjects' consent truly be informed? This is very different from the uncertainty of how a particular patient will respond to a treatment whose efficacy has already been empirically established. If research utilizes control or placebo groups, does it promote their well-being? In research ethics, the principles of respect for autonomy, nonmaleficence, beneficence, and justice apply in ways that are distinct from clinical ethics.

## Early Moral Discussions of Medical Experimentation

The first European moral discourse around medical research arose from religious sources, with the early medieval prohibition on desecrating corpses through dissection, a prohibition that began to be lifted in Italy in the fourteenth century (Ghosh 2015). Historically, there is a blending of therapeutic and experimental purposes: the physician is trying to cure a patient and, along the way, finds out what will help other patients. Sometimes, of course, there is no therapeutic intent. When someone dissects a pig to see how its heart works or performs an autopsy on a human corpse, there is a purely instrumental purpose. Research that uses live human subjects creates unique moral obligations, to ensure that they are not treated merely as means to an end.

It was only in the early and mid-nineteenth century that European and American doctors started to suggest rules governing research that focus on securing the informed consent of research subjects (respect for autonomy), not conducting experiments that cause them harm (nonmaleficence), and benefiting the research subjects themselves (beneficence). An English doctor, Thomas Percival, argued in one of the first texts on medical ethics that physicians should consult with each other on difficult cases, always keeping "the good of the patient [as] the sole object in view" (1803, 37). Although Percival does not distinguish between treatment and research, the consultation he recommends was a precursor to the institutional review boards that now evaluate research proposals. In 1865, Claude Bernard, a preeminent French physiologist, applied this focus on nonmaleficence specifically to medical experimentation: "The principle of medical and surgical morality, therefore, consists in never performing on man an experiment which might be harmful to him to any extent, even though the result might be highly advantageous to science, i.e., to the health of others" (1949, 101). Scientific knowledge could be produced as a side effect of treating patients, but doctors should remain committed to "do no harm," prioritizing individual patients' well-being over the common good.

Respect for the autonomy of research subjects also originated in the early nineteenth century. In 1833, an American army surgeon named William Beaumont wrote a code for researchers that included obtaining consent and suspending the experiment when the subject was harmed or wanted it to stop ("Medical Experimentation" 2004). However, we should understand Beaumont's injunction against the background of his own long-running research on a single subject: Alexis St. Martin, a French-Canadian trader who was accidentally shot in 1822 in the Michigan territory. Beaumont treated St. Martin in his home over the course of ten years, and his abdominal injury healed in such a way that Beaumont could observe the inside of St. Martin's stomach through an inch-wide fistula. During those years, Beaumont performed numerous experiments—often tying a bit of food on a string so that it could be inserted, removed, and observed at various points in the digestive process—that allowed him to publish his *Experiments and Observations on the Gastric Juice and the Physiology of Digestion* (1833). Beaumont did not close the fistula, and his experiments must have caused St. Martin significant pain. Furthermore, St. Martin worked as a servant during these years, so he was economically dependent on Beaumont (Logsdon 2021). This calls into question whether he was truly free to consent to participate.

In these early articulations of researchers' moral obligations, the consent of subjects meant something quite different from what it means now. Subjects were often not informed or were actively misinformed about the risks and benefits of participating in experiments, the distinction between therapeutic and experimental medicine was frequently ignored, and subjects were typically recruited and retained in research by offering them monetary or other incentives, which pressured them, especially if they were poor, to continue even when experiments were painful or inconvenient. Soldiers, people in mental hospitals, children in orphanages, and prisoners were also targeted for experimentation, given how their institutionalization allowed researchers to control their diets and other behaviors.

For instance, extensive research on anti-malarial drugs was conducted during World War II by the U.S. military and the University of Chicago, including the deliberate infection of prisoners at Stateville Penitentiary in Illinois (Miller 2013). Long-term prisoners were recruited into the study through the use of stipends and offers of parole reassessment. Such research was thought to be justified by the need to protect American soldiers abroad—an explicitly utilitarian calculation. For several decades, the project was held up as a model of ethical research, since prisoners were informed about the goals of the research and allowed to withdraw from the study at any point. However, they were also told that they would be "fully cured" of malaria, even though the parasite that causes malaria is notoriously mutable and many strains are drug-resistant ("Prison Official" 1974). This experiment began, in fact, because quinine was losing its efficacy. The research project ended in 1974 as part of a growing wave of criticism of experimentation on prisoners. The early Stateville experiments were referenced by the defense in the Nazi Doctors' Trial as analogous to their own malaria experiments at the Dachau concentration camp.

## Nazi Medical Experiments and the Nuremberg Code

The first attempt at a universal set of principles governing medical research was the **Nuremberg Code**, which was developed out of the so-called Doctors' Trial in Nuremberg, Germany. After World War II, a U.S. military court prosecuted twenty-three high-ranking Nazi doctors and other personnel involved in medical experiments in concentration camps. It is worth remembering that these doctors had taken the Hippocratic Oath, which includes the duty of nonmaleficence. Karl Brandt, personal physician to Adolf Hitler and SS officer overseeing the medical experiments, interpreted the Hippocratic Oath as applying to the German nation as his patient, such that the "degenerate" elements threatening the nation's health needed to be excised. Concentration camp prisoners were excluded from the political status of citizens and the normative status of persons—either by race/ethnicity, political affiliation, sexual orientation, physical or mental disability, or religion. As such, they were seen as instrumentally useful for advancing medical knowledge of human disease and injury but as morally insignificant. Accordingly, the medical experiments conducted at Dachau, Buchenwald, and other camps stand out for their depravity: inmates injected with toxic substances, infants deliberately starved to death, inmates made to stand in freezing water or low-pressure chambers, twins whose organs were sewn together, women sterilized, Roma and Sinti children with noma (a form of gangrene) beheaded, and inmates deliberately infected with malaria, typhus, tuberculosis, and yellow fever. Almost all the research subjects died as a direct result of the experiments.

In 1933, the Nazis had banned vivisection, the use of animals in medical experimentation. In 1943, in a speech arguing that non-Aryan people could be used to fulfill the goals of the Reich, Heinrich Himmler claimed that the prohibition on vivisection demonstrated that Germany was the most civilized of nations:

> Whether 10,000 Russian females fall down from exhaustion while digging an anti-tank ditch interests me only in so far as the anti-tank ditch for Germany is finished. We shall never be rough and heartless when it is not necessary, that is clear. We Germans, who are the only people in the world who have a decent attitude towards animals, will also assume a decent attitude towards these human animals [*Menschentieren*]. But it is a crime against our own blood to worry about them and give them ideals, thus causing our sons and grandsons to have a more difficult time with them. (Himmler 1943)

We should note the moral deflection at work in this short passage, in referring to people as "human animals" and to mass death as "fall[ing] down from exhaustion." This erasure of the boundary between humans and animals serves the moral and political purpose of dehumanization rather than the protection of animals. Again, this logic entails that the suffering of some (especially those framed as unworthy of moral attention) is outweighed by the well-being of present and future persons who deserve support and protection (those framed as worthy of moral attention). The very distinction between Aryans and non-Aryans is a normative judgment masquerading as a biological fact. In sum, at the same time that research on animals was officially banned, human experimentation was accepted because Jews, Roma, and others who were excluded from the German *Volk* were seen as "pathogens"—not even as morally considerable as animals. These experiments were variously driven by military goals, such as how to protect pilots from hypothermia, or by eugenicist ideology, such as how to reduce the reproduction of "undesirables" through sterilization.

At the Doctors' Trial, the defendants argued that their research methods were used in other countries, including the United States, and that no international code of research ethics had been established. There was no such thing as illegal experimental practices, so what they did could not be construed as war crimes. Despite this defense, sixteen of the twenty-three physicians and military officials were convicted and sentenced to death or lengthy prison terms.

To prevent future abuses in medical experimentation, the judges in the Doctors' Trial included in their 1947 decision what has come to be known as the Nuremberg Code, a list of criteria for morally acceptable medical research. The Code originated with six points written by American psychiatrist and neurologist Leo Alexander, a medical advisor to the court during the trial. The court added four more, and the ten points were adopted as part of the verdict. The idea was that these standards should have been followed by the Nazi doctors, and these are the norms that should be followed by future researchers. The ten provisions were drawn in part from the Hippocratic Oath's emphasis on nonmaleficence and beneficence, and from the emerging legal demand for informed consent. Ironically, they were also based on nascent pre-war German medical research guidelines.

The Nuremberg Code begins with Principle 1—"The voluntary consent of the human subject is absolutely essential"—and defines what informed and voluntary consent means (International Military Tribunal 1950, 181). First, people cannot be coerced into serving as experimental subjects. This principle recognizes both overt uses of force and subtle forms of coercion, including deceit and fraud. Fundamentally, a research subject must be able "to make an understanding and enlightened decision" about whether to participate in the research (181). Emphasizing autonomy in this way not only protects potential subjects from abuse but also recognizes the overarching normative justification for this obligation: they are self-determining persons whose control over their own lives needs to be respected.

Experiments should also be necessary "to yield fruitful results for the good of society" (Principle 2), guided by evidence gained from animal research (Principle 3), and designed to "avoid all unnecessary physical and mental suffering and injury" (Principle 4) (International Military Tribunal 1950, 182). Even if test subjects would consent to experiments that are medically unnecessary or unnecessary to perform on humans, such research would be morally wrong. The code prohibits any experiment in which subjects may suffer disability, injury, or death—"except, perhaps, in those experiments where the experimental physicians also serve as subjects" (Principle 5) (182). This exception neatly reminds researchers of the moral status they share with subjects and tests their assessment that an experiment is necessary. The next three principles all concern the proportionality of risk to benefit: the risk posed to subjects should not "exceed . . . the humanitarian importance of the problem to be solved" (Principle 6), researchers should guard against "even remote possibilities of injury, disability, or death" (Principle 7), and research "should be conducted only by scientifically qualified persons" (Principle 8) (182). The code also establishes the right of subjects to withdraw from the research (Principle 9) and the obligation of researchers to suspend it if they realize the risks are too great (Principle 10) (182). That is, the commitment to protecting research subjects' autonomy and well-being is durational—continuing throughout the experiment—rather than a single bureaucratic step. Informed consent is an ongoing process, not just a piece of paper to be signed.

Overall, the Nuremberg Code blends deontological and utilitarian moral intuitions by affirming two fundamental principles of moral decision-making: (1) respecting the autonomy of research subjects, and (2) weighing potential burdens against potential benefits. But it clearly privileges the first principle in arguing that the well-being of research subjects may not be sacrificed for the well-being of others. In the post-war period, the World Medical Association adopted the Declaration of Geneva (1948) and the Declaration of Helsinki (1964), largely following the Nuremberg Code, to provide consistent international standards for medical research.

The Nuremberg Code itself did not become law in the United States or any other country, and due to its unenforceability, it was largely ignored by post-war researchers. American physicians took themselves to be operating in a different moral environment than the Nazi concentration camps: "It was a good code for barbarians but an unnecessary code for ordinary physician-scientists" (Katz 1992, 228). This complacency made possible the abuses of the Tuskegee study, the Willowbrook experiments, and many other unethical studies for several more decades. The cultural authority granted to doctors, especially in the wake of "medical miracles" such as childhood vaccinations and organ transplants, further bolstered paternalistic deference to researchers' methods.

## Post-war Experiments in the U.S.

In 1966, an anesthesiologist named Henry Beecher published an article describing twenty-two examples of American medical studies that were morally problematic for a variety of reasons: they lacked any scientific benefit, they endangered research subjects, or they did not secure fully voluntary and informed consent (Beecher 1966). Two of those twenty-two examples were the Willowbrook hepatitis study and the Jewish Chronic Disease Hospital cancer study. Around the same time, increasing criticism of the Tuskegee syphilis study emerged first internally within the U.S. Public Health Service and then more broadly. In each of these experiments, the research subjects were assumed to be incapable of giving consent. Rather than this functioning as a disqualification for the research, investigators thought it was adequate to decide for them. Research subjects were also exposed to the risk of harm—or the certainty of harm, in the case of the Tuskegee study. All three experiments violated the standards of the Nuremberg Code. These scandals gave rise to the National Commission for the Protection of Human Subjects of Biomedical and Behavioral Research, which published the Belmont Report, the foundation of contemporary U.S. legislation regulating medical research.

### 1. Tuskegee syphilis study (1932–1972)

The U.S. Public Health Service (PHS) study at the Tuskegee Institute in Alabama began in 1932 as an attempt to understand the course of untreated syphilis in six hundred Black men, at a time when no effective treatment for syphilis existed. Each research subject was promised treatment for "bad blood," minimal financial compensation ($1 a year for every year they remained in the study), and burial benefits if their family would consent to an autopsy. The men underwent annual physical examinations and spinal taps. Even after penicillin was discovered to be an effective cure for syphilis in the 1940s, it was withheld from the study participants. A local public health doctor insisted that the infected men be treated (with the methods known in the 1930s) to reduce their bacteria levels just enough that they would not transmit it to others. By the time the experiment was ended in 1972, after a whistleblower in the Public Health Service—Peter Buxtun, a child of Shoah survivors—contacted a journalist, 128 men had died from syphilis or complications from syphilis, 40 of their wives had been infected, and 19 children were born with congenital syphilis.

The study's design was antithetical to the principles of the Nuremberg Code, including:

- Principle 1: The men involved in the study were not asked for voluntary and informed consent. The physicians who conducted the study claimed that the men were incapable of understanding the research. Once questions were raised in the 1960s, they used the concept of **surrogate informed consent**, where the surrogates were the public health officials conducting the study (Jones 1981, 196). The men were not even alerted that they had contracted syphilis, were told they were being treated when in fact treatment was being denied to them, and were not offered information about effective treatments.

- Principle 1: As undereducated and impoverished Black men living in the segregated South, the research subjects had little access to healthcare. The meager offer of examinations by physicians, support from nurses, and basic medication (aspirin), as well as financial compensation and burial benefits, may have had a coercive effect.

- Principles 2 and 6: No scientifically useful knowledge was gained from the study, because no one needed to know the course of partially treated syphilis.

- Principles 4, 5, 6, 7, and 10: The experiment was specifically designed as a "death watch" when effective treatment was available ("Forty Year Death Watch" 1972), rather than avoiding "all unnecessary physical and mental suffering and injury" (International Military Tribunal 1950, 182).

James Jones notes that, despite the participation of many physicians within the Public Health Service over four decades and the publication of scientific reports in medical journals, no moral objections to the study were recorded until 1966, almost twenty years after the Nuremberg Code was written, two years after the Declaration of Helsinki, and the same year that the Public Health Service itself issued ethical guidelines for research funded by its grants (1981, 193). Even when a review board was formed in 1969, the people on the board had some incentive to see the study continue: its members included "PHS officials, medical professors, the state health officer of Alabama, and a senior officer from the Milbank Memorial Fund," which had paid burial stipends to these men for several decades (193). None of the board members were experts in medical ethics, none were Black, and all but one of them had participated in some way in the project (193). It was therefore not an independent review by people who would challenge research methods that had become normalized.

## *2. Willowbrook hepatitis study (1956–1971)*

The Willowbrook hepatitis study similarly targeted a group of subjects who were socially stigmatized and marginalized: children with cognitive disabilities institutionalized at New York's Willowbrook State School. Due to overcrowding and poor hygienic conditions, hepatitis A was endemic when Saul Krugman, a professor of pediatrics at New York University, became the institution's consulting physician. He saw these conditions as an opportunity to test hepatitis vaccines. Consent (or, more properly, permission) was sought from parents, but it was neither informed nor voluntary: Krugman downplayed the risks associated with deliberately exposing children to hepatitis and suggested that taking part in the study would offer "protection" to participants (Rothman and Rothman 1984, 266); and the long waiting list for entry into the school pressured parents into signing consent forms, since that allowed a faster route to acceptance. Krugman came to defend his methods by claiming that children in the institution would inevitably be exposed to hepatitis (a claim later refuted), that his methods would moderate the symptoms, and that his research would result in a vaccine that would prevent disease in the wider population.

Children between the ages of three and eleven were admitted into a special ward of Willowbrook, with some inoculated and others serving as a control group. Some children were exposed to live hepatitis A virus derived from the feces of other Willowbrook patients. Others were injected with live hepatitis B virus, a much more dangerous pathogen that was not endemic at the institution (Halpern 2021, 145–46). These experiments led to a clearer differentiation of hepatitis A and hepatitis B, but concurrent lab research by others led to the same conclusion without endangering human subjects. The study also proved the efficacy of gamma globulin for pre- and post-exposure prophylaxis. Krugman was repeatedly praised for the methods and results of his research, including receiving awards that described it as exemplary (Rothman and Rothman 1984, 260). The moral failures of the Willowbrook experiments resemble those of the Tuskegee study in the sense that physicians could have prevented the spread of hepatitis by inoculating the research subjects with gamma globulin and by instituting stricter hygiene practices. Like the Tuskegee study, the Willowbrook experiments also raise moral questions about when the permission of surrogates (in this case, parents or other guardians) is justified in medical research and when the inability of research subjects to consent on their own behalf means that the research design is problematic.

### 3. Jewish Chronic Disease Hospital cancer study (1963)

In 1963, a physician at the Sloan-Kettering Institute for Cancer Research, Chester Southam, approached the medical director at the Jewish Chronic Disease Hospital, a long-term care facility in Brooklyn, where many patients were physically debilitated and cognitively disabled. Some were Shoah survivors, and some spoke little English. Southam's goal was to see if immunocompromised patients would reject live cancer cells as quickly as healthy volunteers, as an extension of his research on cancer patients and on healthy prisoners in the Ohio State Penitentiary (Katz, Capron, and Glass 1972; Arras 2008). He advised the medical director that no informed consent was necessary because the injection of live cancer cells would have no permanent effect on these patients. The three doctors whom Southam first approached to give the injections refused to do so, objecting that the research subjects could not consent. Southam then asked an unlicensed "house officer," an immigrant from the Philippines, to inject twenty-two debilitated patients with live cancer cells. In later testimony, Southam claimed that "oral consent" was given by each patient: they were told that the injections would test their immunity and that a "small nodule" might grow. The word "cancer" was not used. None of the patients developed cancer as a result of the injections.

The three doctors who refused to participate in the study raised moral objections with the hospital's Grievance Committee, which sided with Southam. Contesting this decision, a hospital board member brought a legal case that found its way to the New York Department of Education, as the regulator of medical licenses. The arguments focused on what kind of informed consent was necessary. Besides the claim that the subjects were unlikely to be harmed, Southam's defense partially echoed that of the Nazi doctors—that he was following standard research practices that allowed physicians to decide how much information to share with research subjects (and patients): "I believe such revelation [use of the word 'cancer'] is generally contraindicated in the best consideration of the patient's welfare and therefore to withhold such emotionally disturbing but medically non-pertinent details (unless requested by the patient) is in the best tradition of responsible clinical practice" (quoted in Katz, Capron, and Glass 1972, 38). It is unclear how a patient (especially one not fluent in English or nonresponsive) could have "requested" details that a physician actively withheld from them.

The New York Board of Regents found that "any fact which might influence the giving or withholding of consent [such as the inclusion of the word 'cancer'] is material," and thus that researchers cannot withhold information based on the paternalistic claim that it might irrationally upset subjects and dissuade them from participating (quoted in Katz, Capron, and Glass 1972, 60). Despite this finding, which resulted in the suspension of Southam's medical license for a year, he was elected president of the American Association for Cancer Research in 1968. This study violated the Nuremberg principles concerning informed consent as well as the principles centered on nonmaleficence: Southam admitted that there was some possibility of the cancer cells spreading within the subjects, and he had seen at least one previous case in which injected cancer cells migrated to the lymph node of a research subject (lymph nodes being a primary way that cancer spreads through the body).

### *4. Other unethical research*

In addition to these three well-publicized experiments that directly led to greater regulation, other twentieth-century experiments violated the

Nuremberg Code by targeting research subjects who could not easily refuse to participate. Military organizations conducted unethical medical research throughout the twentieth century in the name of protecting public health. The Japanese army during World War II tested biological and chemical weapons primarily on Chinese and Soviet prisoners, many of whom died after being deliberately infected with anthrax or cholera. During World War II, the U.S. military exposed sixty thousand American soldiers to mustard gas in various doses, with a particular interest in how people of different races reacted to it (Smith 2008). As part of the Manhattan Project to build a nuclear weapon, the U.S. military conducted tests exposing hospitalized civilians to plutonium without their consent. In 1955, the Atomic Energy Commission tested the effects of radiation by giving 102 Indigenous people in Alaska doses of radioactive iodine without their consent. The Department of Defense sponsored research into whole-body irradiation of cancer patients between 1960 and 1971. Between 1963 and 1969, the U.S. Army sprayed fully staffed military ships with biological and chemical agents (Conahan 1994).

Earlier, we mentioned the malaria experiments at Stateville prison, which were referenced in the defense of Nazi doctors at the Nuremberg trials. U.S. prisoners would continue to be used as "volunteers" for medical research for several decades. For example, dermatological experiments were conducted at Holmesburg Prison in Pennsylvania, which a University of Pennsylvania researcher described as "acres of skin" on which to test household chemicals, chemical weapons such as dioxin, and pharmaceuticals such as Retin-A and anti-viral agents (Hornblum 1998).

Lastly, medical research has increasingly been conducted in developing countries, precisely because U.S. and European regulations are harder to enforce there. Between 1946 and 1948, the U.S. Public Health Service led a study of sexually transmitted diseases in Guatemalan prisons to test the effectiveness of penicillin. Approximately five thousand research subjects were exposed to syphilis and gonorrhea first through infected sex workers and then through direct injections or abrasions. The physician who led this research had participated in the Tuskegee study and deliberately located the research in Guatemala to avoid critical scrutiny and liability (Rodriguez and García 2013). This outsourcing of medical experimentation is often facilitated by economic coercion. Underfunded local public health services may depend on incentives offered by foreign governments or corporations, which pressure them to sacrifice the autonomy and well-being of study participants.

A common thread running through these unethical experiments is the use of research subjects who were socially marginalized or easily controlled: primarily poor Black people, prisoners, soldiers, Indigenous people, people debilitated by chronic illness, people with cognitive disabilities, people in developing countries, and people seeking care at public or teaching hospitals because they could not afford private healthcare. The ethical and political question that demands to be raised in each of these instances is which human beings are seen as morally considerable and which are reduced to lab specimens.

## The Belmont Report and the Common Rule

In response to the scandal caused by the Tuskegee syphilis study, in 1974 Congress formed the National Commission for the Protection of Human Subjects of Biomedical and Behavioral Research, which in 1979 published what has come to be known as the **Belmont Report**, an articulation of principles and corresponding regulations governing all research with human subjects in the United States (National Commission 1979). Although its moral intuitions align with the Nuremberg Code, the Belmont Report identifies three foundational principles that can be used to make judgments about particular cases: respect for persons, beneficence, and justice. The Belmont Report thus codifies a version of principlism as the official regulatory foundation for medical research in the United States—and in fact one of the originators of principlism, Tom Beauchamp, served as a staff member for the Commission that produced the report.

The ethical principles in the Belmont Report guided the U.S. Department of Health and Human Services (HHS) in developing rules for human subjects research in 1981, which applied to all experiments receiving HHS funding. This was superseded in 1991 by the Federal Policy for the Protection of Human Subjects (45 CFR 46, Subpart A). Because fifteen federal departments and agencies include this policy verbatim in their own regulations, it is often called the Common Rule. Subparts B, C, and D cover research on vulnerable populations—respectively, pregnant women and fetuses, prisoners, and children. HHS updated the Common Rule in 2017, and the revised Common Rule now governs medical research using human subjects in all organizations that receive federal funding, including universities (§ 46.122). The Food and Drug Administration (FDA) also requires that any approved drug or device follow requirements in their testing that largely overlap with the Common Rule.

Unlike the Nuremberg Code, the Belmont Report established a mechanism for evaluating the justifiability of research on human subjects in the form of **institutional review boards (IRBs)**, which are formalized by the Common Rule (45 CFR 46.109). IRBs apply the three ethical principles to specific experimental protocols. Each of the three principles has a more concrete area of application: (1) respect for persons is demonstrated through the process of obtaining informed consent, (2) beneficence is demonstrated through an assessment of potential risks and benefits, and (3) justice is demonstrated through an explanation of how research subjects are selected and recruited.

The first principle, respect for persons, establishes the preeminent significance of recognizing the autonomy of research subjects: "Individuals should be treated as autonomous agents," and "persons with diminished autonomy are entitled to protection" (National Commission 1979, 4). This commitment is a restatement of Immanuel Kant's third formulation of the categorical imperative, that humanity should never be treated merely as a means but always also as an end in itself (1996, 4:429). That is, people have the right to determine their purposes for themselves, so they should not be treated as instruments or tools in the service of others' purposes. The Belmont Report distinguishes medical research from medical therapy and requires researchers to make that distinction clear. That is, patients should be informed that the research does not have the primary purpose of treating or curing them, and they should also be informed about possible risks and benefits (including therapeutic benefits) from participating in the research.

Deceiving or coercing someone into giving consent are forms of manipulation that violate this principle. Using deception or incomplete disclosure is prohibited unless it is crucial to achieve the goals of a study—that is, when full knowledge of the study will affect the participants' responses—and the research poses minimal risk. For example, an assistant to the principal investigator (PI) may pose as a test subject so that the PI can gauge the subjects' natural responses to some obnoxious behavior (deception), or they may be asked to rate the credibility of a speaker without knowing that the research question is about measuring racial bias (incomplete disclosure). Participants must be debriefed at the conclusion of the study, including an explanation of why deception or incomplete disclosure was necessary. Other than these specific conditions, which must be approved by an IRB, participants must be fully informed about the purpose and methods of the study, including any risks (45 CFR 46.104).

Informed consent means that the information is not only given to subjects but that it is also given in a language and form that they can comprehend. Ideally, steps would be taken to ensure they have comprehended it. IRBs pay significant attention to how consent is obtained. For example, consent forms must be "in language understandable to the subject or the legally authorized representative" (interpreted to mean no higher than an eighth-grade reading level), they must disclose any possible risks and benefits from participating, and they should make clear that there is no penalty for refusing to participate or withdrawing at any time (45 CFR 46.116). IRBs also build in more stringent guidelines for research subjects whose autonomy is diminished, such as children or people with cognitive disabilities, or who are otherwise more vulnerable to coercion, such as incarcerated people. When college professors are the PIs on a study, IRBs often prohibit them from distributing recruitment materials and consent forms to students in their own classes, since students may feel that their grades will be jeopardized by nonparticipation. An unequal power relationship between the researcher and the subject may create incentives or pressures that are subtly coercive (§ 46.116).

Respect for persons also requires that research subjects' identifiable private information remain confidential (45 CFR 46.111). As we said in Chapter 4, control over one's personal information is an important part of individual autonomy. Since studies may require participants to complete questionnaires about their health history and current conditions or to reveal other things about themselves during the research that they would not want publicized, IRBs often require that investigators assign codes to individual participants so they cannot be associated with the private information. The key matching each code to each subject must be stored separately from the coded data and accessible only to the PI.

The second principle, beneficence, picks up on the utilitarian intuitions of the Nuremberg Code: the research must minimize harm or risk of harm, and the risks must be reasonable in relation to anticipated benefits

(45 CFR 46.111). Risks may include not only physical harms (such as pain, injury, or disease) but also psychological harms (such as anxiety), legal harms (such as revealing that one violated the law), economic harms (such as travel costs to the research site), or social harms (such as embarrassment in front of peers). The primary beneficiaries of research, admittedly, are the people who will take advantage of the knowledge established by the experiment—who will be immunized once the vaccine is discovered and its side effects tested, or whose brains will be imaged by MRIs when those techniques are proven safe. But the Belmont Report obligates researchers to prioritize the well-being of research subjects, both in terms of minimizing the risk of harm and optimizing possible benefits for the subjects themselves. For example, in the early days of the AIDS epidemic, people who were HIV-positive fought to participate in drug trials as a way of possibly extending their own lives as well as contributing to others' future well-being. In discussing the principle of beneficence, the Belmont Report cites the Hippocratic Oath's precept to "do no harm" and Bernard's claim that researchers' obligations to research subjects cannot be outweighed by generalized future benefits (National Commission 1979, 7).

Federal regulations do not require IRBs to evaluate the scientific validity of proposed research because, typically, IRB members do not have the disciplinary background and subject-matter expertise that the investigators do. However, IRBs are obligated to protect subjects against unnecessary risk. If a study is so poorly designed that no useful data will be produced—if the sample size is too small or there are too many confounding variables, for example—then exposing subjects to any amount of risk (or even inconvenience) is unethical. This is one reason why IRBs must include members with scientific backgrounds. When it involves human subjects, bad science is morally wrong.

The third principle, justice, says that the benefits and burdens of research should be equitably distributed. This is relevant at both the individual level and the social level. First, just distribution requires that, everything being equal, participation must be open to all (45 CFR 46.111). In principle, test subjects should reap some benefits from the study, so excluding someone from those benefits is unfair. If a PI wants to exclude potential participants, the burden of proof is on the PI to justify why it is necessary to produce reliable data. Furthermore, on the social level, it would be unjust to have one group bear the burdens while another group gets the benefits—for example, by recruiting impoverished people or citizens of developing countries to test pharmaceuticals that will primarily be used by wealthy people in developed nations. The Tuskegee, Willowbrook, and Jewish Chronic Disease Hospital studies all took advantage of the subjects' marginalized positions when the intended beneficiaries were in the wider population.

Review boards are made up of independent evaluators who ensure that studies adhere to the principles of respect for persons, beneficence, and justice. The Common Rule requires that each IRB must have at least five members with different backgrounds and expertise; it must include at least one scientist, one non-scientist, one person who is not otherwise affiliated with the institution (such as a community member), and people who can represent the interests of research subjects (45 CFR 46.107). From the simplest undergraduate psychology experiment to multi-year pharmaceutical trials, an IRB must approve it or determine it to be exempt before any data can be collected from human subjects. As a rule, peer-reviewed journals will not publish research on human subjects without proof of IRB approval.

There are three levels of review for research protocols on human subjects: full board review, expedited review, or exempt from review (45 CFR 46.109). Research is exempt when there is little to no risk to subjects, and it falls into one of eight categories for exemption—for example, when adults agree to play an online game, and the results are recorded in a way that their identities are not readily discoverable. Under the revised Common Rule, research on children may be exempt only if it involves observed public behavior (without intervention) or educational tests (§ 46.104). If there is a possibility of coercion, participants may be exposed to more than minimal risks, prisoners are being used as test subjects, or confidential or genetic information is involved, research is not exempt. IRBs conduct what is called an expedited review when there is no more than minimal risk of physical or psychological harm to the participants, and the proposed study falls into one of seven categories, such as the collection of blood samples by finger stick or the analysis of materials that were obtained for non-research purposes (e.g., data or specimens collected in the course of medical treatment) (§ 46.110). Research is subject to full board review if it may pose more than minimal risk to subjects and it does not fall into one of the expedited categories. For example, clinical trials with drugs, devices, or new surgical techniques are subject to full board review.

## Contemporary Issues

The core moral commitments articulated in the Belmont Report continue to shape contemporary debates regarding human subjects research: how to use unethically acquired knowledge, how to extend protections to studies (primarily clinical trials) that are not federally funded, whether study participants should be compensated, and how patients can ethically participate in research that blurs the distinction between therapeutic and nontherapeutic purposes.

Concerning the first issue, there is consensus that most of the history of medical research was not governed by anything resembling contemporary regulations. In that sense, current medical knowledge is built on the foundations of unethically acquired information. Some particularly egregious examples stand out against that general background. For instance, the *Topographische Anatomie des Menschen* (*Atlas of Topographical and Applied Human Anatomy*, known as the Pernkopf Atlas) is a four-volume anatomy textbook, originally published between 1937 and 1957, that contains detailed drawings of the human body (Atlas 2001). It was a standard medical textbook for decades and has been translated into many languages. Eduard Pernkopf was dean of the Faculty of Medicine at the University of Vienna for much of the time that he supervised four illustrators who worked on the atlas. All five were allied with the Nazi party, and some of the illustrators incorporated Nazi symbolism into their signatures in the corners of the illustrations. In the 1980s, it was established that many of the cadavers "donated" to the Vienna Anatomical Institute, and possibly used for the anatomical drawings, were political prisoners executed by the Nazi regime as well as patients from public hospitals. The political prisoners almost certainly did not consent to the use of their bodies for this purpose. For these reasons, some scholars have argued that the Pernkopf Atlas should no longer be used in medical education, while others have claimed that the high quality of the illustrations justifies its continued use to train clinicians, who will then help future patients. One problem with refusing to use it is that many current texts have used images or descriptions from it and thus are morally implicated by its provenance. There have been different attempts to reckon with this problematic history. Some medical curricula have replaced this book with more recent texts, and some libraries have chosen to keep the book but include a note at the beginning explaining its origins and condemning the unethical treatment of prisoners. The American Medical Association has taken the position that unethical experiments typically have limited scientific value, but in those rare instances where unethical experiments have yielded useful medical knowledge, that information should be referenced with an explanation of the moral problems with the research, a justification for using it, and an expression of respect for the victims (n.d., 7.2.2).

A second issue concerns corporate funding for research that occurs outside of the U.S. For a treatment to be approved by the FDA, it must go through three phases of testing, with progressively larger groups of test subjects, to determine if it is effective and safe. Each of these phases takes several months to several years. In recent decades, a majority of **clinical trials** have been conducted by private pharmaceutical and medical equipment corporations, and a significant proportion of these trials has shifted to developing countries, where ethical regulations are less likely to be enforced. The Belmont Report and the Common Rule are focused on protecting human subjects within the United States, but the principles of respect for persons, beneficence, and justice call out obligations that researchers have to anyone, regardless of national boundaries or citizenship. Extending those considerations beyond the borders of the United States and other wealthy countries has become the focus of ethical discussion over the last few decades.

The principle of justice, in particular, challenges researchers not to disproportionately burden people in poorer countries to develop medicines or technologies that will primarily benefit people in wealthier countries. For instance, clinical trials of HIV anti-retroviral treatments were largely conducted in sub-Saharan Africa, and there was a concern that when the drugs were available, they would be too expensive for most communities in which they were originally tested. Concerted efforts by government and nongovernmental agencies have helped to address that ethical concern (Weigmann 2015). However, pharmaceutical companies generally focus their efforts on developing medicines that will eventually turn a profit, which means that so-called diseases of prosperity—heart disease, cancer, diabetes—tend to be targeted by clinical trials more frequently than diseases that primarily impact the Global South. The World Health Organization (n.d.) maintains a list of twenty "neglected tropical diseases"— such as dengue, leprosy, and schistosomiasis—that receive little research attention but collectively affect one billion people. Not only how medical research projects are designed but which ones are funded may reflect whose autonomy and well-being are seen as worth protecting.

A third issue is whether compensating research subjects interferes with voluntary, informed consent. Sometimes poverty or lack of access to quality healthcare generates coercive conditions under which subjects only appear to be freely consenting. On the other hand, compensation may seem justified in the sense that research subjects are giving up their time and privacy and, in some cases, are taking risks to participate in research. If compensation is appropriate, how much should test subjects receive? Do researchers working in lower- and middle-income communities have an obligation to provide ancillary care—that is, medical care to research subjects who are not receiving adequate healthcare—even if it is irrelevant to the objectives of the study? Are researchers responsible for long-term care after the study is completed, including access to the medicine or procedure that the participants helped to test (Millum 2020)?

A final issue concerns patient well-being. Although there is some debate about standards of evidence in medical experimentation (e.g., Worrall 2007), the gold standard for clinical trials is the **randomized controlled trial**, in which research subjects are divided into groups, at least one of which receives the medication or procedure being tested and at least one of which receives the existing medication or procedure (if any). Subjects do not know into which of those groups they fall. The ethical problem is that patients who are sick and have been referred to the clinical trial by a physician—for instance, patients whose cancer has not responded well to existing chemotherapies—have an interest in receiving an experimental treatment. Do such trials violate the principle of beneficence, since the subjects receiving the standard treatment do not receive any potential benefits from the experimental treatment, even if these trials meet the requirements of informed consent and their randomization supports the principle of justice? The Belmont Report's emphasis on separating therapeutic interventions from medical research is significant here: subjects are entitled to a research design that maximizes possible benefits, but part of the goal of research entails risk, including the risk that one will be assigned to a control group that receives the current treatment only, which may be less effective. Recognizing this problem, the FDA has authorized an exception to its usual process of approving medical products (drugs or medical devices). **Compassionate use** or expanded access is a way for patients "with a serious or immediately life-threatening disease or condition" to gain access to experimental treatments outside of clinical trials and before they have been approved for the general public (U.S. Food and Drug Administration 2024).

The concept of **equipoise** has played a crucial role in this debate. In the original account developed by Charles Fried in 1974, the idea was that the physician who referred a patient to a clinical trial must be uncertain as to which treatment would be most beneficial. In that case, referral to a randomized trial would not deviate from the duty to care for the patient (Fried 1974). Variants of equipoise have been discussed in the decades since, including the idea that the whole medical community might be uncertain as to the proper treatment for patients, which serves as the impetus for research in the first place (Freedman 1987). It is important to note that the condition of equipoise limits the use of placebos in clinical trials since, by definition, placebos will have no direct medical benefit. In situations where there is not an available treatment that is known to be better than a placebo, its use may still be consistent with equipoise because some people may derive indirect benefits from placebos, such as pain relief, and the tested treatment may carry the risk of harm. This debate once more raises the question of the relationship between medical treatment and medical research, and the duties of the clinical physician as opposed to the physician-researcher.

## Conclusion: The Legacy of Paternalism

Just as paternalism has been overthrown as the dominant clinician-patient model, so too the paternalistic authority invested in researchers has been questioned. This shift has opened up a number of ethical debates that focus on researchers' obligations to test subjects as morally considerable agents rather than specimens to be sacrificed for the benefit of a wider population or future generations. Although it falls outside the scope of this book, some of the principles used to govern experimentation on human subjects have also started to be used in debates concerning experimentation on nonhuman animals. Critics of animal experimentation give different arguments, including deontological (based on animal rights) and utilitarian (based on animal welfare) reasoning, for extending the bounds of moral considerability beyond our own species (see Regan 2004; Singer 2023).

The history of medical experimentation largely serves as a warning about the dangers of ignoring our obligations to those whose interests we tend to disregard, even with the best of intentions, and also as a warning about the dangers of assuming we have progressed beyond the atrocities of the past.

## REFERENCES

American Medical Association. n.d. "Code of Medical Ethics." Accessed January 15, 2025. https://code-medical-ethics.ama-assn.org/.

Arras, John D. 2008. "The Jewish Chronic Disease Hospital Case." In *The Oxford Textbook of Clinical Research Ethics*, edited by Ezekiel J. Emanuel, Christine C. Grady, Robert A. Crouch, Reidar K. Lie, Franklin G. Miller, and David D. Wendler, 73–79. New York: Oxford University Press. doi:10.1093/oso/9780195168655.003.0007.

Atlas, Michel C. 2001. "Ethics and Access to Teaching Materials in the Medical Library: The Case of the Pernkopf Atlas." *Bulletin of the Medical Library Association* 89, no. 1 (January): 51–58.

Beecher, Henry K. 1966. "Ethics and Clinical Research." *New England Journal of Medicine* 274, no. 24 (June 16): 1354–60. doi:10.1056/NEJM196606162742405.

Bernard, Claude. 1949. *An Introduction to the Study of Experimental Medicine*. Translated by Henry Copley Greene. New York: Schuman.

Conahan, Frank C. 1994. *Human Experimentation: An Overview on Cold War Era Programs*. Washington, DC: U.S. General Accounting Office.

"The Forty Year Death Watch." 1972. *Medical World News*. August 18: 15–17.

Freedman, Benjamin. 1987. "Equipoise and the Ethics of Clinical Research." *New England Journal of Medicine* 317, no. 3 (July 16): 141–45. doi:10.1056/NEJM198707163170304.

Fried, Charles. 1974. *Medical Experimentation: Personal Integrity and Social Policy*. Amsterdam: North Holland.

Ghosh, Sanjib Kumar. 2015. "Human Cadaveric Dissection: A Historical Account from Ancient Greece to the Modern Era." *Anatomy & Cell Biology* 48, no. 3 (September): 153–69. doi:10.5115/acb.2015.48.3.153.

Halpern, Sydney A. 2021. *Dangerous Medicine: The Story behind Human Experiments with Hepatitis*. New Haven, CT: Yale University Press.

Himmler, Heinrich. 1943. "Excerpt from Himmler's Speech to the SS-*Gruppenführer* at Posen (October 4, 1943)." German History in Documents. https://ghdi.ghi-dc.org/sub_document.cfm?document_id=1513.

Hornblum, Allen M. 1998. *Acres of Skin: Human Experiments at Holmesburg Prison*. New York: Routledge.

International Military Tribunal. 1950. *Trials of War Criminals before the Nuernberg Military Tribunals under Control Council Law No. 10 Nuernberg, October 1946–April 1949*. Vol. 2. Washington, DC: Government Printing Office.

Jones, James H. 1981. *Bad Blood: The Tuskegee Syphilis Experiment*. New York: Free Press.

Kant, Immanuel. 1996. *Groundwork of the Metaphysics of Morals*. In *Practical Philosophy*, translated and edited by Mary J. Gregor, 41–108. Cambridge: Cambridge University Press.

Katz, Jay. 1992. "The Consent Principle in the Nuremberg Code: Its Significance Then and Now." In *The Nazi Doctors and the Nuremberg Code: Human Rights in Human Experimentation*, edited by George J. Annas and Michael A. Grodin, 227–39. New York: Oxford University Press. doi:10.1093/oso/9780195070422.003.0013.

Katz, Jay, Alexander Morgan Capron, and Eleanor Swift Glass, eds. 1972. "The Jewish Chronic Disease Hospital Case." In *Experimentation with Human Beings: The Authority of the Investigator, Subject, Professions, and State in the Human Experimentation Process*, 9–65. New York: Russell Sage Foundation. https://www.russellsage.org/publications/experimentation-human-beings.

Logsdon, Stephen. 2021. "William Beaumont's Momentous and Unethical Experiments." Washington University School of Medicine in St. Louis, Bernard Becker Medical Library. August 26. https://becker.wustl.edu/news/william-beaumonts-momentous-and-unethical-experiments/.

"Medical Experimentation." 2004. In *Encyclopedia of Genocide and Crimes against Humanity*, edited by Dinah L. Shelton, 669–75. New York: Macmillan.

Miller, Franklin G. 2013. "The Stateville Penitentiary Malaria Experiments: A Case Study in Retrospective Ethical Assessment." *Perspectives in Biology and Medicine* 56, no. 4 (Autumn): 548–67. doi:10.1353/pbm.2013.0035.

Millum, Joseph. 2020. "International Clinical Research and Justice in the *Belmont Report*." *Perspectives in Biology and Medicine* 63, no. 2 (Spring): 374–88. doi:10.1353/pbm.2020.0025.

National Commission for the Protection of Human Subjects of Biomedical and Behavioral Research. 1979. *The Belmont Report: Ethical Principles and Guidelines for the Protection of Human Subjects of Research*. Washington, DC: U.S. Department of Health and Human Services. https://www.hhs.gov/ohrp/regulations-and-policy/belmont-report/read-the-belmont-report/index.html.

Percival, Thomas. 1803. *Medical Ethics; or, A Code of Institutes and Precepts, Adapted to the Professional Conduct of Physicians and Surgeons*. Manchester: Russell.

"Prison Official in Illinois Halts Malaria Research on Inmates." 1974. *New York Times*. April 28, 50. https://www.nytimes.com/1974/04/28/archives/prison-official-in-illinois-halts-malaria-research-on-inmates.html.

Regan, Tom. 2004. *The Case for Animal Rights*. Rev. ed. Berkeley: University of California Press.

Rodriguez, Michael A., and Robert García. 2013. "First, Do No Harm: The US Sexually Transmitted Disease Experiments in Guatemala." *American Journal of Public Health* 103, no. 12 (December): 2122–26. doi:10.2105/AJPH.2013.301520.

Rothman, David J., and Sheila Rothman. 1984. *The Willowbrook Wars: Bringing the Mentally Disabled into the Community*. New York: Harper & Row.

Singer, Peter. 2023. *Animal Liberation Now*. New York: HarperCollins.

Smith, Susan L. 2008. "Mustard Gas and American Race-Based Human Experimentation in World War II." *Journal of Law, Medicine & Ethics* 36, no. 3 (Fall): 517–21. doi:10.1111/j.1748-720X.2008.299.x.

U.S. Food and Drug Administration. 2024. "Expanded Access." Last modified February 28, 2024. https://www.fda.gov/news-events/public-health-focus/expanded-access.

Weigmann, Katrin. 2015. "The Ethics of Global Clinical Trials." *EMBO Reports* 16, no. 5 (May 1): 566–70. doi:10.15252/embr.201540398.

World Health Organization. n.d. "Neglected Tropical Diseases." Accessed January 15, 2025. https://www.who.int/health-topics/neglected-tropical-diseases#tab=tab_1.

Worrall, John. 2007. "Evidence in Medicine and Evidence-Based Medicine." *Philosophy Compass* 2, no. 6 (November): 981–1022. doi:10.1111/j.1747-9991.2007.00106.x.

## Further Reading

Angell, Marcia. 2008. "Industry-Sponsored Clinical Research: A Broken System." *JAMA: Journal of the American Medical Association* 300, no. 9 (September 3): 1069–71. doi:10.1001/jama.300.9.1069.

> Argues that industry-sponsored medical research, which makes up the majority of research conducted in the United States and globally, should be more carefully regulated to prevent companies from publishing selective results. Prior to the 1980s, academic researchers had more independence in testing the efficacy and side effects of pharmaceuticals, but for-profit companies have increasingly designed the studies, interpreted the results, and decided whether those results should be published.

Annas, George J., and Michael A. Grodin, eds. 1992. *The Nazi Doctors and the Nuremberg Code: Human Rights in Human Experimentation.* New York: Oxford University Press. doi:10.1093/oso/9780195070422.001.0001.

> An edited volume that considers the lasting impact of Nazi experimentation and the Nuremberg Code. Various contributors provide historical, legal, and ethical perspectives on this document, as well as a consideration of its influence on more recent attempts to articulate the ethics of medical experimentation.

Council for International Organizations of Medical Sciences. 2016. *International Ethical Guidelines for Health-Related Research Involving Humans.* Geneva: CIOMS. doi:10.56759/rgxl7405.

> A set of principles governing medical research developed by the World Health Organization and the Council for International Organizations of Medical Sciences. This document is largely aligned with the Belmont Report but includes specific guidelines that attempt to grapple with subsequent debates, such as the possibility of subtle forms of coercion in the consent process.

Field, Marilyn J., and Richard E. Behrman, eds. 2004. *The Ethical Conduct of Clinical Research Involving Children.* Washington, DC: National Academies Press. https://nap.nationalacademies.org/catalog/10958/ethical-conduct-of-clinical-research-involving-children.

> A report compiled by the Committee on Clinical Research Involving Children at the Institute of Medicine of the National Academies that explores why research on children is both necessary and more ethically complex than research on adults. The authors examine the ethical and legal dimensions of research on children and consider how to promote well-being and respect autonomy. The committee links the protection of children in research to other vulnerable populations and to basic ethical principles that apply to all research subjects.

Foster, Claire. 2001. *The Ethics of Medical Research on Humans.* Cambridge: Cambridge University Press. doi:10.1017/CBO9780511545498.

> A philosophical consideration of the ethics of medical research, focusing on goal-based, duty-based, and rights-based approaches. In the process of evaluating these approaches, Foster discusses a range of practical and theoretical issues through a consideration of case studies: the distinction between therapy and research, what counts as informed consent, and the purpose of medical research.

Halpern, Sydney A. 2004. *Lesser Harms: The Morality of Risk in Medical Research.* Chicago: University of Chicago Press.

> A history of medical experimentation in the United States in the twentieth century, particularly focused on vaccine trials starting in the 1930s. The book includes a history of immunization and the "logic of risk" used to justify such research. Halpern contrasts this approach with the ethical guidelines for research developed in response to public scandals.

Petryna, Adriana. 2009. *When Experiments Travel: Clinical Trials and the Global Search for Human Subjects.* Princeton, NJ: Princeton University Press.

> An examination of how clinical trials have become globalized. The book describes the economic incentives for this outsourcing and how medical industries intersect with local healthcare institutions. Petryna argues that our current understanding of informed consent inadequately protects research subjects.

Vollmann, Jochen, and Rolf Winau. 1996. "Informed Consent in Human Experimentation before the Nuremberg Code." *BMJ* 313, no. 7070 (December 7): 1445–47. doi:10.1136/bmj.313.7070.1445.

> Provides a historical perspective on nineteenth- and early twentieth-century ethical debates around medical experimentation. This tradition is important in part because the defendants at the Doctors' Trial in Nuremberg claimed that there were no explicit ethical codes regulating research on human subjects and that their practices followed experimental norms in Germany and elsewhere. The authors demonstrate that the demand for informed consent from experimental subjects emerged much earlier than the post-war period.

Wertheimer, Alan. 2010. *Rethinking the Ethics of Clinical Research: Widening the Lens.* Oxford: Oxford University Press. doi:10.1093/acprof:oso/9780199743513.001.0001.

> A philosophical evaluation of medical research, starting with the idea that experimentation on human subjects primarily benefits others: How then can research not exploit those subjects? Wertheimer compares the regulations around human experimentation with the kinds of instrumentalization experienced by human beings in other contexts, such as dangerous professions. He considers informed consent, pediatric research, incentives to participate in research, and research in developing countries.

World Medical Association. 2013. *WMA Declaration of Helsinki—Ethical Principles for Medical Research Involving Human Subjects.* https://www.wma.net/policies-post/wma-declaration-of-helsinki-ethical-principles-for-medical-research-involving-human-subjects/.

A set of international principles guiding medical research on human subjects. First adopted in 1964 and updated nine times since, the Declaration of Helsinki builds on the Nuremberg Code but provides more detailed regulations, including those governing informed consent, the structure of research ethics committees, confidentiality, the weighing of risks and benefits, public registration of the study and dissemination of research results, and protection of vulnerable groups.

# CONCLUSION
## Reflective Equilibrium, between Medicine and Philosophy

The moral issues raised in the practice of medicine point to crucial elements of what it means to be human. Although much of the Western philosophical and political tradition has imagined a sovereign, rational subject as the default, medical care is often sought at moments when autonomous decision-making is compromised—due to, for instance, the cognitive limitations of very young patients or the urgency with which choices must be made, in a climate of anxiety and uncertainty. Thus, many of the debates in medical ethics tackle the question of how to respect patient autonomy when it is limited by various conditions. Philosophically, we must pay attention to a more nuanced picture of who and what we are: embodied, aging, mortal beings who can sometimes articulate our purposes but who often make decisions with limited information, cognitive bias, and incomplete understanding of the situations in which we find ourselves—as patients and clinicians.

Recent work in the field of medicine, as well as sociology and public health, supports treating patients as whole persons. That means recognizing the links between psychological health and physical health—for example, how anxiety and depression can exacerbate or act as risk factors for cardiovascular disease, diabetes, and a weaker immune system. Additionally, individual patients need to be understood and treated as interpersonal selves, embedded in family relationships that impact their physical health and decision-making, and shaped by their location in social and economic systems. Reproductive ethics, pediatric ethics, disability ethics, and ethics at the end of life reckon with a spectrum of autonomy, including emerging or future autonomy, rather than a simple binary between autonomy and heteronomy. The contemporary focus on adverse childhood events, such as growing up with an adult dealing with addiction or mental health issues, reflects this shift toward understanding the patient in longitudinal and holistic ways. Palliative care specialists, among others, also model how to attend to a patient's core values and sense of purpose in their lives, as a way to promote self-determination more substantively than the ritual of signing a consent form.

Similarly, the principles of nonmaleficence and beneficence appeal to a commonsense notion of well-being. But it is often difficult to specify what attending to a patient's welfare means. Should clinicians prioritize their longevity? Quality of life? The individual patient's wishes as described in a substantive advance directive or as voiced by a proxy? Their current best interests? And who gets to assess or predict their quality of life, interpret their wishes, or judge their best interests? What do we do when family members and clinicians disagree? As the preceding chapters show, two simple starting points of medical ethics—respecting autonomy and promoting well-being—frequently conflict, complicating judgments we make in the clinical space, in public health, and in research. Finally, when we go beyond our obligations to isolated patients and consider all persons, our commitment to justice means that we have to distribute medical resources equitably, however we define that, and take into account links between medical care and wider hierarchies that impact the social determinants of health.

Running through many of these debates is the problem of who should count as a person, or who is morally considerable. There are fundamental disagreements about how to draw that line because it would require us to reach consensus on what is essential to personhood—a question that must be normatively rather than empirically settled and that touches on people's core philosophical and religious beliefs. Our inability to definitively answer this question arises most pointedly in debates around pregnancy and reproduction, but also when people suffer serious cognitive impairments. When does personhood begin, and under what circumstances should we say that a human being is no longer a person?

It would make the discussions of ethics committees, families, legislators, and clinicians much easier if all these questions could be answered cleanly and objectively, on the model of geometrical proofs. Medical ethics is a domain in which judgment is necessary precisely because we have different kinds of obligations, represented by the four principles (respect for autonomy, nonmaleficence, beneficence, and justice) and perhaps other obligations such as care or the rule of rescue. In specific scenarios, we are obligated in highly variable ways. It is through dialogue or internal reflection, not the application of an algorithm, that we recognize what is legitimate in competing moral claims and we attempt to capture those intuitions in our practical conclusions. There is no way to eliminate entirely the messiness of normative judgment, even if there are ways to structure our moral reasoning so that we can more consistently identify what is significant in a given case.

Cultivating the skills of moral reasoning allows us to evaluate the implications of new medical advancements, which typically develop faster than we can reach ethical consensus and create regulations. We can make designer babies, electronically monitor people's everyday decisions around diet and exercise, and extend the lives of those who are permanently unconscious almost indefinitely, but should we? Support for medical experimentation (financial and otherwise) may be driven by a desire for innovation or profit rather than moral concern. Training in medical ethics can mitigate our cultural tendency to trust that technological progress inevitably leads to social justice or a better quality of life. It can attune us to the moral implications of those innovations by appealing to enduring principles and historical precedents, even as we test those principles in light of particular cases—the process of reflective equilibrium.

Another way to approach these topics is to ask abstract philosophical questions with deeply practical consequences: What is the purpose of medicine? Is it set by the desires and priorities of the patient or by whoever is authorizing payment for the medical service? Should it primarily serve individual or collective interests? Is the purpose constant and universal, or are there many purposes that vary according to different cultural, religious, or individual values? How we conceive of the goal (or goals) of medicine shapes what is morally permissible and impermissible. For instance, if the role of clinicians is to heal patients, then medical aid in dying is unjustifiable. By contrast, if the role of clinicians is to help patients understand their options, articulate their priorities, and then act on those decisions, end-of-life care will prioritize patient autonomy rather than, by default, prolonging life.

It is important to reflect critically on what medicine should accomplish because clinicians receive messages about its purpose during their medical education not only explicitly but also through watching mentors make decisions and interact with patients. How clinicians conceive of what they are doing informs nearly every aspect of the profession. Ideally, then, medical ethics education would not be confined to discussing case studies in one part of the curriculum but would include regular evaluation of clinical practices and the deeper commitments they express and reinforce. It should also draw on the work of philosophers, historians, sociologists, and those working in medical humanities, who can help medical students get beyond specialized technical training to a broader consideration of their obligations to individual patients and society as a whole. Medical ethics should also be integrated into the ordinary practice of medicine, which may help alleviate moral distress by encouraging clinicians to articulate their values and by promoting institutional practices that respect practitioners as moral agents.

While healthcare practitioners and institutions need to learn from bioethicists, theorists in turn need to understand the business of healthcare and why clinicians experience moral distress, among other issues. How are the four principles of biomedical ethics lived out in particular cases? Can the healthcare industry and individual clinicians do what we want them to, given the many pressures they face? Scholars should consider the economic conditions that shape the clinician-patient relationship, how public policy impacts healthcare institutions, which medical studies are funded, and why clinical trials are conducted globally.

In these debates and others to come, medical ethics illuminates how philosophy, in its humanistic orientation, intersects with the increasingly technical focus and specialization of medicine over the last several decades. Philosophers and other medical ethicists are trained to draw attention to what it means to be human, what our obligations to each other are, and how to temper our biases and assumptions. Case studies and other experiences of practitioners have much to add to these reflections. In the dialogue between theory and practice, we can continue to build a more just healthcare system.

# INDEX

abortion, 115–48
  Hippocratic Oath and, 62–63, 131–32
  legality of
    in U.S., 79, 100, 121–31, 157–58, 182, 228–29, 347–48
    exceptions to abortion bans, 24, 115–16, 133–36
    fetal heartbeat laws, 118, 135
    fetal personhood laws, 118–19, 124, 127, 129–30, 158
    outside of U.S., 138–40
  morality of, 116–21, 154, 157, 168
    arguments against, 117–19, 120–21, 132
    arguments for, 119–20, 121, 132–33
    violinist example, 120
  selective reduction, 157
  *See also* conscientious refusal; disability-selective abortion; privacy, right to: regarding abortion and reproduction
advance directive. *See* proxy directive; substantive directive
Affordable Care Act, 65, 130, 261–62
Alexander, Leo, 410
allocation of medical resources, 36, 267, 278–309
  fair innings, 283, 285–86, 300
  Fair Priority Model, 300–301
  first-come, first-served, 26, 280–81, 282, 285, 294, 297
  instrumental value, 281, 284–85
  lottery, 280–82, 284
  macroallocation vs. microallocation, 256
  prioritarianism, 281
  prognosis or life years, 279–80, 281, 284, 290–92, 296, 297–98
  vs. rationing, 256–57
  reciprocity, 281, 284, 291
  save the most lives, 281, 284, 293, 296, 298–99
  sickest first, 281, 282–83, 290
  youngest first, 281–84, 291
Allow Natural Death order. *See* Do Not Resuscitate order
American Medical Association, 93, 132–33, 234, 235, 245, 258, 324, 424
amputation, voluntary 81–82
Aquinas, Thomas, 127
Aristotle, 26, 127, 132, 265
artificial insemination. *See* intrauterine insemination
assent. *See* informed consent: vs. assent
assisted reproductive technology, defined, 155
autonomy, 61–88
  clinician, 99–100, 133, 159–60, 378, 383, 387–88
  conditions of, 10
  constraints on, 74–77, 197, 228, 236, 366–67, 420, 433
  defined, 10, 68–69, 217, 385
  emerging, 80, 179, 339–44, 346, 347–48, 353, 359–60, 366, 433
  future (of fetuses), 150, 154, 177–78, 433

vs. heteronomy, 68, 347, 433
vs. liberty, 10–11, 71, 73–77, 179
limited familial, 211
parental, 342–45, 349–51, 353, 357
principle of respect for, 8–13, 20, 24–26, 31, 33–35, 36, 68–71, 90–93, 94, 95–96, 149, 153–55, 176, 200, 206, 209, 211, 227–29, 234–35, 239, 240–47, 266, 271, 293, 316, 318, 340, 349, 353, 354, 357, 359, 363, 376, 389–92, 405–7, 410–11, 419, 434–35
procreative, 125, 139–40, 150, 152–53, 159–62, 165–66, 177, 183, 209
prospective, 207–10, 211–16, 218
relational, 32, 79–80
*See also* informed consent; mental health: autonomy; procreative autonomy, right to

Baby Doe, 345
Baby M, 162, 166
Belmont Report, 7, 70, 73–74, 290, 317, 360, 362, 412, 418–25
beneficence, 15–19
vs. nonmaleficence, 13–14, 16
positive, 15–16
principle of, 7–8, 13, 25, 26, 31, 34–35, 46, 62, 82, 90–92, 94, 149, 153, 177, 200, 205, 217–18, 235, 236–37, 239, 241, 242–45, 247, 339–40, 342–45, 349–51, 352–54, 357, 359, 363, 366, 389–90, 391–92, 406–7, 410, 418–19, 420–22, 424–25, 434
procreative, 160, 173, 177
specific vs. general, 16
Bentham, Jeremy, 286, 291
best interests standard, 200–202, 344

Beveridge Model, 258
bioethics, defined, 1
Bismarck Model, 261
British Medical Association, 93, 225, 234
burnout, 27, 103–5, 395
*See also* moral distress; moral injury
*Buzzanca v. Buzzanca*, 161

*Canterbury v. Spence*, 71, 73
capacity, 10–11, 26, 28, 29, 70–71, 78, 205, 211, 213, 231, 245, 247, 347–48, 356, 359, 366–67
defined, 198
incapacitated patients, 12, 199–205, 206, 207–8, 214, 217
*See also* competence: vs. capacity
care ethics, 32–33, 266, 384–86
Cass Review, 358
casuistry or case-based reasoning, 3, 35–37, 79
categorical imperative, 10–11, 44
formula of the end in itself, 419
procedure, 32
Catholic Church, 126–27, 160, 164, 183, 203, 205, 217–18
Centers for Medicare and Medicaid Services, 46, 51, 54–55, 104, 259, 263
character, moral, 7–8, 26–27
Charter of Fundamental Rights of the European Union, 163
circumcision and genital cutting, 288–89, 354–55
clinical trial. *See* experimentation: clinical trials
clinician-patient relationship, 61–88, 89–114, 233–35, 321–25, 340–44, 383–86
deliberative model, 78

engineering model, 72
informative model, 72–73, 75, 77–78
interpretive model, 77–78
legalistic model, 72
practical reasoning model, 78
*See also* paternalism
*Cobbs v. Grant*, 67, 71
collective responsibility, 43–60
commodification, 80, 183
   of babies, 165–67
   of stem cells, 182
   of women, 165–67
common morality, 3, 8–9, 22–23, 28, 33–37
Common Rule, 418–19, 422, 424
compassion, 15, 26–27, 77, 205, 218, 237–39
   fatigue, 396
compassionate use, 425–26
compelling state interest, 123, 125, 161
competence, 11, 68–69, 161, 230, 232, 348
   vs. capacity, 197–99
   defined, 11, 198
   incompetent patients, 197–99, 200–207, 209, 213–15, 317, 340–41, 360
   pre-competence, 339
   *See also* capacity; mental health: competence
confidentiality, patient, 11–12, 63, 69, 95–99, 104, 152, 153–54, 339, 386, 420, 422
   *See also* mental health: confidentiality
*Conroy, In the Matter of Claire C.*, 200–201
conscientious objection. *See* conscientious refusal
conscientious refusal, 99–101, 116, 133, 141

consent. *See* informed consent
consequentialism, 13, 90–91, 94, 96, 179, 242, 265–66, 268, 344–45
   *See also* utilitarianism
cost-benefit analysis, 17–18, 19
cost-effectiveness analysis, 17, 18–19, 286–89
COVID-19 pandemic, 91–92, 292, 311–12, 350, 393, 395
   treatment distribution, 292–98
   vaccine distribution, 18–19, 256, 284, 298–301
"crack babies," 150–51, 154
CRISPR, 175
*Cruzan v. Director, Missouri Department of Health*, 71, 81, 204, 206–7, 226

Daniels, Norman, 22, 265–67
death, cerebral vs. whole-brain, 204
death with dignity. *See* medical aid in dying; Oregon Death with Dignity Act
deception, 35–36, 72, 90
   of pediatric patients, 341, 353–54, 365
   in research, 410, 419–20
   *See also* truth-telling
Declaration of Geneva, 411
Declaration of Helsinki, 411, 414
dementia, 10, 28, 77, 81, 140, 198–99, 205–6, 213
deontological ethics, 2, 8, 90, 94, 95–96, 268, 284, 344–45, 411, 426
desires, first- and second-order, 74, 81
*Diagnostic and Statistical Manual of Mental Disorders*, 355–57
Dickey-Wicker Amendment, 181–82
disability, 28, 29, 76, 77, 81, 140, 178, 198, 202, 340, 351, 385, 395, 405, 414, 415, 418, 420

vs. handicap, 169, 238
stigma against, 19, 159–60, 168–71, 174, 176, 177, 205, 217–18, 235–38, 289, 294, 319–20, 345, 360, 363, 409
value-neutral model of, 168–69
disability paradox, 168
disability-adjusted life year, 288–89
disability-selective abortion, 167–75
disorders of sex development, 341, 351–55
See also intersex
distribution principle, 20, 264
Do Not Resuscitate order, 202, 209–10, 345
*Dobbs v. Jackson Women's Health Organization*, 115, 119, 127, 128–30, 133, 161, 170
doctrine of double effect, 241, 245–46
Du Bois, W. E. B., 310–11
duty to warn/protect, 97–98
Dworkin, Ronald, 122–27, 228–29, 241, 243, 269–70

electronic health records, 50, 52, 72, 97, 102, 103–4, 323, 328
embryos, 28, 30, 117–19, 138, 140, 155–60, 166–67, 179–83
vs. fetuses, 116
See also experimentation: on embryos; in vitro fertilization: moral status of embryos in
Emergency Medical Treatment and Labor Act, 260–61, 263
epistemic injustice, 325, 342, 378–82, 387, 393
equipoise, 426
errors, medical, 47–55
disclosure of, 93–95
ethics of care. See care ethics

eugenics, 170, 174–75, 177–79, 218, 236–37, 314, 320, 410
liberal, 177
European Convention on Bioethics, 163
European Convention on Human Rights, 99
euthanasia, 23, 218, 225, 229, 233, 237, 244
active, 15, 206, 225, 226, 234–37, 242, 246
legality of, 225–26, 230–32, 236
passive, 15, 225, 226, 245–47
voluntary vs. nonvoluntary vs. involuntary, 225
See also medical aid in dying: vs. euthanasia; withholding treatment: vs. euthanasia
expanded access. See compassionate use
experimentation, 8, 12, 34, 179, 351, 405–32, 435
on animals, 29–30, 155, 182, 315, 360, 405, 409–10, 411, 426
clinical trials, 34, 361, 422, 423, 424–26
on embryos, 158–59, 176, 179–83
on enslaved people, 314–16
history of, 62, 70, 137, 314–20, 406–10, 412–18
minimal risk, 361–62, 419, 422
pediatric, 178, 340–41, 359–63
on prisoners, 314, 317–18, 408, 409, 415, 417–18, 422, 423–24
racism in, 137, 312, 314–20, 328, 387–88, 410, 412–14, 417
randomized controlled trials, 73, 425–26
therapeutic vs. nontherapeutic, 360, 406, 408

*See also* Common Rule; mental health: in research subjects; Nazi Germany: human experimentation; stem cell research

Faden, Ruth, 22, 265–66, 267
Federal Policy for the Protection of Human Subjects. *See* Common Rule
female genital cutting. *See* circumcision and genital cutting
fetal endangerment laws, 150–53
  *See also* pregnancy, criminalization of
Flexner Report, 324
focal virtues, 26–27, 77
Four Box Method, 36–37
free-market healthcare, 257, 258–61, 263
futile treatment. *See* overtreatment

gender dysphoria, 355–59
  gender identity disorder, 355
  gender incongruence, 355–56, 358
genetic enhancement, 175–79
  vs. genetic therapy, 175–76
  somatic vs. germline, 176
Gilligan, Carol, 32, 384–85
Gillon, Raanan, 31
"God Committee," 2, 279–80, 298
*Gonzales v. Oregon*, 230
*Griswold v. Connecticut*, 123, 161
guardian ad litem, 152, 199

harm principle, 20, 64, 117, 119, 121, 123, 137–38, 344, 346
healer, physician's role as, 233–35, 244, 245
  *See also* medicine, purpose of
health, right to, 264–65, 267
health insurance marketplaces, 262
Health Insurance Portability and Accountability Act, 95–96, 99

healthcare, right to, 22, 100–101, 263–67, 386
  vs. entitlement, 263–64, 266
  vs. privilege, 263–64
  statist/nationalist view vs. global/cosmopolitan view, 22
Hippocratic Oath, 2, 14, 31, 62–63, 66–67, 69, 75–76, 90, 95, 131–32, 233–34, 408–10, 421
Holmesburg Prison, 317–18, 417
hospice care, 92, 215, 227, 228, 239, 322, 392

in vitro fertilization, 155–60, 178
  history of, 155
  legal debates, 157–58, 180–83
  moral status of embryos in, 157–59
  process, 155–56
incompetent patients. *See* competence
individual mandate. *See* Affordable Care Act
informed consent, 2, 11–12, 34, 70–73, 82, 164, 176, 179, 180, 182, 198–99, 211, 213, 240, 339–40, 359–60, 389, 406–7, 410, 411, 419–20, 425
  vs. assent, 340–41, 347, 351, 361–62
  contemporaneous, 180–81
  elements of, 11–12
  surrogate, 413
  violations of, 316–18, 412–13, 415–16
  *See also* parental permission
informed permission. *See* parental permission
institutional review board, 5, 181, 360–61, 407, 419–22
interpretivism, 122–25
intersex, 341, 349, 351–54
  *See also* disorders of sex development
intrauterine insemination, 155, 161–62

Jehovah's Witnesses, blood transfusions, 68, 346
Jewish Chronic Disease Hospital cancer study, 317, 412, 415–16, 422
Joint Commission, 46, 47, 93
justice
   capability theory, 22, 265, 267
   egalitarian theory, 22, 265–67
   as fairness, 20–22, 264, 282
   libertarian theory, 259
   principle of, 3, 7, 8, 13, 19–22, 25–26, 28, 34–35, 36, 68, 73, 80, 94, 122, 153, 155, 178–79, 257–71, 278, 283, 290–91, 292–94, 296, 349–51, 364–65, 366, 376, 406, 418, 419, 420–22, 424–25, 434–35
   well-being theory, 22, 265–66
   *See also* epistemic injustice

Kant, Immanuel, 2, 10–11, 15–16, 32, 44, 68, 74, 165, 169, 177–78, 281, 284, 302, 344, 363, 419
killing vs. letting die, 15, 224, 246–47
   *See also* euthanasia: passive; withholding treatment

Lacks, Henrietta, 317
Letchworth Village polio study, 360
liberty principle, 20, 264
licensure, 24, 45–46, 51–52, 100, 134, 258–59, 324
limited-objective standard, 201
   *See also* competence: incompetent patients
living will. *See* substantive directive
lying. *See* deception; truth-telling

mature minors, 26, 341, 347–48, 362
maximin principle, 21–22

medical aid in dying, 224–54
   defined, 224–26
   vs. euthanasia, 225–26
   legality of
      in U.S., 76–77, 100, 225–30, 235–36, 240–43
      outside of U.S., 230–32
   morality of, 15, 68, 288, 435
      arguments against, 232–39
      arguments for, 239–45, 246–47
   *See also* slippery slopes: empirical; slippery slopes: theoretical
medical ethics, defined, 1–2
medicine, purpose of, 224, 229–30, 232–35, 244–45, 246, 377, 383–86, 405–6, 435–36
   *See also* healer, physician's role as
mental health, 28, 63, 90, 92, 136, 138–39, 206, 229, 231–32, 234–36, 383, 385, 433
   autonomy, 10, 73–74, 81–82, 390–92
   competence, 76–77, 227
   confidentiality, 96–99
   pediatric, 166, 341–43, 347, 353, 355–59, 365–66
   racial disparity, 312, 326–27
   in research subjects, 411, 421–22
   *See also* burnout; gender dysphoria; moral distress; moral injury
Mid-Staffordshire Hospital, 388
Mill, John Stuart, 2, 13, 15–16, 64, 117, 123, 266, 302
Mills, Charles W., 315–16
moral considerability/status, 1, 4, 8–9, 26, 28–31, 116, 120, 123–24, 149–50, 154, 158–59, 174, 180, 183, 315–16, 319, 397, 405–6, 410–11, 418, 426–27, 434

moral distress, 27, 89–90, 101–5, 381–82, 393–96, 436
  vs. burnout, 27, 103, 395
  *See also* burnout; moral injury
moral imperialism, 33–35
moral injury, 103, 395
  *See also* burnout; moral distress
moral status. *See* moral considerability/status
multi-payer healthcare, 22, 261–63

narrative ethics, 35–36
National Commission for the Protection of Human Subjects of Biomedical and Behavioral Research, 7, 412, 418
  *See also* Belmont Report
National Health Insurance Model, 257–58
National Organ Transplant Act, 290
Natural Death Act, 229
Nazi Germany, 170, 423
  Doctors' Trial, 408–10
  human experimentation, 62, 314, 327, 412, 416, 417
  T4 program, 236–37
  *See also* eugenics
newborn screening, 351
Nightingale, Florence, 377–78
nonmaleficence, principle of, 8, 13–16, 25–26, 30, 31, 34, 36, 46, 62, 68, 94, 149, 153–55, 176, 177, 200–201, 366, 391–92, 406–7, 408, 410, 416, 434
Nuremberg Code, 2, 70, 73, 316, 327, 360, 362, 408–14, 416–17, 418–19, 420–21
Nussbaum, Martha, 22, 265, 267

objectification. *See* commodification
opportunity
  fair equality of, 22, 264, 266, 282, 285
  normal range, 265, 268
ordinary vs. extraordinary care, 15, 203, 208, 363
Oregon Death with Dignity Act, 100, 226–28, 229–30, 240, 242–43
organ donation, 25–26, 80, 204, 206, 289–91
organs for transplant, allocation of, 25–26, 278, 283–84, 289–92, 312–13, 363–64
  *See also* UNOS points system
original position, 20–21, 264
originalism, 127–29
overtreatment, 73, 81, 214, 216, 344–46

palliative care, 15, 208, 236, 365–66, 394, 433–34
  sedation, 245
parental permission, 340–41, 348, 351, 359–60, 361–62, 414–15
  vs. parental consent, 340
parenthood, conceptions of, 170–71
parents, role of, 340–44
paternalism, 11, 34, 62–70, 72, 76, 160, 164, 339, 378, 380, 389, 426–27
  arguments against, 66–70, 77–78
  arguments for, 62–66, 75, 391
  defined, 63–64
  history of, 62–63, 205, 341–42, 359–60, 363, 382, 412, 416
  types of, 64–65, 243
patient advocacy, 5, 152, 154–55, 182, 328, 344, 347, 359, 366, 382–83, 386–87, 389, 390, 394

patient privacy. *See* confidentiality, patient
Patient Self-Determination Act, 207, 226
pediatric patients/subjects. *See* autonomy: emerging; deception: of pediatric patients; experimentation: pediatric; mature minors; mental health: pediatric; newborn screening; vaccination: childhood
Pernkopf Atlas, 423–24
persistent vegetative state, 25–26, 28, 198, 200, 202–8, 212
personhood, 67, 69, 116, 166, 204, 213, 310, 315–16, 323, 328, 434
    constitutional, 123–24, 127, 129–30
    fetal, 117–21, 126–27, 129–30, 153–54, 157–59, 174, 179–80
    vs. humanity, 119
    *See also* abortion: legality of: fetal personhood laws; subpersons
Physician (or Portable) Orders for Life-Sustaining Treatment, 209–10
physician-assisted suicide. *See* medical aid in dying
*Planned Parenthood v. Casey*, 126, 228–29
Plato, 19, 132, 183
potentiality, 28–29, 119–21, 125–26, 158–59, 183
    active vs. passive, 159
Powers, Madison, 22, 265–66, 267
pregnancy, criminalization of, 150–55
prenatal screening, 167–68, 170–71, 173
President's Commission for the Study of Ethical Problems in Medicine and Biomedical and Behavioral Research, 266–68, 345
President's Commission on the Health Needs of the Nation, 266–67
Price Transparency Rule, 259
prima facie duties, 8–9, 15, 32, 55, 90–92, 97–98, 284
principlism, 7–42, 285–86, 418
    alternatives to, 35–37
    defined, 7–8
    four principles plus scope version, 31
    objections to, 31–35
privacy, right to
    regarding abortion and reproduction, 122, 126–28, 130–31, 133, 140, 161–62, 228–29
    regarding personal information, 14, 95–99, 153, 351, 386, 420
    *See also* confidentiality, patient
procreative autonomy, right to, 125, 183
procreative beneficence, 160, 173, 177
proxy, 199–203, 209–11, 215–18, 226, 245, 247, 339–40, 434
    defined, 199
proxy directive, 207, 210–11, 216–18
prudent insurance test, 269
pure-objective standard, 201–2
    *See also* competence: incompetent patients

quality-adjusted life year, 18–19, 286–89, 295

racism in medicine, 310–37, 363–65, 412–14
    disparities in health outcomes, 137, 169, 310–14, 321–28, 363–64

implicit bias, 280, 291, 293–94, 311–12, 318–21, 323–24, 325, 328, 364–65
mistrust of healthcare professionals, 137, 311, 319–22, 324–25, 328, 365
*See also* experimentation: racism in; mental health: racial disparity; weathering
rationing. *See* allocation of medical resources: vs. rationing
Rawls, John, 19–22, 264–65, 267, 282, 302
reflective equilibrium, 2, 9, 25, 32, 302, 435
Reproductive Privacy Act, 100, 115
research. *See* experimentation
right to health. *See* health, right to
right to healthcare. *See* healthcare, right to
right to privacy. *See* privacy, right to
right to procreative autonomy. *See* procreative autonomy, right to
Rivers, Eunice, 387
*Roe v. Wade*, 122–24, 125–30, 132–33, 136
Ross, W. D., 8–9, 14, 15, 16, 32, 284
rule of rescue, 17, 260–61, 283, 434

Scalia, Antonin, 127–28
Schiavo, Terri, 202–5, 217–18
*Schloendorff v. Society of New York Hospital*, 71
Sen, Amartya, 22, 265, 267
sentience, 28–30, 119, 158
shortage of clinicians, 100, 102–4, 255, 388
Singer, Peter, 16–17, 30, 426
single-payer healthcare, 257–58, 259, 261, 263

site-neutral payments, 270–71
slippery slopes, 178, 232–33
  empirical, 236–39, 243–44
  theoretical, 235–36, 239, 242–43
*Smith v. Seibly*, 348
social determinants of health, 151, 264, 267, 321, 325–27, 347, 366–67, 387, 434
Social Vulnerability Index, 296
socialized medicine, 22, 257–58, 263
Stateville Penitentiary experiments, 408, 417
stem cell research, 175, 179–83
stereotype threat, 323–24
sterilization, forced, 123, 218, 237, 320–21, 409–10
strict scrutiny test, 124–25, 126
subjective standard, 201
  *See also* competence: incompetent patients
subpersons, 315–18, 320, 323
substantive directive, 207–18, 434
substituted judgment standard, 200–202, 204, 214, 216–17
surrogate, medical. *See* proxy
surrogate hierarchy, 199–200
surrogate motherhood, 160–67
  commercial vs. altruistic, 162–64, 165
  legality of, 161–63
  *See also* Baby M; commodification: of babies; commodification: of women

*Tarasoff v. Regents of the University of California*, 97–99
team-based care model, 47, 52, 54, 104–5
textualism, 127–29

transgender care, 101, 156
    for minors, 355–59, 391, 394
    *See also* gender dysphoria
transhumanism, 178–79
transparency, duty of, 35, 48, 89, 90–93, 292–93
triage, 282–83, 388
    committees, 256, 285, 292–98
    defined, 279
truth-telling, 34–35, 75–76, 90–93, 94–96, 212–13, 365
    *See also* deception; errors, medical: disclosure of
Tuskegee syphilis study, 137, 316–17, 319–20, 387, 412–15, 417, 418, 422

undertreatment, 214, 236, 323, 325, 344–46
Universal Declaration of Human Rights, 264
UNOS points system, 289–92, 302
    *See also* organs for transplant, allocation of
unresponsive wakefulness syndrome. *See* persistent vegetative state
U.S. Constitution, 121–31, 170, 228, 241–42, 262, 320, 357
    First Amendment, 125
    Fourteenth Amendment, 71, 123–24, 126–29, 133, 228
    Ninth Amendment, 126
utilitarianism, 2, 8, 13, 16, 29, 32, 95, 201, 259–60, 265–66, 281–82, 284–85, 288, 291, 295, 362, 388, 406, 408, 411, 420–21, 426
principle of utility, 13

vaccination, 16, 65, 256, 287–88, 320, 324
    childhood, 64, 66, 349–51, 412
    hesitancy/refusal, 350–51
    research, 317, 349, 359–60, 362, 414–15, 421
    *See also* COVID-19 pandemic: vaccine distribution
*Vacco v. Quill*, 228
Vaught, RaDonda, 48–55, 93
veil of ignorance, 20–21, 264
*Volk v. DeMeerleer*, 98–99

Warnock Report, 158, 163–64, 182
*Washington v. Glucksberg*, 129, 228–29
weathering, 326–28, 365
willingness to pay, 18
Willowbrook State School hepatitis study, 412, 414–15, 422
withholding treatment, 201, 205–6, 232, 240, 245, 247, 345
    vs. euthanasia, 225–26, 246
    vs. withdrawing treatment, 15, 34, 208, 217–18, 241
    *See also* euthanasia: passive
World Health Organization, 47, 264, 288, 300–301, 322, 356, 424
World Medical Association, 95, 234, 411